KNOW YOUR MEDICINE

The Irish Guide to Non-Prescription Medicines

GW00371053

Editor: Ann-Marie Hardiman

Production: John Dunleavy

Publisher: Graham Cooke

Medical Editor: Professor Graham Shaw

Design: Kim Perry

Sub-editor: Tim Ilsley

Managing Director: Christopher Goodey

Editorial Director: Maura Henderson

This Irish Guide to Non-Prescription Medicines has been produced by Eireann Healthcare Publications, 25-26 Windsor Place, Dublin 2.   Tel: (01) 475 3300 Fax: (01) 475 3311 Email: ahardiman@eireannpublications.ie

First published in 2001.

ISSN No 16491254

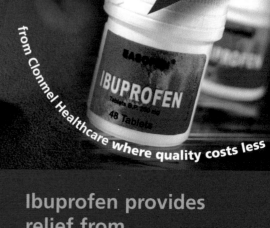
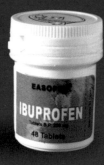

CONTENTS

PREFACE

Over the counter (OTC) medicines make a significant contribution to the nation's health. They are rightly seen by the Government as a means whereby simple ailments can be treated effectively, thus relieving the Health Services of the burden of dealing with such ailments. This ensures that scarce public resources are used to treat the more serious types of illness. Confidence in the OTC approach is leading to an increasing number of medicines – which were once available only on prescription – becoming available through pharmacies.

The variety of OTC medicines offered for sale today can be bewildering, even for health service professionals. This little book has been compiled to offer guidance and advice which will help the consumer find a way through the OTC maze. Its unique feature – in keeping with the information age in which we live – is that it provides detailed information on many of the medicines offered for sale, including a description of their active ingredients.

It should be emphasised that the book is intended to help the reader to make an informed choice. It is not a substitute for professional advice and readers are advised to consult their pharmacist if they have any concerns.

I am indebted to Eireann Healthcare Publications for their foresight in recognising the need for this book.

Professor Graham G Shaw
Medical Editor
Professor of Pharmacology
Trinity College Dublin

INTRODUCTION

While OTC medicines can be very effective, there are four important rules to remember:

- They are not a substitute for prescription medicines
- They are intended for short-term use only
- When symptoms are prolonged, frequent in occurrence or severe, seek medical advice immediately
- If taking prescription medicines, seek the advice of a pharmacist before taking any OTC medicine.

Any product that claims to be useful in treating an illness is defined as a medicine. The Irish Medicines Board, the State Agency that licenses medicines used in Ireland, assesses each of these products and evaluates its quality, safety and effectiveness. When satisfied it issues a Product Authorisation number. This number, called the PA number, appears on the package of the product. This book only includes those medicines which have a PA number, since this guarantees that they have been expertly and independently reviewed, both in their manufacture and in relation to their medical use.

There are some exceptions to this rule. Nutritional products which do not make a medical claim do not require an Authorisation. Vitamin products are also regarded as nutritionals if the vitamin content is equal to or less than the recommended dietary allowance. Nutritional products may state a claim that they make a contribution to general health, but they may not suggest that they are effective in the treatment of disease. Nutritionals have been allocated their own section in this book.

Some skin moisturising products (emollients), which are listed in the Skin Care chapter, also do not require a product authorisation. Once again, this is because they do not claim to treat an illness.

You will find the products listed according to the disorders they are intended to treat. Some will appear in more than one category, because they are used to treat more than one disorder.

There are thousands of active ingredients. It is not possible to describe every one, but all the more commonly used ingredients are described. All medicines have side effects. You will also find information on the more common and serious side effects, together with the most important precautions and warnings. This information provides an excellent guide for the layperson but it is not comprehensive. So, once again, remember that your pharmacist is the person to consult if you have any doubts or questions.

Know Your Medicine is an educational and information tool for Irish consumers. The content has been dictated with this in mind. Eireann Healthcare Publications is an independent publishing company, and information contained within product listings in this publication is at the discretion of Eireann Healthcare Publications, its editorial staff, and the medical editor, Professor Graham Shaw.

GLOSSARY OF SYMBOLS

In *Know Your Medicine*, we want to make it as easy as possible for you to find at a glance all the information you need about the OTC medicines you may need. Therefore, in every product listing, each section is represented by a symbol. Here is a glossary of what each symbol means:

☐ A description of the medicine – e.g. whether it's a tablet, capsule, liquid or powder – and what kind of packaging it comes in.

☑ A list of the more important, or active, ingredients in the medicine.

☐ What you should take the medicine for.

☑ The correct and safe dosage to take.

☐ Special precautions and warnings regarding each medicine, i.e. situations where it might be advisable to take a different medicine, or to ask your doctor or pharmacist for advice.

TYPES OF MEDICINE

The most common way of taking medicines is by mouth. Liquid medicines may be prepared by dissolving or dispersing the medicine in water or the medicine may be supplied in liquid form, e.g. as a cough mixture. This type of medicine presents the active ingredients in their most easily absorbed form, especially if the ingredients are fully dissolved. This may be an advantage if a rapid effect is wanted.

The most widely used type of medicine is the so-called "solid oral dosage form". These come in several varieties:

- Tablets – made by compressing granules under high pressure – are the most frequently used medicine. They are generally intended to dissolve in the stomach within a few minutes so they are slightly slower to act than soluble medicines. If you have difficulty in swallowing tablets, you might find that oval or oblong shaped tablets are easier to swallow. Alternatively, you might try capsules.

- Capsules are made by filling a gelatin shell with powder or granules. Capsules may be a little slower to dissolve than tablets but they are good for disguising ingredients that have an unpleasant taste and they are easy to swallow. Do not try to open capsules.

- Lozenges are designed to dissolve very slowly in the mouth. They are intended to release the active ingredients slowly and they are suitable for throat or mouth problems where prolonged contact is useful.

- Pills are made by allowing a wet mass to dry out and harden. Pills are very slow to break up in the body and they are hardly ever used now. The oral contraceptive 'pill' is actually a tablet.

- Other types of medicine are particularly useful for a local action on various areas of the body, e.g. sprays or nose or eye drops.

- Suppositories are torpedo shaped and are intended to be inserted into the rectum. They are made of a wax that slowly melts and releases the active ingredients. In Continental Europe many people use suppositories in preference to tablets and they are widely available.

- Pessaries are tablets that are intended to be inserted into the vagina.

Special Precautions

Because of their size, babies and young infants require much lower doses of medicines than adults, so medicines intended for adults are usually not suitable for children.

As a general rule, more powerful medicines are not given to babies or young infants except under medical supervision because children of this age may be more sensitive than adults to unwanted effects. Even when products intended for babies and infants are available, the dosage instructions given on the product should be carefully followed.

Babies are often more susceptible to illness than adults and are likely to become seriously ill faster. If your baby cries for a prolonged period, has a raised temperature, is pale, fails to thrive or will not accept feed, or forcibly vomits regularly after feeding, seek medical advice. Some regurgitation of food after a feed, possibly during winding, is common and should not cause alarm. This may be caused by air intake during bottle-feeding and is often associated with the use of an incorrect size or type of teat.

COLDS AND COUGHS

Cough mixtures for infants are simple syrup-based medicines (**linctuses**) containing **guaiphenesin** which helps to loosen phlegm. Nasal drops containing a **decongestant, xylometazoline**, are available for the relief of a stuffy nose (see **Coughs/Colds** for further information). These preparations are only suitable for children aged two years or over except under medical advice and supervision.

Capsules containing various **aromatic oils** which release a vapour may provide some relief of stuffy nose in younger infants but are not suitable for babies under three months old. These should only be put on the baby's bedding, not onto the skin. A similar product, a **vapour rub**, can be applied to the skin but should not be put in the nostrils.

KARVOL
Boots Healthcare Ltd

PA No: 43/4/1

■ Packs of 10 capsules.

■ Chlorbutol 2.25mg, menthol 35.55mg, pine oil sylvestris 9mg, pumilio pine oil 103.05mg, terpineol 66.6mg, thymol 3.15mg.

■ For the relief of symptoms of nasal congestion and head colds.

■ Adults: Snip tip off capsule. Dab contents onto bedding or handkerchief and inhale the vapour freely. Or, squeeze contents into hot water and inhale vapour.

Children: Dab contents onto handkerchief in the vicinity but out of reach of the child.

■ Not recommended for children under 3 months.

Avoid contact with eyes and skin.

Pharmacy only: Yes

SNUFFLEBABE DECONGESTANT
Intrapharma/Dugdale/J Pickles Healthcare

PA No: N/A

■ 24g of cream.

■ Menthol, eucalyptus and thyme oils.

■ Chest rub for children to provide relief from upper respiratory congestion.

Pharmacy only: Yes

Always Read The Label

TIXYLIX CHESTY COUGH
Novartis Consumer Health

PA No: 30/22/1

◻100ml bottle containing a clear, sugar-free linctus with a blackcurrant flavour.

☑Guaiphenesin 50mg per 5ml.

▨Symptomatic relief of chesty coughs. Helps loosen mucus to make breathing easier.

▨Under 2 yrs: On medical advice. 2-5 yrs: 5ml given 4 hourly. 6-10 yrs: 5-10ml given 4 hourly.

Pharmacy only: Yes

COLIC

Bouts of crying, especially in the early evening, which are difficult to console, accompanied by drawing the knees up to the chin and by reddening of the face, are the usual signs of colic. Colic occurs in babies between one and four months old. You should be reassured that colic is temporary. It is not clear exactly what causes colic but it is often thought to be caused by intestinal pain, spasm or wind. If you are bottle-feeding your baby, check that you are using a suitable teat.

Treatment

Colic is traditionally treated using **gripe water**, containing **dill oil** which helps to bring up wind. The more recently introduced **dimethicone** also helps to reduce wind by causing air bubbles to join together so that they may be more easily removed on winding.

Colic has also been attributed to a temporary reaction to **lactose** in milk that will disappear as the infant matures. The addition of a **lactase enzyme** to milk feed which breaks down some of the lactose to other sugars may be worth a try if other measures are ineffective.

COLIEF® INFANT DROPS
Clonmel Healthcare Ltd

PA No: N/A

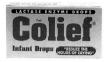

◻7ml drops.

☑Lactase enzyme.

▨For the relief of colic associated with lactose intolerance.

▨Infants from birth onwards: Add 2 drops to cooled baby's bottle. Refrigerate for 4 hrs.

Reheat and use as normal.

Pharmacy only: Yes

DENTINOX INFANT COLIC DROPS
DDD Ltd

PA No: 302/3/1

◻100ml bottle containing translucent, white, emulsified liquid with aroma of dill.

☑Activated dimethicone 21mg per 2.5ml dose.

▨For the relief of wind and griping pains caused by accumulation of ingested air.

▨Infants from birth onwards: 2.5ml with or after each feed.

▨If symptoms persist, seek medical advice.

Pharmacy only: Yes

Always Consult Your Pharmacist

"REDUCE THE HOURS OF CRYING"

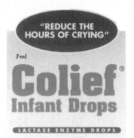
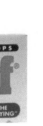
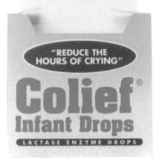

The active ingredient in Colief ® is lactase, a safe enzyme which occurs naturally within the body. Milk, dairy products, breast milk and infant formulas contain a complex sugar called lactose. Lactese is the enzyme our bodies normally produce to break down this lactose into the simple sugars glucose and galactose, so that we can absorb it. Undigested lactose in foods can cause temporary digestive discomfort, bloatedness and wind. This is sometimes the result of transient lactrose intolerance which may be an important factor in some babies with Colic.

Colief ® Infant Drops, added to babies usual milk reduce the levels of lactose by breaking it down into glucose and galactose before the baby is fed. Studies have shown that the hours of crying may be greatly reduced when babies are fed with milk treated with Colief ®.

Colief ® is a safe natural product and full instructions are given with the product. It is available without prescription from your pharmacy. If you are happy that your baby is thriving and without illness, but it has been concluded that your child has colic don't despair. The condition while unpleasant will usually have resolved itself by the time the child is three months old.

We have received many calls from people who tell us that they are very grateful to Colief ® for making their lives more bearable during this time. Always consult your GP or Public Health Nurse if your child is ill.

If you have any queries on the product, please contact our free phone number 1800 522 8243.

Colief®

LACTASE ENZYME DROPS

Colief® is manufactured for Crosscare Ltd., Broomhill Road, Tallaght, Dublin 24 and distributed in Ireland by Clonmel Healthcare Ltd., Waterford Road, Clonmel, Co Tipperary

INFACOL
Pharmax Ltd

PA No: 100/41/1

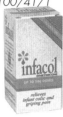

◾50ml bottle containing a white, orange-flavoured liquid.

◾Simethicone 40mg/ml.

❓For the relief of infant colic and griping pain.

◾Children: 0.5ml before each feed. If necessary this may be increased to 1ml.

Pharmacy only: Yes

MILKAID®
Crosscare Ltd

PA No: N/A

◾Packs of 120 capsules.

◾Lactase enzyme.

❓To aid digestion of milk and dairy foods.

◾Adults: 2-3 capsules immediately before meals.

Children: Dosage available upon request.

❗Use with caution in diabetics

as lactase makes the sugar in milk more available.

Pharmacy Only: Yes

WOODWARDS GRIPE WATER
SSL Healthcare Ireland Ltd

PA No: 618/20/1

◾150ml bottle of clear liquid.

◾Terpeneless dill seed oil

0.69mg, sodium bicarbonate 52.5mg.

❓Relieves wind pains and minor tummy upsets in babies and young children, particularly at the difficult period when they are cutting teeth.

◾Children: 1-6 months: 5ml. 6 months-1 yr: 10ml. Doses may be given during or after each feed. Maximum 6 doses in 24 hrs.

❗Do not give to infants under 1 month old.

Pharmacy only: No

If Symptoms Persist Consult Your Doctor

CONSTIPATION

Babies and infants should only occasionally require a **laxative** and routine use of laxatives is not encouraged. For occasional constipation in infants, a suppository containing **glycerin** – a natural substance that softens the motions and lubricates their passage – is the appropriate form of treatment.

BABYLAX
Pharma Global Ltd

PA No: 141/15/1

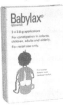

Faecal softener/lubricant.

Glycerol 1.8g, benzalkonium chloride 0.36g; 3.6g solution in rectal applicator.

Constipation in adults, the elderly and children of any age.

Adults and the elderly: 1-2 applicators.

Children: Under 3 months: $\frac{1}{2}$-1 applicator. 3 months-6 yrs: 1 applicator. Over 6 yrs: 1-2 applicators.

For single use only.

Pharmacy only: Yes

NAPPY RASH

Nappy rash is a form of irritant **eczema** that produces a large bright red rash in the napkin area. This often looks much worse than it is. It happens when the baby's skin is exposed to moisture and to the ammonia that is formed by bacteria from urine. Nappy rash may be prevented by leaving the nappy off (easier said than done!), by frequent changing and by use of a nappy that draws moisture away. Applying a thin layer of a barrier cream containing a **silicone (dimethicone)** or an oily material such as **lanolin** to the skin after changing is helpful. Some products for nappy rash prevention contain **antibacterials** such as **benzalkonium**, **cetrimide** etc. (see **Antiseptics** in the main **Skin Care** section). **Zinc oxide** has a long history of use as a soothing and protective agent.

Caution

If nappy rash is severe, it may become infected with the yeast, **Candida**. An anti-yeast agent, **clotrimazole**, is available in cream form. This type of rash should be treated under medical supervision.

Precautions and Warnings

• Do not use **hydrocortisone** cream to treat skin conditions in babies or infants unless under strict medical supervision.

CALDEASE
Roche Consumer Health

PA No: 72/7/1

30g tube of nappy rash ointment.

Zinc oxide 15%, cod liver oil 15%.

For treatment of nappy rash, minor skin irritations, superficial wounds and burns.

Children: Apply to affected area as required.

Pharmacy only: Yes

CALDESENE
Roche Consumer Health

PA No: 72/2/1

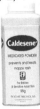

⬛55g tin of antifungal, antibacterial powder.

✔Calcium undecylenate.

❓For treatment and prevention of nappy rash, prickly heat and chafing.

Pharmacy only: Yes

CANESTEN 1% CREAM
Bayer Ltd

PA No: 21/4/2

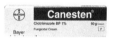

⬛20g or 50g tubes containing a white cream base.

✔Clotrimazole 1% w/w.

❓For treatment of fungal and candidal skin infections including candidal nappy rash, vulvitis and balanitis.

✔Adults and children: Apply thinly 2-3 times daily rubbing in gently.

Pharmacy only: Yes

DRAPOLENE CREAM
Pfizer/Warner Lambert Consumer Healthcare

PA No: 823/7/1

⬛100g tube containing a smooth, homogeneous, pink, water-miscible cream.

✔Benzalkonium chloride solution 0.02% w/w (equivalent to benzalkonium chloride 0.01% w/w), cetrimide 0.2% w/w in a water base.

❓For the prevention and treatment of nappy rash and in the treatment of minor wounds and burns.

✔Children: Nappy rash: After thorough cleansing and drying the cream should be applied at each nappy change with particular care to skin folds. Other conditions: Apply twice daily or as indicated.

Pharmacy only: Yes

MORHULIN OINTMENT
SSL Healthcare Ireland Ltd

PA No: 618/6/1

⬛50g tube of ointment.

✔Zinc oxide 38% w/w, cod liver oil 11.4% w/w.

❓For the treatment of minor wounds, minor excoriations, pressure sores, varicose ulcers, eczema and nappy rash.

✔Adults and children: Apply to the affected area as required.

Pharmacy only: No

SNUFFLEBABE MEDICATED NAPPY CREAM
Intrapharma/Dugdale/J Pickles Healthcare

PA No: N/A

⬛Cream.

✔Benzyl benzoate, zinc oxide and lanolin.

❓Hypoallergenic/mild astringent stopping organisms that can cause nappy rash.

Pharmacy only: Yes

Always Consult Your Pharmacist

SNUFFLEBABE ZINC & CASTOR OIL CREAM
Intrapharma/Dugdale/J Pickles Healthcare

PA No: N/A

☐Cream.

🔲Zinc oxide in a blend of castor and peanut oils and natural beeswax.

☑For external use only.

Pharmacy only: Yes

SUDOCREM
Tosara Products Ltd

PA No: 247/1/1

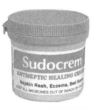

🔲25g, 60g, 125g and 400g containers or 30g tube of cream emulsion.

🔲Zinc oxide 15.25%, lanolin (hypoallergenic) 4.00%, benzyl benzoate 1.01%, benzyl cinnamate 0.15%, benzyl alcohol 0.39%.

🔲For the treatment of nappy rash, bedsores, minor burns,

eczema, acne, chilblains, surface wounds and sunburn.

🔲Adults: Apply in a thin layer as required.

Children: As adult dose.

🔲For external use only.

Pharmacy only: No

VASOGEN CREAM
Pharmax Ltd

PA No: 601/1

🔲50g or 100g tubes of topical cream.

🔲Dimethicone 20.0% w/w, zinc oxide 7.5% w/w, calamine 1.5% w/w.

🔲Prevention and treatment of nappy rash and bedsores. Local protection of skin around stoma

after ileostomy and colostomy.

🔲Adults: Apply in thin layer as required.

Children: As adult dose.

Pharmacy only: Yes

If Symptoms Persist Consult Your Doctor

PAIN AND TEETHING

The most frequently used pain reliever in babies and infants is **paracetamol**. It also reduces the fever that may accompany infections such as colds or flu. Paracetamol is a safe painkiller when used correctly, but it is very important that the correct dosage is strictly observed. See the main sections on **General Pain Relief** and **Colds/Coughs** for further information.

If inflammation is a problem, for example if a child suffers a sprain or strain, **ibuprofen** is a painkiller that has the same effects as paracetamol but also reduces inflammation. Ibuprofen should not be given to a child who has asthma.

Caution

Aspirin is not suitable for children under 12 because of its association with a serious toxic reaction, known as **Reyes syndrome**.

Teething pain can be relieved by applying a gel to the gum area because pain relievers can penetrate the soft gum tissue. You may be aware that **salicylate**, which is used in this gel form, is similar chemically to aspirin. However, there are differences in its action and a link with Reyes syndrome has not been established when salicylate is used in this way.

A sedative, **diphenhydramine**, is present in some medicines for short-term use to relieve sleeplessness. It is unsuitable for babies under three months old and should not be used on a routine or long-term basis. See **Hayfever** for further information.

Precautions and Warnings

- Observe dosage instructions carefully
- Aspirin is not suitable for children under 12 years
- Do not give ibuprofen if your child has asthma
- Do not give analgesics on a routine basis
- See General Pain Relief for further information on precautions and warnings.

BONJELA
Reckitt Benckiser

PA No: 979/1/1

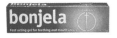

▣ 15g tube of colourless gel with an aniseed flavour.

☑ Choline salicylate 8.7% w/w, cetalkonium chloride 0.01% w/w.

❓ For the relief of pain and discomfort of common mouth ulcers, cold sores, denture sore spots and pain due to orthodontic devices in children. It aids healing of ulcers and sore spots due to dentures in adults and orthodontic devices in children.

☑ Adults: Dry affected site. Apply 1cm of gel onto sore area. The dose may be repeated every 3 hrs.

Children: Over 4 months: Dry affected site. Apply 0.5cm of gel onto sore area. The dose may be repeated every 4 hrs.

❗ Maximum 6 doses in 24 hrs.

Pharmacy only: Yes

Always Read The Label

CALPOL 6+ SUGAR/COLOUR FREE SUSPENSION

Pfizer/Warner Lambert Consumer Healthcare

PA No: 823/10/4

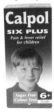

70ml bottle containing an off-white suspension with an odour of strawberries.

Paracetamol 250mg per 5ml.

For the management of pain and fever associated with such conditions as colds, flu, headaches and toothache.

Children 6-12 yrs: 1-2 x 5ml spoonfuls.

Adults and children over 12 yrs: 2-4 x 5ml spoonfuls.

Children 3 months-under 6 yrs: Calpol Infant Suspension is recommended.

Pharmacy only: Yes

CALPOL 6+ SUSPENSION

Pfizer/Warner Lambert Consumer Healthcare

PA No: 823/10/3

70ml bottle containing an orange-coloured suspension with an odour of oranges.

Paracetamol 250mg per 5ml.

For the management of pain and fever associated with such conditions as colds, flu, headaches and toothache.

Children 6-12 yrs: 1-2 x 5ml spoonfuls.

Adults and children over 12 yrs: 2-4 x 5ml spoonfuls.

Children 3 months-under 6 yrs: Calpol Infant Suspension is recommended.

Pharmacy only: Yes

CALPOL INFANT SUSPENSION

Pfizer/Warner Lambert Consumer Healthcare

PA No: 823/10/2

70ml or 140ml bottles containing a viscous, pink suspension with a strawberry odour and taste.

Paracetamol 120mg per 5ml.

For the management of pain and fever associated with colds, flu, high temperature, headaches and teething.

Three months - under 1 yr: $\frac{1}{2}$ (2.5ml) -1 x 5ml spoonful.

1 yr to under 6 yrs: 1-2 x 5ml spoonfuls.

Under 3 months: 2.5ml for fever following vaccination at 2 months, otherwise use only under medical supervision.

Pharmacy only: Yes

CALPOL INFANT SUSPENSION SUGAR FREE

Pfizer/Warner Lambert Consumer Healthcare

PA No: 823/10/5

140ml bottle containing an off-white suspension with strawberry odour.

Paracetamol 120mg per 5ml.

For the management of pain and fever associated with colds, flu, high temperature, headaches and teething.

Three months - under 1 yr: $\frac{1}{2}$ (2.5ml) -1 x 5ml spoonful.

1 yr to under 6 yrs: 1-2 x 5ml spoonfuls.

Under 3 months: 2.5ml for fever following vaccination at 2 months, otherwise use only under medical supervision.

Pharmacy only: Yes

Always Consult Your Pharmacist

CALPOL SACHETS
**Pfizer/Warner Lambert
Consumer Healthcare**

PA No: 823/10/5, 823/10/2

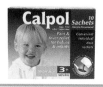

◻Packs of 10 x 5ml sachets.

☑Paracetamol 120mg per 5ml.

◪Children under 3 months: 2 x 5ml. 3 months: 1 x 2.5ml to 1 x 5ml spoonful. 1yr - under 6 yrs: 1-2 x 5ml spoonfuls.

❗Do not give with any other paracetamol-containing products.

Pharmacy only: No

DISPROL PARACETAMOL SUSPENSION
Reckitt Benckiser

PA No: 979/8/1

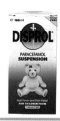

◻100ml bottle containing a sugar-free, banana-flavoured suspension.

☑Paracetamol 120mg per 5ml.

▣For the management of pain and fever associated with headaches, toothache, common colds, influenza and musculoskeletal pain.

◪Children: 6-12 yrs: 10-20ml every 4 hrs.

1-6 yrs: 5-10ml every 4 hrs.

3-12 months: 2.5-5ml every 4 hrs.

❗Maximum 4 doses in 24 hrs.

Do not continue dosing for more than 3 days without consulting a doctor.

Pharmacy only: Yes

DISPROL SOLUBLE PARACETAMOL TABLETS
Reckitt Benckiser

PA No: 979/8/2

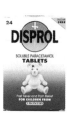

◻Foil packs of 24 sugar-free, white, circular, fruit-flavoured, soluble tablets.

☑Paracetamol 120mg.

▣For the management of pain and fever associated with headaches, toothache, common colds, influenza and musculoskeletal pain.

◪Children: Take tablets dissolved in water or fruit juice. 6-12 yrs: 2-4 tablets every 4 hrs. Do not take more than 16 tablets in 24 hrs.

1-6 yrs: 1-2 tablets every 4 hrs. Do not take more than 8 tablets in 24 hrs.

3-12 months: $\frac{1}{2}$-1 tablet every 4 hrs. Do not take more than 4 tablets in 24 hrs.

❗Do not continue dosing for more than 3 days without consulting a doctor.

Pharmacy only: Yes

If Symptoms Persist Consult Your Doctor

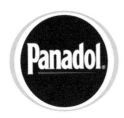 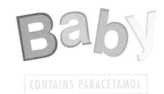

CONTAINS PARACETAMOL

Nothing acts faster[1,2] to relieve pain and fever.

- Panadol Baby is a sugar-free paracetamol suspension specifically for children from 2 months upwards.

- It contains paracetamol; so it acts fast[2].
  Paracetamol is a safe medication when used at the recommended dose[3], and it is not associated with gastrointestinal bleeding in children. [4,5]

- Importantly, paracetamol is well tolerated when given with many other childrens' medications including antibiotics and asthma medicines.

Why recommend anything else for childrens' pain and fever?

Effective relief from:

- HIGH TEMPERATURE
- TEETHING PAIN
- SORE THROAT
- COLD & FLU SYMPTOMS
- TOOTHACHE

Suitable for children as young as 2 months

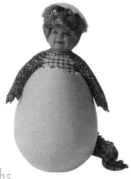

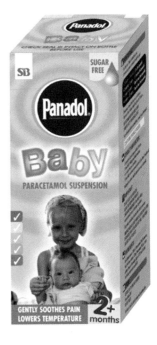

References:
1. Walson PD et al. AJDC May 1992; 146: 626-632
2. Schachtel BP, Thoden WR, Clin Pharmac. Ther May 1993; 53: 593-601
3. Cranswick N, Coghlan D. Paracetamol efficacy and safety in children - the forst 40 years. American Journal of Therapeutics 2000;7: 135-141.
4. Lesko SM, Mitchell AA. An assessment of the safety of paediatric ibuprofen: a practitioner-based randomized clinical trial. The Journal of the American Medical Association 1995; 929-933.
5. Lesko SM, Mitchell AA. The safety of acetaminophen and ibuprofen among children younger than two years old. Paediatrics 1999; 104: e39.

Full prescribing information available on request.   CONTAINS PARACETAMOL   Always read the label

PA No. 678/39/3 GlaxoSmithKline Consumer Healthcare, Corrig Ave, Dun Laoghaire, Co Dublin

DOZOL
Ricesteele Manufacturing

PA No: 95/4/1

📦30ml or 100ml bottles containing an amber liquid with caramel odour.

💊Paracetamol 120mg/5ml, diphenhydramine hydrochloride 12.5mg/5ml.

❓Relief of teething pains, irritability after injections, feverishness, aches or pains, colds, flu, sleeplessness associated with above.

📋Children: Over 6 yrs: 10-20ml 3 times daily. 1-6 yrs: 5-10ml 3-4 times daily. 3-12 months: 5ml 3-4 times daily.

❗May cause drowsiness. Large doses of antihistamines may cause fits in epileptics. This product should be administered with caution to patients with known liver or kidney impairment.

Pharmacy only: Yes

MEDINOL UNDER 6
SSL Healthcare Ireland Ltd

PA No: 258/15/1

📦70ml or 140ml bottles containing a strawberry-flavoured, sugar- and colour-free suspension.

💊120mg paracetamol per 5ml dose.

❓For the treatment of mild to moderate pain and fever.

📋Children over 5 yrs: 3-4 x 5ml spoonfuls 3-4 times daily.

Children 1-5 yrs: 1-2 x 5ml spoonfuls 3-4 times daily.

3 months-1 yr: ½-1 x 5ml spoonfuls 3-4 times daily.

❗Do not repeat dose more frequently than every 4 hrs. Do not take more than 4 doses in 24 hrs. In other cases use only under medical supervision. Not to be given to infants under 2 months except on medical advice.

Pharmacy only: Yes

NUROFEN FOR CHILDREN
Boots Healthcare Ltd

PA No: 43/6/5

📦100ml or 150ml bottles containing an orange-flavoured, sugar-free and colour-free suspension.

💊Ibuprofen 100mg per 5ml.

❓Reduction in temperature and relief of pain associated with teething and toothache, earache, sore throat, headache, minor sprains and strains and cold and flu symptoms.

📋Babies 6-12 months: 2.5ml 3-4 times daily.

Children 1-3 yrs: 5ml 3 times daily.

Children 4-6 yrs: 7.5ml 3 times daily.

Children 7-9 yrs: 10ml 3 times daily.

Children 10-12 yrs: 15ml 3 times daily.

❗Do not exceed the stated dose.

Do not repeat dose more frequently than 4 hourly.

Pharmacy only: Yes

PANADOL BABY
GlaxoSmithKline

PA No: 678/39/3

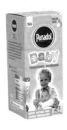

📦100ml bottle containing a sugar-free, strawberry-flavoured suspension.

💊Paracetamol Ph Eur 120mg per 5ml.

❓For the relief of teething pain, sore throat, toothache, and the feverishness of colds, flu, measles, whooping cough, mumps and chickenpox.

📋Children: 6-12 yrs: 10-20ml. 1-6 yrs: 5-10ml. 3 months-1 yr: 2.5-5ml. 2-3 months: 2.5ml. Repeat every 4 hrs to a maximum of 4 doses in 24 hrs.

❗Do not exceed the stated dose.

Do not take with any other paracetamol-containing product.

Not suitable for babies under 2 months.

Pharmacy only: Yes

Always Read The Label

PARALINK PARACETAMOL SOLUTION
Ricesteele Manufacturing

PA No: 95/7/1

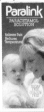

100ml bottle containing a colourless liquid with raspberry odour and taste.

Paracetamol 120mg per 5ml.

For treatment of pain and fever.

Children: 6 yrs and over: 10-20ml. 1-5 yrs: 5-10ml. 3 months-1 yr: 5ml. Doses may be given 3-4 times daily.

The product should be administered with caution to patients with known liver or kidney impairment.

Pharmacy only: Yes

PARALINK PARACETAMOL SUPPOSITORIES
Ricesteele Manufacturing

PA No: 180mg: 95/7/2; 500mg: 95/7/4

Packs of 10 white, tapered, cylindrical suppositories.

Paracetamol 180mg, 500mg.

For treatment of pain and fever associated with such conditions as common cold, flu, headaches, rheumatism, teething and post-operative pain.

Adults and children over 12 yrs: 1-2 suppositories (500mg) every 6 hrs.

Children: 6-12 yrs: 1 suppository (500mg) every 6 hrs. 3-6 yrs: 1½ suppositories (180mg) every 6 hrs. 1-3 yrs: 1 suppository (180mg) every 6 hrs. 3 months-1 yr: ½ suppository (180mg) every 6 hrs.

Suppositories should be administered with caution to patients with known liver or kidney impairment.

Pharmacy only: Yes

PARAPAED 6+
Pinewood Healthcare

PA No: 281/2/3

70ml bottle containing an orange-coloured oral suspension with an odour and flavour of orange.

5ml contains 250mg of paracetamol Ph Eur.

For pain and fever in the treatment of teething pain, toothache, colds, flu and post-immunisation fever.

Adults and children over 12 yrs: 60mg/kg bodyweight.

Children 6-12 yrs: 1-2 x 5ml tsps, 3-4 times daily.

Not recommended for children under 6 yrs.

Do not use if you are hypersensitive to paracetamol or any of its constituents. Special precautions if liver or kidney function is impaired.

Pharmacy only: Yes

PARAPAED JUNIOR
Pinewood Healthcare

PA No: 281/2/1

70ml or 140ml amber glass bottles containing a pink suspension with cherry odour and flavour.

Each 5ml contains paracetamol Ph Eur 120mg.

For pain and fever in the treatment of teething pain, toothache, headache, colds and flu.

Children 3 months-1 yr: ½-1 x 5ml tsp 3-4 times daily.

Children 1-6 yrs: 1-2 x 5ml tsp 3-4 times daily.

Children 6-12 yrs: 2-4 x 5ml tsp 3-4 times daily.

Do not use if liver or kidney function is impaired.

Pharmacy only: Yes

Always Consult Your Pharmacist

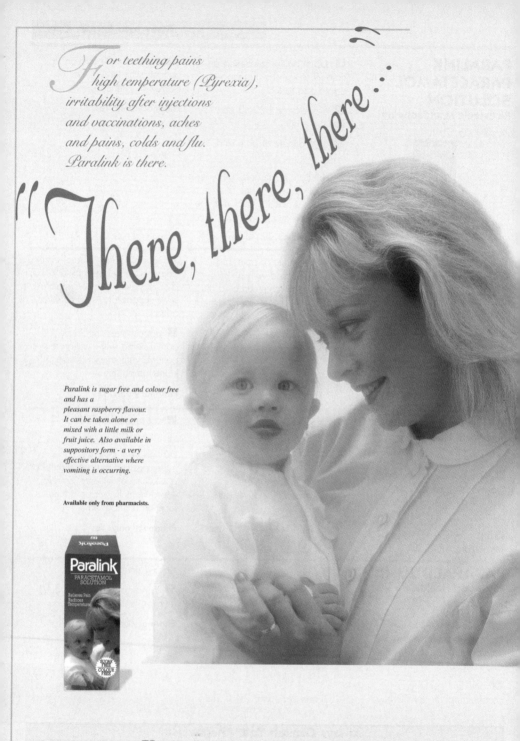

For teething pains
high temperature (Pyrexia),
irritability after injections
and vaccinations, aches
and pains, colds and flu.
Paralink is there.

"There, there, there..."

Paralink is sugar free and colour free
and has a
pleasant raspberry flavour.
It can be taken alone or
mixed with a little milk or
fruit juice. Also available in
suppository form - a very
effective alternative where
vomiting is occurring.

Available only from pharmacists.

TEE JEL TEETHING GEL

SSL Healthcare Ireland Ltd

PA No: 618/5/1

🔲10g tube of gel.

🔲Cetalkonium chloride 0.01% w/w, choline salicylate 8.7 % w/w.

🔲Treatment of pain and minor infections in and around the mouth, including mouth ulcers, infant teething and stomatitis.

🔲Adults and children over 2 yrs: Approx 1cm of gel should be massaged onto the affected area every 3-4 hrs as required.

Children: 4 months-2 yrs: Approx 0.5cm of gel should be massaged onto the affected area every 3-4 hrs as required.

🔲Not to be used in children under 4 months.

Pharmacy only: No

TEEDEX

Ricesteele Manufacturing

PA No: 95/3/1

🔲100ml bottle containing a red liquid with raspberry odour.

🔲Paracetamol 120mg, diphenhydramine hydrochloride 12.5mg per 5ml.

🔲Relief of teething pains, irritability associated with injections or feverishness.

🔲Children: Over 6 yrs: 10-20ml 3 times daily. 1-6 yrs: 5-10ml 3-4 times daily. 3-12 months: 5ml 3-4 times daily.

🔲May cause drowsiness.

The product should be administered with caution to patients with known liver or kidney impairment.

Large doses of antihistamines may cause fits in epileptics.

Pharmacy only: Yes

If Symptoms Persist Consult Your Doctor

SKIN AND SCALP

Cradle Cap

Cradle cap is a form of **dermatitis** (see main **Skin Care** section) that results in the top of the baby's scalp becoming covered in greasy yellow scales. These scales are not removed by normal washing. It usually first occurs in babies before they reach three months old but it generally improves with time. If only a small area is affected, a simple remedy such as a nightly application of **olive oil** or a **baby oil** preparation may be sufficient to clear it. If it is more extensive, then use of a mild shampoo containing **salicylic acid** and/or **coal tar** is usually effective. See **Hair and Scalp** for further information.

Dermatitis, Eczema and Dry Skin

Dermatitis and **eczema** are essentially the same thing. Eczema and dry skin are treated using **moisturising agents (emollients)** that include oily materials, especially **liquid paraffin** and **soft paraffin** or other natural oils, which hydrate and soften the skin. There are many preparations of this type that can be applied directly to the skin or added to the bath. It is important to note that not all of these products are medicines, and so they do not require a product authorisation (PA) number from the Irish Medicines Board (see **Introduction**). If you are not sure which product to choose, ask your pharmacist's advice.

A form of allergic eczema (**atopic eczema**) is possible in infants where there is a family history of asthma, hayfever or hives. This often starts in babies as a rash on the cheeks and upper body and it settles later in childhood on the backs of the knees and the fronts of the elbows, wrists and ankles. This is treated by using the oily preparations mentioned above.

Thrush

Our immune system, which defends our bodies against infection, is often not fully developed in babies and this may lead to the yeast infection in the mouth known as thrush. Thrush appears as creamy-white raised patches on the tongue or cheeks. In very young babies, thrush is best treated under medical supervision. For infants aged one and over, a gel containing the anti-yeast agent **miconazole**, is an effective treatment. For further information see **Mouth Care**.

AVENT BABY BODY & HAIR WASH
E J Bodkin & Co Ltd

PA No: N/A

▢ 250ml plastic container of golden-coloured bath additive.

▢ Formulation of milk proteins, amino acids and water lily extracts. Tear-free, hypoallergenic, clinically proven to be mild, pH balanced.

▢ Low lather, all-over shampoo mildly cleanses without removing the skin and hair's natural oils.

▢ Children: Add a few drops to baby's bath water.

Pharmacy only: Yes

AVENT BABY BOTTOM BALM
E J Bodkin & Co Ltd

PA No: N/A

▢ 125ml plastic container of light, white, water-resistant cream, naturally perfumed.

▢ Milk proteins, amino acids as the base ingredient with allantoin, camomile, calendula and shea butter. Hypoallergenic, clinically proven to be mild, pH balanced.

▢ Helps calm irritated skin, soothes and moisturises.

▢ Children: At each nappy change or as often as required.

▢ Will not cure nappy rash.

Pharmacy only: Yes

Always Read The Label

AVENT BABY CLEANSER AND MOISTURISER
E J Bodkin & Co Ltd

PA No: N/A

☐200ml plastic container of white, naturally perfumed lotion.

☑Milk proteins, amino acids as the base ingredient with avocado oil and shea butter. Hypoallergenic, clinically proven to be mild, pH balanced.

☐Lotion cleanses, moisturises and protects baby skin between baths. Removes dry patches.

☑Children: As often as required.

Pharmacy only: Yes

BABY NATURALS BABY BARRIER CREAM
Power Health Products Ltd

PA No: N/A

☐125ml tub of white, opaque cream. Not tested on animals.

☑Aloe vera and chamomile extract, vegetable oil, cetearyle alcohol, ceteareth-20, glyceryl monostearate, dimethicone, parabens phenoxyethanol, imidazolidinyl urea, mixed tocopherals, de-ionised water, natural fragrance.

☑Smooth gently on at each nappy change.

Pharmacy only: Yes

BABY NATURALS BABY OIL
Power Health Products Ltd

PA No: N/A

☐250ml plastic container of golden yellow, clear oil. Not tested on animals.

☑Aloe vera and chamomile extract, vegetable oil, isopropyl palmitate, natural fragrance and preservative.

☑Apply gently to the skin as required.

Pharmacy only: Yes

BABY NATURALS BUBBLE BATH
Power Health Products Ltd

PA No: N/A

☐250ml bottle of colourless liquid. Not tested on animals.

☑Aloe vera and chamomile extract, sodium laureth sulphate, cocoamidoprophyl betaine, PER-7 glyceryl cocoate, citric acid, de-ionised water, natural fragrance and preservative.

☑Pour small amount into running water or add to warm water and agitate by hand.

Pharmacy only: Yes

BABY NATURALS LOTION
Power Health Products Ltd

PA No: N/A

☐250ml white plastic bottle of white, opaque cream. Not tested on animals.

☑Aloe vera and chamomile extract, vegetable oil, glycerin, stearic acid, cetearyle alcohol, ceteareth-20, glyceryl stearate, triethanolamine, hydroxyethylcellulose, de-ionised water, natural fragrance and preservative.

Pharmacy only: Yes

BABY NATURALS SCALP OIL
Power Health Products Ltd

PA No: N/A

☐White plastic container of golden yellow oil. Not tested on animals.

☑Macadamia nut oil, calendula oil, wheatgerm oil, aloe vera oil, chamomile extract, capric/caprylic triglyceride, polysorbate 20, natural fragrance.

☑Apply a few drops to the scalp and gently massage in. Leave for a few minutes and then shampoo the hair as normal. Reapply as necessary.

☒Avoid contact with eyes.

Pharmacy only: Yes

Always Consult Your Pharmacist

BABY NATURALS SHAMPOO
Power Health Products Ltd

PA No: N/A

▭ 250ml bottle of colourless liquid. Not tested on animals.

▯ Aloe vera and chamomile extract, sodium laureth sulphate, cocoamidopropyl betaine, PEG-7 glyceryl cocoate, citric acid, de-ionised water, natural fragrance and preservative.

▯ Wet the hair and gently massage a little shampoo onto the hair and scalp. Rinse thoroughly with warm water.

Pharmacy only: Yes

BALNEUM PLUS BATH TREATMENT
Boots Healthcare Ltd

PA No: 54/74/1

▭ 150ml bottle of liquid bath treatment.

▯ Soya oil 82.95% w/w, lauromacrogols 15% w/w.

▯ Provides relief from pruritus. It is recommended for the treatment of dry skin conditions including those associated with eczema and dermatitis where pruritus is also experienced.

▯ Adults: Shake bottle before use. Pour 3 capfuls into a full bath of water as water is running and soak for at least 10 mins. May also be used in the shower with a flannel or sponge. Rinse and pat dry with a towel.

Children: Add 1 capful to bath while water is running and soak for at least 10 mins. Rinse and pat dry with a towel.

Babies and infants: Daily application is recommended.

Pharmacy only: Yes

CAPASAL THERAPEUTIC SHAMPOO
Dermal Laboratories

PA No: 278/16/1

▭ 100ml or 250ml bottles of golden brown, therapeutic shampoo.

▯ Salicylic acid 0.5% w/w, coconut oil 1.0% w/w, distilled coal tar 1.0% w/w.

▯ For the treatment of dry, scaly scalp conditions such as seborrhoeic eczema, seborrhoeic dermatitis, dandruff, psoriasis and cradle cap in children. It may also be used to remove previous scalp applications.

▯ Children: Use a small amount, sufficient to produce a lather, which should then be washed off immediately with warm water, and the scalp gently patted dry. Can be used daily until condition clears.

▯ Discontinue if any irritation occurs. Avoid contact with eyes.

Pharmacy only: Yes

DENTINOX CRADLE CAP SHAMPOO
DDD Ltd

PA No: 302/11/1

▭ 125ml plastic bottle of clear, orange shampoo.

▯ Sodium lauryl ether sulphosuccinate 6% w/w, sodium lauryl ether sulphate 2.7% w/w.

▯ For the treatment of infant cradle cap and general care of infant scalp and hair.

▯ Children: Infants from birth onwards: 2 shampoos of 2-3ml repeated at each bath.

▯ Avoid contact with eyes.

Pharmacy only: Yes

E45 BATH
Boots Healthcare Ltd

PA No: N/A

▭ 250ml bottle of colourless, semi-dispersing bath oil.

▯ White oil 90.95% w/w and cetyl dimethicone 5% w/w.

▯ To soothe and moisturise dry skin. It helps prevent dry skin by retaining the skin's natural moisture.

E45 Emollient Bath Oil is also recommended for bathing more serious dry skin conditions.

▯ Adults: 15ml poured into warm bath water or applied on a wet sponge if showering.

Children: Pour 5-10mls into a small bath of warm water.

Pharmacy only: Yes

If Symptoms Persist Consult Your Doctor

E45 CREAM
Boots Healthcare Ltd

PA No: 43/7/1

50g, 125g or 500g containers of cream.

☑Hypoallergenic anhydrous lanolin 1.0% w/w, light liquid paraffin 12.6% w/w, white soft paraffin 14.5% w/w, cetyl alcohol, citric acid, monohydrate, sodium lauryl sulphate, sodium hydroxide, methyl hydroxybenzoate, propyl hydroxybenzoate.

☑For the symptomatic relief of dry skin conditions, including

flaking, itching, chapped skin, eczema and contact dermatitis.

☑Adults and children: Apply to affected area 2-3 times daily.

Pharmacy only: Yes

E45 LOTION
Boots Healthcare Ltd

PA No: N/A

200ml of lotion.

☑White, soft paraffin 10% w/w, light liquid paraffin 4.0%

w/w, hypoallergenic anhydrous lanolin 1.0% w/w.

☑Soothes and softens dry skin.

☑Adults and children: Use frequently on face, hands and body.

Pharmacy only: Yes

E45 WASH
Boots Healthcare Ltd

PA No: N/A

250ml pump of white, creamy liquid emulsion.

☑Paraffinum liquidum,

petrolatum, cetyl dimethicone, cera microcrystallina.

☑To clean and moisturise dry skin without changing normal skin pH. It helps prevent dry skin by retaining the skin's natural moisture.

Also recommended instead of soap for washing more serious dry skin conditions.

Pharmacy only: Yes

EMULSIDERM EMOLLIENT
Dermal Laboratories

PA No: 278/8/1

300ml or 1 litre bottles of pale blue/green liquid emulsion, with a measuring cap.

☑Benzalkonium chloride 0.5%, liquid paraffin 25%, isopropyl myristate 25%.

☑For the treatment of dry skin conditions, including those associated with dermatitis and

psoriasis. It permits rehydration of the keratin by replacing lost lipids, and its antibacterial properties assist in overcoming *Staphylococcus aureus*, the pathogen which often complicates atopic eczema and associated pruritus.

☑Adults and children: Shake bottle before use. Add 7-30ml to a bath of warm water. Soak for 5-10 mins. Pat dry. For application to the skin: Rub a small amount of undiluted emollient into the dry areas of

skin until absorbed.

Pharmacy only: Yes

Always Read The Label

JOHNSON'S BABY BEDTIME BATH
Johnson & Johnson

PA No: N/A

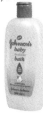

300ml or 500ml bottles of baby bedtime bath.

Add NO MORE TEARS® baby bath to warm water to release aroma of lavender and other natural extracts such as camomile.

Mild enough for new-born babies.

Pharmacy only: No

JOHNSON'S BABY TOP-TO-TOE WASH
Johnson & Johnson

PA No: N/A

500ml pump action bottle.

Suitable for direct application to the skin, for use as a foaming bath and for washing baby's hair. Milder than baby soap and mild enough for new-borns.

Pharmacy only: No

JOHNSON'S NURSING PADS
Johnson & Johnson

PA No: N/A

Carton - 30 pads per c/s.

For breastfeeding mums experiencing leakage between feeds, which may cause discomfort.

Pharmacy only: No

NIVEA CREME
Beiersdorf Ireland Ltd

PA No: N/A

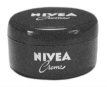

25ml, 50ml, 200ml, or 500ml pot and 100ml tube.

Aqua (water), paraffinum liquidum, cera microcristallina, glycerin, ceresin, isohexadecane, lanolin alcohol (eucerit), paraffin, magnesium sulphate, decyl oleate, octyldodecanol, aluminium stearates, panthenol, citric acid, magnesium stearate, parfum (fragrance).

To prevent dry skin conditions resulting in such diseases as eczema and psoriasis, and to help maintain healthy skin.

Moisturises, nourishes and protects dry, rough and chapped skin.

Suitable for all ages.

Pharmacy only: No

OILATUM CREAM
Stiefel Laboratories (Ireland) Ltd

PA No: 144/23/2

40g tube of emollient cream.

Arachis oil 21%.

Oilatum Cream is an emollient cream used in the treatment of dry, sensitive skin conditions, including ichthyosis. It coats the skin with a moisture-retaining film. Suitable for people allergic to lanolin.

Apply to the affected area, and rub in well. Use as often as required or as directed by doctor. Oilatum Cream is particularly effective when applied after washing.

Contains arachis oil.

Pharmacy only: Yes

Always Consult Your Pharmacist

OILATUM EMOLLIENT
Stiefel Laboratories (Ireland) Ltd

PA No: 144/22/1

150ml, 250ml or 500ml bottles of water dispersible bath emollient.

Light liquid paraffin 63.4%.

Oilatum Emollient is a bath emollient for eczema and dry skin conditions. Its dual action provides soothing rehydration and helps prevent further drying. It disperses in bath water giving a milky bath which also cleanses, so no soap is required.

Adults and children: Add 1-3 capfuls to a 20cm bath. Soak for 10-20 mins. Pat skin dry using a soft, clean towel. For maximum benefit use twice daily.

Infants: Add ½-2 capfuls to a small bath of water. Apply gently over body with a sponge. Pat skin dry using a soft, clean towel. For maximum benefit use twice daily.

Always use with water; either add to the bath or apply to wet skin. Take care to avoid slipping in the bath.

Pharmacy only: Yes

OILATUM JUNIOR
Stiefel Laboratories (Ireland) Ltd

PA No: 144/22/4

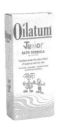

150ml or 300ml bottles of colour-free, fragrance-free emollient bath additive for children.

Light liquid paraffin 63.4%.

For children with eczema and other dry skin conditions. It has a dual action which: i) soothes and rehydrates the skin to provide relief, and ii) helps protect against further drying.

Infants: ½-2 capfuls to a small bath of water. Apply gently over body with a sponge. Pat skin dry using a soft, clean towel. For maximum benefit use twice daily.

Children: 1-3 capfuls to a 20cm bath. Soak for 10-20 mins. Pat skin dry using a soft, clean towel. For maximum benefit use twice daily.

Always use with water; either add to the bath or apply to wet skin. Take care to avoid slipping in the bath.

Pharmacy only: Yes

OILATUM SOAP
Stiefel Laboratories (Ireland) Ltd

PA No: 144/22/3

100g bar of mild cleanser for dry, sensitive skin.

Light liquid paraffin 7.5%.

To cleanse skin gently without causing dryness. Leaves a protective layer on the skin after washing to protect against any further moisture loss.

Adults and children: Use as ordinary soap for washing, bathing and showering.

Pharmacy only: Yes

SNUFFLEBABE CRADLE CAP CREAM
Intrapharma/Dugdale/J Pickles Healthcare

PA No: N/A

30g cream.

1.5% salicylic acid.

To soften and loosen flakes of skin, also has an antifungal and anti-yeast action.

Pharmacy only: Yes

If Symptoms Persist Consult Your Doctor

SNUFFLEBABE MOISTURISING E CREAM
Intrapharma/Dugdale/J Pickles Healthcare

PA No: N/A

◻150g cream.

◪Aloe vera, lanolin, dimethicone and glyceryl lanolate.

Pharmacy only: Yes

SNUFFLEBABE WHITE PETROLEUM JELLY
Intrapharma/Dugdale/J Pickles Healthcare

PA No: N/A

◻Petroleum jelly.

◪White soft paraffin BP.

Pharmacy only: Yes

TONICS AND VITAMIN SUPPLEMENTS

Vitamin supplements and tonics containing vitamins are available for children. It is important that dosage instructions are strictly observed and more than one such preparation should not be given. Infant feeds contain all the necessary nutrients in a balanced proportion. After weaning, a properly balanced diet will provide all the nutrients that are necessary. See **Tonics** and **Nutritionals** for further information.

ABIDEC DROPS
Pfizer/Warner Lambert Consumer Healthcare

PA No: 823/30/1

◻25ml bottle and dropper graduated at 0.3ml and 0.6ml. Contains a clear, yellow liquid with a characteristic odour and taste.

◪Vitamin A 4,000IU, thiamine hydrochloride 1mg, riboflavine 0.4mg, pyridoxine hydrochloride 0.5mg, ascorbic acid 50mg, calciferol 400IU, nicotinamide 5mg per 0.6 ml.

❓For the prevention of vitamin deficiencies.

▨Children: 1-12 yrs: 0.6ml daily. Under 1 yr: 0.3ml daily.

Pharmacy only: Yes

Always Read The Label

SANATOGEN BABY SYRUP
Roche Consumer Health

PA No: N/A

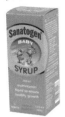

200ml bottle of orange-flavoured, sugar-free syrup.

10ml contains: Vitamin A 350µg, vitamin D 7µg, vitamin E 4mg, vitamin C 50mg, thiamin (vitamin B1) 0.6mg, riboflavin (vitamin B2) 0.8mg, niacin 10mg, vitamin B6 0.7mg, pantothenic acid 2.66mg.

Balanced formula of vitamins specially tailored for children from 1 month to 5 yrs to help maintain health.

Children: 1-6 months: $\frac{1}{2}$ x 5ml spoonful daily, 6 months – 1 yr: 1 x 5ml spoonful daily, 1-5 yrs: 2 x 5ml spoonfuls daily.

Taking more than the recommended dose may be harmful. Keep out of reach of children.

Pharmacy only: Yes

SEVEN SEAS HALIBORANGE MULTIVITAMIN ORANGE FLAVOURED LIQUID
Seven Seas Ireland Ltd

PA No: N/A

250ml bottle of orange-flavoured liquid.

Vitamin C (ascorbic acid) 15mg, vitamin E (dl-alpha-tocopheryl acetate) 3mg, vitamin B1 (thiamine hydrochloride), vitamin B2 (riboflavine) 0.4mg, vitamin B6 (pyridoxine hydrochloride) 0.6mg, nicotinic acid (niacin) 5mg, vitamin D 5µg, pantothenic acid 3mg, vitamin A 200µg.

Multivitamin supplement.

Adults: 10ml daily.

Children: Over 6 yrs: 10ml daily. 6 months-6 yrs: 5ml daily. Under 6 months: Mix dose into milk or diluted fruit juices.

Pharmacy only: Yes

SEVEN SEAS MINADEX MULTIVITAMIN SYRUP
Seven Seas Ireland Ltd

PA No: 416/6/1

150ml bottle of orange-flavoured syrup.

Vitamin C (ascorbic acid) 35mg, vitamin E (dl-alpha-tocopheryl acetate) 3mg, vitamin B1 (thiamine hydrochloride) 1.4mg, vitamin B2 (pyridoxine hydrochloride) 0.7mg, nicotinamide 18mg, vitamin A acetate 4,000IU, vitamin D3 (cholecalciferol) 400IU.

For the prevention of vitamin A, B group, C, D and E deficiency and for use during convalescence from debilitating illness.

Children: From 6 months: 10ml daily mixed in feed or a drink.

Pharmacy only: Yes

SEVEN SEAS MINADEX ORANGE FLAVOUR TONIC
Seven Seas Ireland Ltd

PA No: 417/7/1

200ml or 400ml bottles of orange-flavoured, oil-in-water emulsion.

Vitamin A palmitate 650IU, manganese sulphate monohydrate 0.38mg, copper sulphate 0.5mg, calcium glycerophosphate 11.25mg, potassium glycerophosphate solution 2.25mg, vitamin D2 (ergocalciferol) 65IU, ferric ammonium citrate 12mg.

Vitamin and mineral supplement, particularly during and after illness.

Adults: 10ml 3 times daily.

Children: 3-12 yrs: 5ml 3 times daily. 6 months-3 yrs: 5ml twice daily.

Not recommended for children under 6 months.

Pharmacy only: Yes

COUGHS AND COLDS

COLDS AND FLU

Colds and influenza (flu) are often confused but symptoms of the common cold usually appear quickly and consist of a tickling sensation in the nose resulting in sneezing, a sore throat and a stuffy nose with a watery discharge. After a day or two the discharge from the nose usually becomes green or yellow. This happens as a result of secondary infection. For the same reason, colds may be followed by inflammation of the sinuses (sinusitis), ear infection or bronchitis. Allergies can result in symptoms similar to those seen in the early stages of a cold.

Flu is a more serious illness causing fever, generalised aches and pains and often a harsh dry cough. If you have flu you should follow the traditional advice. If you go to bed and keep warm symptoms will usually subside within three to five days. However, the feeling of being run down and lifeless, which is a key symptom of flu, may persist for several weeks in some people. Secondary infection after flu often leads to bronchitis and sometimes even to pneumonia, so early medical advice should be sought if you start to wheeze or if you have any difficulty in breathing.

Colds and flu are caused by **viruses** that are spread by droplet infection (fine moist particles produced by coughing or sneezing). Flu in particular occurs in epidemics, usually in winter, and the viruses that cause it (**myxoviruses**) change in type from year to year depending on the part of the world where the outbreak occurs. Our ability to travel across the world in a few hours has enhanced the spread of flu. If you are elderly or have heart disease or any serious illness, prevention is better than cure. Once-yearly immunisation – specially developed to protect against the flu virus strains likely to be present at the time – is strongly recommended. Elderly people, or those considered to be at high risk, are entitled to receive flu vaccination free of charge. You should consult your doctor for further information.

COLD AND FLU TREATMENT

OTC treatment for colds and flu is 'symptomatic'. That is to say that the medicines used merely suppress the various symptoms without altering the underlying cause of the illness. Some prescription medicines that directly attack the viruses which cause colds and flu, are now available. So anyone in the groups at special risk who is affected, should visit their doctor.

Painkillers, especially **paracetamol** (see earlier), are often included in medicines for colds and flu because they relieve symptoms such as aches and pains and fever. As mentioned in the **General Pain Relief** section, it is important to ensure that two medicines containing paracetamol are not taken at the same time.

Decongestants (including **pseudoephedrine**, **phenylephrine** and **phenyl-propanolamine**) are used to dry up excessive secretions from the nose. They work by constricting the blood vessels in the nose, which reduces the volume of the mucus-producing membranes. This improves air flow. **Oxymetazoline** and **xylometazoline** in nasal sprays work in the same way.

Antihistamines (**diphenhydramine**, **triprolidine**, **brompheniramine**, **promethazine**, **methoxyphenamine**) also dry up nasal secretions. They are particularly useful if you have trouble sleeping, but they are sedatives. You should avoid these substances if you have to do anything that requires alertness and good co-ordination, such as driving or operating machinery. You should also be aware that the stronger sedative antihistamines have been used by drug abusers.

Vitamin C (**ascorbic acid**) is sometimes included in cold relief products, although there is little good evidence to show that it helps to cure a cold.

If Symptoms Persist Consult Your Doctor

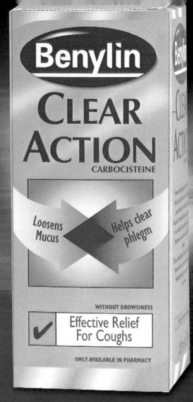

ACTION HERO

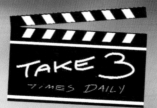

Now appearing in your local pharmacy: the new action hero cough bottle from Benylin. New Benylin Clear Action is strong enough to tackle even the toughest thick chesty coughs with stubborn phlegm. Benylin Clear Action works with your body deep in the lungs to loosen the grip of thick mucus, relieving your cough and making your breathing feel easier. Keep a bottle handy so you can be a hero to your family.

  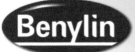

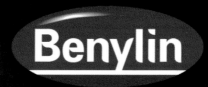

Benylin

THE EFFECTIVE RANGE FOR COUGHS, COLDS AND FLU.

BENYLIN ADULT COUGH RANGE

Benylin Traditional
Contains Diphenhydramine and Menthol. Indicated for the symptomatic relief of non-productive cough and of allergic conditions and reactions.

Benylin Non-drowsy for Chesty Cough
Contains Guaifenesin and Menthol. Indicated for the symptomatic relief of chesty cough (with phlegm/mucus) without causing drowsiness.

Benylin Dry Cough
Contains Dextromethorphan, Diphenhydramine and Menthol. Indicated for the treatment of non-productive, dry, irritating coughs.

Benylin Non-drowsy for Dry Cough
Contains Dextromethorphan. Indicated for the treatment of non-productive, dry, irritating coughs without causing drowsiness.

Benylin with Codeine
Contains Diphenhydramine, Codeine phosphate and Menthol. Indicated for the treatment of persistent, dry, irritating coughs.

Benylin Clear Action
Contains the mucolytic carbocisteine which helps restore mucus to its normal consistency. Indicated for the relief of a thick productive cough.

BENYLIN CHILDREN'S COUGH RANGE

Benylin Children's Chesty Cough
Contains Guaifenesin. Indicated for the relief of chesty coughs (with phlegm/mucus) without causing drowsiness.

Benylin Children's Coughs & Colds
Contains Dextromethorphan and Triprolidine. Indicated for the symptoms of coughs, colds and flu, catarrh and watery eyes.

COLDS AND FLU

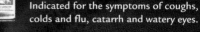

Benylin Day & Night
Indicated for relief from the symptoms of colds and flu such as nasal congestion, aches and pains.

The day tablet contains Paracetamol and Pseudoephedrine and is Non - Drowsy The night tablet contains Paracetamol and Diphenhydramine which aids restful sleep.

Benylin 4 Flu
Four way action to give relief for the symptoms of congestion, fever, pain and cough.

Contains three active ingredients
- Paracetamol (pain and fever)
- Diphenhydramine (anti-tussive)
- Pseudoephedrine (decongestant)

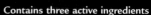

Available in liquid (200ml) and tablet (24's)

Warner Lambert Consumer Healthcare

Precautions and Warnings
- If you are being treated with a monoamine oxidase inhibitor or MAOI (usually used for depression), it is imperative to avoid decongestants. Your doctor will warn you about this
- If you have high blood pressure or diabetes it is prudent to avoid medicines containing oral decongestants (those intended to be taken by mouth)
- Some medicines for high blood pressure (ACE inhibitors) may produce a persistent dry cough that is usually worse at night. See your doctor if this is a problem
- Do not use nasal sprays containing decongestants for more than a few days at a time as prolonged use may cause rebound stuffiness and eventually damage the nasal membranes
- Do not take antihistamines if you intend to drive or if your occupation requires you to stay alert, e.g. in order to operate machinery
- Avoid alcohol if you are taking an **antihistamine**, as it strongly increases the antihistamine's sedative effect
- If you have glaucoma or if you have prostate or bladder problems avoid antihistamines
- Avoid **carbocysteine** if you have had an ulcer.

ACTIFED TABLETS
Pfizer/Warner Lambert Consumer Healthcare

PA No: 823/6/3

Packs of 12 white, uncoated, biconvex tablets.

Pseudoephedrine hydrochloride 60.0mg, triprolidine hydrochloride

2.5mg.

Contains a decongestant to provide relief from nasal congestion and blocked sinuses. Also contains an antihistamine to relieve the symptoms of allergies such as sneezing and a runny nose.

Adults: 1 tablet 3 times daily.

Children: Over 12 yrs: 1 tablet 3 times daily.

Pharmacy only: Yes

ADVIL COLD AND FLU
Whitehall Laboratories Ltd

PA No: 172/24/1

Blister packs containing 10 or 20 oval-shaped, butterscotch-coloured, sugar-coated tablets imprinted 'Advil cold and flu'.

Ibuprofen 200mg, pseudoephedrine HCl 30mg.

For relief of the symptoms associated with the common cold and influenza including blocked sinuses.

Adults and young persons over 12 yrs: 1 or 2 tablets should be taken every 4-6 hrs. No more than 6 tablets to be taken in 24 hrs.

Children under 12 yrs: Not recommended.

Not to be taken by patients with stomach ulcers or those allergic to aspirin or other similar medicines.

Patients who are pregnant, breastfeeding, elderly, have asthma or are receiving regular treatment should consult the doctor before taking Advil Cold and Flu.

Pharmacy only: Yes

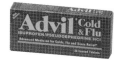

Always Read The Label

ANADIN ANALGESIC TABLETS
Whitehall Laboratories Ltd

PA No: 172/04/5

▢Packs of 6, 12 or 24 white, capsule-shaped tablets embossed 'ANADIN'.

☑Aspirin 325mg, caffeine 15mg, quinine sulphate 1mg.

▨For the relief of pain such as headache, toothache etc. and for the relief of cold symptoms.

☑Adults: 2 tablets every 3-4 hrs if necessary. Maximum of 6 doses (12 tablets) in 24 hrs.

Children (over 12 yrs): 1 tablet every 3-4 hrs.

▉Not to be given to children under 12 yrs except on medical advice.

Prolonged use can be harmful. If symptoms persist or if taking any other medication consult physician.

Do not exceed the stated dose.

Not to be taken by patients with stomach ulcers or those allergic to aspirin or other similar medicines.

Patients who are pregnant, breastfeeding, elderly, have asthma or are receiving regular treatment should consult the doctor before taking Anadin.

Pharmacy only: No

ANADIN EXTRA
Whitehall Laboratories Ltd

PA No: 172/18/1

▢Packs of 8, 12 or 24 white, film-coated, capsule-shaped, cylindrical tablets with a breakbar on one side and 'AE' in the other.

☑Aspirin 300mg, paracetamol 200mg, caffeine 45mg.

▨For the relief of headache, neuralgia, neck pain, rheumatism, toothache, period pain and symptoms of the common cold and flu.

☑Adults: 1-2 tablets every 4 hrs. Maximum 6 tablets in 24 hrs.

Children: Over 12 yrs: 1-2 tablets every 4 hrs. Maximum 6 tablets in 24 hrs.

▉Not to be given to children under 12 except on medical advice.

Prolonged use can be harmful. If symptoms persist or if taking any other medication consult physician.

Do not exceed the stated dose.

Do not take with any other paracetamol-containing products.

Not to be taken by patients with stomach ulcers or those allergic to aspirin or other similar medicines.

Patients who are pregnant, breastfeeding, elderly, have asthma or are receiving regular treatment should consult the doctor before taking Anadin Extra.

Pharmacy only: No

BEECHAMS FLU-PLUS
GlaxoSmithKline

PA No: 678/44/1

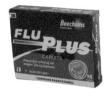

▢Packs of 16 caplets.

☑Paracetamol Ph Eur 500mg, caffeine 25mg, phenylephrine hydrochloride Ph Eur 5mg, ascorbic acid Ph Eur 30mg per capsule.

▨For relief of all major flu symptoms.

☑Adults and children aged 12 yrs and over: Take 2 caplets every 4 hrs as required. Do not take any more than 8 caplets in 24 hrs.

▉Not suitable for children under 12 yrs.

Do not exceed the stated dose.

Do not take with any other paracetamol-containing product.

Pharmacy only: Yes

Always Consult Your Pharmacist

BEECHAMS HOT BLACKCURRANT
GlaxoSmithKline

PA No: 678/11/2

Packs of 5 sachets of blackcurrant-flavoured powder.

Paracetamol Ph Eur 600mg, vitamin C Ph Eur 40mg per sachet.

For the relief of cold and flu symptoms.

Adults: 1 sachet every 4 hrs. Maximum 6 sachets in 24 hrs.

Not suitable for children under 12 yrs.

Do not exceed the stated dose.

Do not take with any other paracetamol-containing product.

Pharmacy only: No

BEECHAMS HOT LEMON
GlaxoSmithKline

PA No: 678/11/1

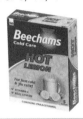

Packs of 5 or 10 sachets of lemon-flavoured powder.

Paracetamol Ph Eur 600mg, vitamin C Ph Eur 40mg per sachet.

For the relief of cold and flu symptoms.

Adults: 1 sachet every 4 hrs. Maximum 6 sachets in 24 hrs.

Not suitable for children under 12 yrs.

Do not exceed the stated dose.

Do not take with any other paracetamol-containing product.

Pharmacy only: No

BEECHAMS HOT LEMON WITH HONEY
GlaxoSmithKline

PA No: 678/11/3

Packs of 5 sachets of lemon and honey-flavoured powder.

Paracetamol Ph Eur 600mg, vitamin C Ph Eur 40mg per sachet.

For the relief of cold and flu symptoms.

Adults: 1 sachet every 4 hrs. Maximum 6 sachets in 24 hrs.

Not recommended for children under 12 yrs.

Do not exceed the stated dose.

Do not take with any other paracetamol-containing product.

Pharmacy only: No

BEECHAMS VENOS EXPECTORANT
GlaxoSmithKline

PA No: 379/14/2

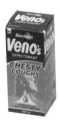

100ml or 160ml bottles of menthol-flavoured liquid.

Guaiphenesin BP 100mg, liquid glucose BPC 3g, treacle 1.35g per 5ml.

For the relief of chesty coughs.

Adults: 10ml every 2-3 hrs.

Children: 3-12 yrs: 5ml every 2-3 hrs.

Not recommended for children under 3 yrs.

Pharmacy only: No

If Symptoms Persist Consult Your Doctor

BEECHAMS VENOS HONEY & LEMON
GlaxoSmithKline

PA No: 379/7/1

▣100ml or 160ml bottles of yellow, honey and lemon-flavoured liquid with added menthol.

▪Lemon juice 1ml, honey 0.25g, ammonium chloride BP 0.03g, ipecacuanha liquid extract BP 0.003ml, liquid glucose 4g per 5ml.

▪Relieves dry and tickly coughs, soothes and protects sore, irritated throat. Does not cause drowsiness.

▪Adults: 15ml every 2-3 hrs. Maximum 8 doses in 24 hrs.

Children: 6-12 yrs: 10ml every 2-3 hrs. Maximum 6 doses in 24 hrs.

1-6 yrs: 5ml every 2-3 hrs. Maximum 4 doses in 24 hrs.

▪Not recommended for children under 1 yr.

Pharmacy only: No

BENYLIN 4 FLU LIQUID 200ML
Pfizer/Warner Lambert Consumer Healthcare

PA No: 823/34/1

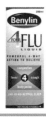

▣200ml bottle of orange oral solution.

▪Each 20ml contains paracetamol Ph Eur 1,000mg, pseudoephedrine hydrochloride BP 45mg, diphenhydramine hydrochloride Ph Eur 25mg.

▪Formulated to relieve the four main symptoms of flu; fever, aches and pains, nasal congestion and coughing.

▪Adults, elderly and children over 12 yrs: 20ml (2 x 10ml measuring cup doses or 4 x 5ml spoonfuls) 4 times daily.

Children 6-12 yrs: 10ml (1 measuring 10ml cup dose or 2 x 5ml spoonfuls) 4 times daily.

▪Not recommended for children under 6 yrs.

Pharmacy only: Yes

BENYLIN 4 FLU TABLETS
Pfizer/Warner Lambert Consumer Healthcare

PA No: 823/34/2

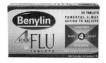

▣Packs of 24 orange, film-coated tablets.

▪Each tablet contains paracetamol Ph Eur 500mg, pseudoephedrine hydrochloride BP 22.5mg, diphenhydramine hydrochloride Ph Eur 12.5mg.

▪Formulated to relieve the four main symptoms of flu; fever, aches and pains, nasal congestion and coughing.

▪Adults, elderly and children over 12 yrs: 2 tablets 4 times daily.

Children 6-12 yrs: 1 tablet 4 times daily.

▪Not recommended for children under 6 yrs.

Pharmacy only: Yes

Always Read The Label

BENYLIN CHILDREN'S COUGHS AND COLDS MEDICINE
Pfizer/Warner Lambert Consumer Healthcare

PA No: 823/1/1

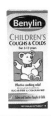

📺 125ml bottle containing a clear, colourless oral solution.

🔋 Each 5ml contains dextromethorphan hydrobromide Ph Eur 5mg, triprolidine hydrochloride 0.625mg.

▦ Relieves the symptoms of dry coughs and colds, catarrh and watery eyes. Sugar and colour free.

✓ Children aged 6-12 yrs: 2 × 5ml spoonfuls 3 or 4 times daily. Maximum daily dose 40ml.

Children aged 2-6 yrs: 1 × 5ml spoonful 3 or 4 times daily. Maximum daily dose 20ml.

❗ Children under 2 yrs: Not recommended except on the advice of the doctor.

Pharmacy only: Yes

CLEARWAY INHALANT OIL
E J Bodkin & Co Ltd

PA No: N/A

📺 10ml glass bottle dispenser of blended natural aromatic plant oils.

🔋 Menthol BP (5% w/w), eucalyptus oil BP (35% w/w), wintergreen oil BPC (7% w/w), fractionated coconut oil (53% w/w).

▦ To relieve symptoms of catarrh, blocked sinuses, coughs and colds.

✓ Adults: Fill cup to ²/₃ level with very hot water and add 2-5 drops of inhalant oil. Inhale deeply up to 4 or 5 times.

Children: For children over 2 yrs, use no more than 2 drops of inhalant added to hot rather than very hot water, under close adult supervision.

❗ Not for use by asthmatics or children under 2 yrs.

Pharmacy only: Yes

CLEARWAY STEAM INHALER & INHALANT OIL
E J Bodkin & Co Ltd

PA No: N/A

📺 Green, two-handled, plastic steam inhaler cup with soft transparent PVC nose/mouth mask. Sold in conjunction with natural decongestant inhalant oil.

🔋 Inhalant oil: Menthol BP (5% w/w), eucalyptus oil BP (35% w/w), wintergreen oil BPC (7% w/w), fractionated coconut oil (53% w/w).

▦ To relieve symptoms of catarrh, blocked sinuses, coughs and colds. Steam inhalation traditionally used to relieve croup. Speech therapists use to hydrate vocal chords.

✓ Adults: Fill cup to ²/₃ level with very hot water and add 2-5 drops of inhalant oil. Inhale deeply up to 4 or 5 times.

Children: For children over 2 yrs, use no more than 2 drops of inhalant added to hot rather than very hot water, under close adult supervision.

❗ Inhalant oil not for use by asthmatics or children under 2 yrs. To avoid scalding, do not tilt the inhaler during use.

Pharmacy only: Yes

Always Consult Your Pharmacist

DAY AND NIGHT COLD AND FLU RELIEF

Pfizer/Warner Lambert Consumer Healthcare

PA No: 823/19/1

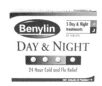

5 day treatment pack containing 15 round, amber tablets for daytime use and 5 round, blue tablets for use at night.

Day tablet: Paracetamol 500mg, phenylpropanolamine 25mg.

Night tablet: Paracetamol 500mg, diphenhydramine 25mg.

For the relief of cold and flu symptoms such as nasal congestion and aches and pains.

Adults and children: 1 amber tablet to be taken in the morning, at midday and in the afternoon. 1 blue tablet to be taken at night.

Pharmacy only: Yes

DAY NURSE CAPSULES

GlaxoSmithKline

PA No: 678/13/1

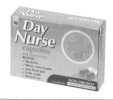

Packs of 20 capsules.

Paracetamol Ph Eur 500mg, phenylpropanolamine hydrochloride Ph Eur 12.5mg, dextromethorphan hydrobromide Ph Eur 7.5mg.

For the relief of tickly cough, sore throat pain, blocked nose and aches associated with colds and flu.

Adults: 2 capsules every 4 hrs. Maximum 8 capsules in 24 hrs.

Adults/children over 16 yrs who take Night Nurse before bed should take no more than 6 capsules in 24 hrs.

Children: 6-12 yrs: 1 capsule every 4 hrs. Maximum 4 capsules in 24 hrs. Not suitable for children under 6 yrs.

Do not exceed the stated dose.

Do not take with any other paracetamol-containing product.

Does not cause drowsiness.

Pharmacy only: Yes

DRISTAN NASAL SPRAY

Whitehall Laboratories Ltd

PA No: 172/07/1

15ml bottle containing a colourless, aqueous solution with a characteristic odour.

Oxymetazoline hydrochloride 0.05% w/w.

Nasal decongestant for relief of the symptoms of acute rhinitis in head cold, hayfever, catarrh and nasal congestion.

Adults: 1-2 sprays up each nostril every 8-10 hrs. Maximum 4 sprays per nostril in 24 hrs.

Children: 6-16 yrs: Spray once lightly in each nostril every 8-10 hrs. Maximum 2 sprays per nostril in 24 hrs.

Do not use for more than 7 days. Consult doctor before use if receiving medication, if pregnant or breastfeeding.

Pharmacy only: Yes

If Symptoms Persist Consult Your Doctor

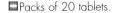

ILVICO
Merck Consumer Healthcare

PA No: 417/10/1

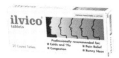

🔲Packs of 20 tablets.

🔳Brompheniramine hydrogen maleate 3mg, calcium ascorbate 2 H2O 36mg, caffeine monohydrate 10mg, paracetamol 250mg.

❓For the relief of common cold and influenza symptoms. It is also of value when used as additional therapy in upper respiratory tract infections. Helps relieve a range of symptoms including fever, congestion and allergic reaction.

📝Adults: 1-2 coated tablets 3 times daily.

Elderly: 1 coated tablet 2-4 times daily.

Children: 6-12 yrs: 1 coated tablet 2-4 times daily.

❗Not recommended for children under 6 yrs. Ilvico should not be taken by patients known to have brain damage or epilepsy.

Pharmacy only: Yes

LEMSIP COLD AND FLU HEADCOLD
Reckitt Benckiser

PA No: 979/14/1

🔲Cartons of 5 or 10 sachets of pale yellow, lemon and menthol-flavoured powder.

🔳Paracetamol 600mg, ascorbic acid 46mg.

❓For the relief of the symptoms of colds and flu.

📝Adults: 1 sachet every 4 hrs. Maximum 6 doses in 24 hrs.

❗Not suitable for children.

Do not take any medicine containing paracetamol within 4 hrs of taking Lemsip.

Pharmacy only: No

LEMSIP COLD AND FLU MAX STRENGTH
Reckitt Benckiser

PA No: 979/14/2

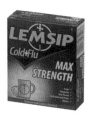

🔲Cartons of 5 sachets of pale yellow, lemon-flavoured powder.

🔳Paracetamol Ph Eur 1,000mg, ascorbic acid 100mg.

❓Relief of cold and flu symptoms.

📝Adults and children over 12 yrs: 1 sachet every 4 hrs. Do not exceed 4 sachets in 24 hrs.

❗Not recommended for children under 12 yrs.

Do not take any medicine

containing paracetamol within 4 hrs of taking Lemsip.

Pharmacy only: No

Always Read The Label

LEMSIP COLD AND FLU ORIGINAL LEMON
Reckitt Benckiser

PA No: 979/13/1

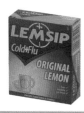

▣Cartons of 5 or 10 sachets of pale yellow, lemon-flavoured powder.

▨Paracetamol 600mg, sodium citrate 462mg, ascorbic acid 9.23mg.

▣For the relief of the symptoms of colds and flu.

▨Adults: 1 sachet every 4 hrs. Maximum 6 doses in 24 hrs.

❶Not suitable for children.

Do not take any medicine

containing paracetamol within 4 hrs of taking Lemsip.

Pharmacy only: No

LEMSIP PHARMACY BLACKCURRANT WITH PHENYLEPHRINE
Reckitt Benckiser

PA No: 979/13/2

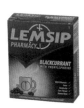

▣Cartons of 5 sachets of blackcurrant-flavoured powder taken as a hot drink.

▨Paracetamol Ph Eur 650mg, phenylephrine HCl BP 10mg, vitamin C Ph Eur 50mg.

▣For the relief of the symptoms of colds and flu.

▨Adults and children 12 yrs and over: 1 sachet every 4 hrs. Maximum 4 sachets in 24 hrs.

❶Do not give to children under 12 yrs.

Do not take any medicine containing paracetamol or a

decongestant within 4 hrs of taking Lemsip.

Pharmacy only: Yes

LEMSIP PHARMACY FLU STRENGTH
Reckitt Benckiser

PA No: 979/14/3

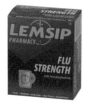

▣Cartons of 10 sachets of pale yellow, lemon-flavoured powder.

▨Paracetamol 1,000mg, pseudoephedrine hydrochloride 60mg, ascorbic acid 100mg.

▣For the relief of severe cold and flu symptoms.

▨Adults: 1 sachet every 4 hrs. Maximum 3 doses in 24 hrs.

❶Children: Not suitable.

Do not take any medicine

containing paracetamol or a decongestant within 4 hrs of taking Lemsip.

Pharmacy only: Yes

Always Consult Your Pharmacist

MEDINOL OVER 6
SSL Healthcare Ireland Ltd

PA No: 258/45/1

Strawberry-flavoured, sugar- and colour-free suspension.

250mg paracetamol per 5ml dose.

For the relief of pain and fever associated with such conditions as common cold, influenza, headaches and sore throats.

Adults, the elderly and children over 12 yrs: 2-4 x 5ml spoonfuls 4 times daily.

Children 6-12 yrs: 1-2 x 5ml spoonfuls 4 times daily.

Do not repeat dose more frequently than every 4 hrs. Do not take more than 4 doses in 24 hrs. Not to be given to children under 6 yrs.

Pharmacy only: Yes

NIGHT NURSE CAPSULES
GlaxoSmithKline

PA No: 678/21/2

Cartons of 10 capsules.

Paracetamol Ph Eur 500mg, promethazine hydrochloride Ph

Eur 10mg, dextromethorphan hydrobromide Ph Eur 7.5mg per capsule.

For the relief of tickly cough, sore throat pain, runny nose and aches associated with colds and flu.

Adults: 2 capsules before

bedtime.

Not suitable for children under 16 yrs.

Do not exceed the stated dose. Do not take with any other paracetamol-containing product. May cause drowsiness.

Pharmacy only: Yes

NIGHT NURSE COLD REMEDY LIQUID
GlaxoSmithKline

PA No: 678/14/1

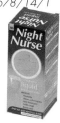

160ml bottle containing green syrup.

Paracetamol BP 1,000mg, promethazine hydrochloride BP 20mg, dextromethorphan hydrobromide BP 15mg per 20ml.

For the relief of tickly cough, runny nose, sore throat pain and aches associated with colds and flu.

Adults and children 16 yrs

and over: 20ml before bedtime.

Under 16 yrs: Only as directed by doctor.

Do not exceed the stated dose.

Do not take with any other paracetamol-containing product. May cause drowsiness.

Pharmacy only: Yes

NUROFEN COLD & FLU
Boots Healthcare Ltd

PA No: 43/12/1

Packs of 12 or 24 round, biconvex, yellow, film-coated tablets; embossed 'N'.

Ibuprofen 200mg, pseudoephedrine hydrochloride 30mg.

For fast, effective relief of

symptoms of colds and flu including aches and pains, headache, fever. Eases the pain of sore throat, plus a decongestant for blocked nose and sinuses.

Adults and children 12 yrs and over: Swallow 2 tablets with water, then, if necessary, take 1-2 tablets every 4 hrs. Do not exceed 6 tablets in 24 hrs.

Do not take Nurofen Cold & Flu if you have or ever had a

stomach ulcer or other digestive system disorder, if you are allergic to any of the ingredients, to aspirin or to any other NSAIDs.

Consult your doctor before use if you are pregnant, breastfeeding, elderly, asthmatic, on any regular medication or treatment, if you have heart ptoblems, high blood pressure, diabetes, glaucoma, thyroid or prostate problems.

Pharmacy only: Yes

If Symptoms Persist Consult Your Doctor

OTRIVINE ADULT MEASURED DOSE SINUSITIS SPRAY
Novartis Consumer Health

PA No: 30/26/4

🔲 10 ml bottle of nasal spray.

▪️ Xylometazoline hydrochloride 0.1% w/v.

❔ For the symptomatic relief of acute rhinitis in allergic or upper respiratory tract infections (including the common cold or influenza) and sinusitis.

✅ Adults: 1 application in each nostril 1-3 times daily.

❗ Not recommended for children under 12 yrs.

Do not use for more than 7 consecutive days.

Pharmacy only: Yes

OTRIVINE ADULT NASAL DROPS
Novartis Consumer Health

PA No: 30/26/1

🔲 10ml bottle containing a clear, colourless, odourless solution.

▪️ Xylometazoline hydrochloride 0.1% w/v.

❔ For the symptomatic relief of acute rhinitis in allergic or upper respiratory tract infections (including the common cold or influenza).

✅ Adults: 2 or 3 drops in each nostril 2-3 times daily.

❗ Not recommended for children under 12 yrs.

Do not use for more than 7 consecutive days.

Pharmacy only: Yes

OTRIVINE ADULT NASAL SPRAY
Novartis Consumer Health

PA No: 30/26/2

🔲 10ml bottle containing a clear, colourless, odourless solution.

▪️ Xylometazoline hydrochloride 0.1% w/v.

❔ For the symptomatic relief of acute rhinitis in allergic or upper respiratory tract infections (including the common cold or influenza).

✅ Adults: 1-2 applications in each nostril 2-3 times daily.

❗ Not recommended for children under 12 yrs.

Do not use for more than 7 consecutive days.

Pharmacy only: Yes

SEVEN SEAS HÖFELS GARLIC & PARSLEY ONE-A-DAY
Seven Seas Ireland Ltd

PA No: 616/2/1

🔲 Pack of 30 green, round, biconvex, sugar-coated tablets.

▪️ Garlic oil 15mg.

❔ Herbal remedy for the relief of catarrh and symptoms of rhinitis and common colds.

✅ Adults: 1 tablet daily.

Children: Over 7 yrs: 1 tablet daily.

Pharmacy only: Yes

SEVEN SEAS HÖFELS GARLIC PEARLES ONE-A-DAY
Seven Seas Ireland Ltd

PA No: 616/1/2

🔲 Pack of 30 clear, oval, gelatin capsules.

▪️ Garlic oil 2mg.

❔ Herbal remedy for the relief of catarrh, rhinitis, common cold and troublesome coughing, as in flu attacks.

✅ Adults: 1 capsule daily before a meal or prior to retiring.

Children: Over 7 yrs: 1 capsule daily before a meal or prior to retiring.

Pharmacy only: Yes

Always Read The Label

TRAMIL
Whitehall Laboratories Ltd
PA No: 172/09/1

☐Blister packs of 12 or 24 hard, gelatin capsules with blue cap and yellow body, containing a white, free-flowing powder/ granule mix. The word 'Tramil' is printed longitudinally on both cap and body.

☑Paracetamol 500mg, caffeine 32mg.

❓For the treatment of pain and fever, headache, migraine, neuralgia, colds and influenza, period and dental pain.

☑Adults: 1-2 capsules which may be repeated every 4 hrs as necessary. Maximum 8 capsules in 24 hrs.

❗Do not exceed the stated dose.

Do not take with any other paracetamol-containing products.

Pharmacy only: No

UNIFLU PLUS
Unigreg
PA No: 81/2/1

☐Packs of 12 or 24 tablets. Two tablet formulation. Uniflu: Lilac oblong s/c tablet. Gregovite C: Yellow tablet.

☑Paracetamol 500mg, caffeine 30mg, diphenhydramine HCL 15mg, phenylephrene HCL 10mg, codeine phosphate 10mg, vitamin C 300mg.

☑Adults: 1 tablet of each type

every 6 hrs.

Children: 1 tablet of each type every 8 hrs.

❓For the symptomatic relief of colds.

Pharmacy only: Yes

UNIFLU WITH GREGOVITE 'C'
Unigreg
PA No: 81/1/1

☐Packs of 12 or 24 tablets. Two types per pack: Uniflu: lilac, oblong, sugar-coated tablet; Gregovite 'C': yellow

tablet.

☑Uniflu: Paracetamol 500mg, caffeine 30mg, diphenhydramine hydrochloride 15mg, phenylephrine hydrochloride 10mg. Gregovite 'C': Ascorbic acid 300mg.

❓Symptomatic relief of colds and flu.

☑Adults: 1 tablet of each type every 6 hrs.

Children: 1 tablet of each type every 8 hrs.

❗Not recommended for children under 12 yrs.

Maximum 4 doses in 24 hrs.

Pharmacy only: Yes

Always Consult Your Pharmacist

COUGHS

Cough is usually simply described according to whether it is dry or chesty, that is, whether or not phlegm (sputum) is being produced. The colour of the phlegm is important. If you are coughing up green or yellow phlegm, it indicates that an infection is present and medical advice should be sought. The presence of blood or any unusual colour in the phlegm also calls for medical advice. If your cough lasts more than a week or so it also makes sense to visit your doctor.

Cough Treatment

A dry cough is best treated with a simple cough suppressing medicine. Such medicines usually take the form of a syrupy mixture (**linctus**) because the syrup may help to soothe an irritated throat. Lozenges have the same effect. Cough suppressants commonly used include **dextromethorphan**, **codeine** (see **Pain Relief**) and **pholcodine**. These agents help you to control your cough but remember that codeine and pholcodine can be addictive.

If you have a chesty cough you may benefit from the use of an agent that makes it easier to bring up phlegm (an **expectorant**). Examples of expectorants include **guaiphenesin**, **ipecacuanha**, and **ammonium chloride**. An alternative way of making the phlegm easier to cough up is to use a substance that makes it thinner (a **mucolytic**). **Carbocysteine** works in this way.

Antihistamines in cough mixtures serve the same purpose as they do in cold remedies (see above) and the same precautions apply.

Because coughs and colds may occur at the same time, some medicines contain a mixture of ingredients that is intended to treat both conditions.

ACTIFED CHESTY NON-DROWSY
Pfizer/Warner Lambert Consumer Healthcare

PA No: 823/2/1

◨100ml bottle of clear, orange-red, cherry-flavoured syrup.

◨Pseudoephedrine hydrochloride BP 30mg, guaiphenesin BP 100mg.

◨Contains a decongestant to provide relief from nasal congestion and blocked sinuses. Also contains an expectorant to relieve a chesty cough without causing drowsiness.

◨Adults: 10ml 3 times daily.

Children over 12 yrs: 10ml 3 times daily.

Children 6-12 yrs: 5ml 3 times daily.

Children 2-5 yrs: 2.5ml 3 times daily.

◨Children under 2 yrs: Not recommended.

Pharmacy only: Yes

ACTIFED COMPOUND LINCTUS
Pfizer/Warner Lambert Consumer Healthcare

PA No: 823/6/1

◨100ml bottle containing a clear, bright red, blackberry-flavoured syrup.

◨Triprolidine hydrochloride 1.25mg, pseudoephedrine hydrochloride 30mg, dextromethorphan hydrobromide 10mg per 5ml.

◨Contains a decongestant to provide relief from nasal congestion and blocked sinuses. Also contains an antitussive to relieve a dry, irritating cough.

◨Adults: 10ml 3 times daily.

Children: Over 12 yrs: 10ml 3 times daily. 6-12 yrs: 5ml 3 times daily. 2-5 yrs: 2.5ml 3 times daily.

◨Not recommended for children under 2 yrs.

Pharmacy only: Yes

If Symptoms Persist Consult Your Doctor

ACTIFED SYRUP
Pfizer/Warner Lambert Consumer Healthcare

PA No: 823/6/2

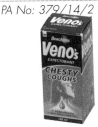100ml bottle containing a clear, yellow syrup.

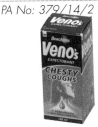Triprolidine hydrochloride 1.25mg, pseudoephedrine hydrochloride 30mg, syrup base per 5ml.

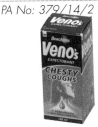Contains a decongestant to provide relief from nasal congestion and blocked sinuses. Also contains an antihistamine to relieve the symptoms of allergies such as sneezing and a runny nose. Suitable for children 2 yrs and upwards.

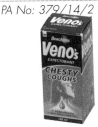Adults: 10ml 3 times daily.

Children: Over 12 yrs: 10ml 3 times daily. 6-12 yrs: 5ml 3 times daily. 2-5 yrs: 2.5ml 3 times daily.

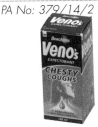Not recommended for children under 2 yrs.

Pharmacy only: Yes

BEECHAMS VENOS EXPECTORANT
GlaxoSmithKline

PA No: 379/14/2

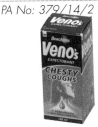

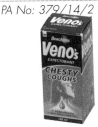100 or 160ml bottles containing a menthol-flavoured liquid.

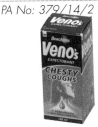Guaiphenesin BP 100mg, liquid glucose BPC 3g, treacle 1.35g per 5ml.

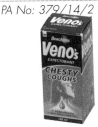For the relief of chesty coughs.

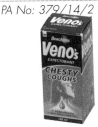Adults: 10ml every 2-3 hrs.

Children: 3-12 yrs: 5ml every 2-3 hrs.

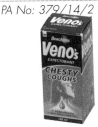Not recommended for children under 3 yrs.

Pharmacy only: No

BEECHAMS VENOS HONEY & LEMON
GlaxoSmithKline

PA No: 379/7/1

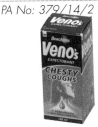100 or 160ml bottles of yellow, honey and lemon-flavoured liquid with added menthol.

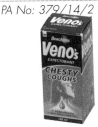Lemon juice 1ml, honey 0.25g, ammonium chloride BP 0.03g, ipecacuanha liquid extract BP 0.003ml, liquid glucose BPC 4g per 5ml.

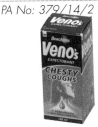Relieves dry and tickly coughs, soothes and protects sore, irritated throat. Does not cause drowsiness.

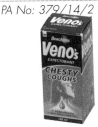Adults: 15ml every 2-3 hrs.

Maximum 8 doses in 24 hrs.

Children: 6-12 yrs: 10ml every 2-3 hrs. Maximum 6 doses in 24 hrs.

1-6 yrs: 5ml every 2-3 hrs. Maximum 4 doses in 24 hrs.

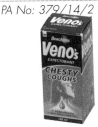Not recommended for children under 1 yr.

Pharmacy only: No

BENYLIN CHESTY NON-DROWSY
Pfizer/Warner Lambert Consumer Healthcare

PA No: 823/20/1

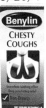

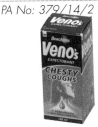125ml bottle of clear, red syrup.

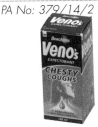Guaiphenesin 100mg, L-menthol 1.1mg per 5ml.

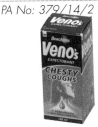Contains an expectorant to relieve the symptoms of chesty coughs. Also loosens phlegm and clears bronchial and nasal congestion.

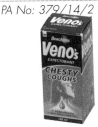Adults: 10ml 4 times daily.

Children: 6-12 yrs: 5ml 4 times daily.

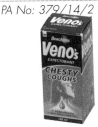Not recommended for children under 6 yrs.

Pharmacy only: Yes

BENYLIN CHILDREN'S CHESTY COUGHS
Pfizer/Warner Lambert Consumer Healthcare

PA No: 823/31/1

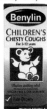

▣125ml bottle of syrup.

◨50mg guaiphenesin per 5ml.

⬚Relieves the symptoms of chesty coughs without causing drowsiness. Sugar and colour free.

◪Children: 6-12 yrs: 10ml 4 times daily.

2-5 yrs: 5ml 4 times daily.

Pharmacy only: Yes

BENYLIN CHILDREN'S COUGHS AND COLDS MEDICINE
Pfizer/Warner Lambert Consumer Healthcare

PA No: 823/1/1

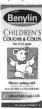

▣125ml bottle of clear, colourless oral solution.

◨Each 5ml contains dextromethorphan hydrobromide Ph Eur 5mg, triprolidine hydrochloride 0.625mg.

⬚Relieves the symptoms of dry coughs and colds, catarrh and watery eyes. Sugar and colour free.

◪Children aged 6-12 yrs: 2 x 5ml spoonfuls 3 or 4 times daily. Maximum daily dose 40ml.

Children aged 2-6 yrs: 1 x 5ml spoonful 3 or 4 times daily. Maximum daily dose 20ml.

▣Children under 2 yrs: Not recommended except on the advice of the doctor.

Pharmacy only: Yes

BENYLIN CLEAR ACTION 125ML/300ML
Pfizer/Warner Lambert Consumer Healthcare

PA No: 823/25/2

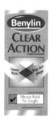

▣125ml or 300ml bottle of light yellow, clear syrup with taste and odour of punch.

◨Carbocysteine 250ml per 5ml.

⬚For treatment of heavy cough accompanied by mucus. Liquifies mucus, allowing the cough to clear the chest.

◪Adults: 15ml 3 times daily initially, then 10ml 3 times daily after a satisfactory response.

Children: 6-12 yrs: 5ml 3 times

daily. Under 6 yrs: 5-10ml daily in divided doses.

▣Not recommended for children under 2 yrs.

Pharmacy only: Yes

Always Consult Your Pharmacist

BENYLIN DRY COUGHS
Pfizer/Warner Lambert Consumer Healthcare

PA No: 823/14/1

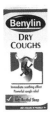

◻ 125ml bottle of clear, red syrup.

◩ Diphenhydramine hydrochloride 14mg, dextromethorphan hydrobromide 6.5mg, menthol 1.1mg.

❓ Soothes and relieves a dry, irritating cough.

✎ Adults: 10ml 3-4 times daily.

Children: 6-12 yrs: 5ml 3-4 times daily.

❗ Not recommended for children under 6 yrs.

Pharmacy only: Yes

BENYLIN DRY (NON-DROWSY)
Pfizer/Warner Lambert Consumer Healthcare

PA No: 823/29/1

◻ 125ml bottle of amber syrup.

◩ Dextromethorphan hydrobromide 7.5mg per 5ml.

❓ Soothes and relieves a dry, irritating cough without causing drowsiness.

✎ Adults: 10ml 3-4 times daily.

Children: 6-12 yrs: 5ml 3-4 times daily.

❗ Not recommended for children under 6 yrs.

Pharmacy only: Yes

BENYLIN TRADITIONAL
Pfizer/Warner Lambert Consumer Healthcare

PA No: 823/17/1

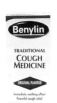

◻ 125ml bottle of menthol-flavoured, red syrup.

◩ Diphenhydramine hydrochloride 14mg, levomenthol 1.1mg.

❓ Symptomatic relief of an irritating cough, aiding a restful night's sleep.

✎ Adults: 5-10ml 3-4 times daily.

Children: 6-12 yrs: 5ml 3-4 times daily.

❗ Not recommended for children under 6 yrs.

Pharmacy only: Yes

If Symptoms Persist Consult Your Doctor

BENYLIN WITH CODEINE
Pfizer/Warner Lambert Consumer Healthcare

PA No: 823/11/1

▣125ml bottle of clear, red syrup.

☑Diphenhydramine hydrochloride 14mg, codeine phosphate 5.70mg, L-menthol 1.1mg.

▣For the treatment of dry irritating cough.

▣Adults: 10ml 3-4 times daily.

Children: 6-12 yrs: 5ml 3-4 times daily.

❗Not recommended for children under 6 yrs.

Pharmacy only: Yes

BRONALIN EXPECTORANT LINCTUS
SSL Healthcare Ireland Ltd

PA No: 258/20/1

▣100ml bottle of linctus.

☑Ammonium chloride 135mg, sodium citrate 57mg, diphenhydramine hydrochloride 14mg.

▣Symptomatic relief of deep, chesty coughs and colds.

▣Adults: 5-10ml 3-4 times daily.

Children: 6-12 yrs: 5ml 3-4 times daily.

❗Not recommended for children under 6 yrs.

Pharmacy only: Yes

CASACOL
Helsinn Birex Pharmaceuticals

PA No: 294/1/1

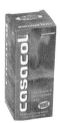

▣125ml bottle of expectorant/decongestant.

☑Methoxyphenamine HCl 20mg, guaiphenesin 100mg, sodium citrate 200mg.

▣For the treatment of cough associated with the common cold.

▣Adults: 5-10ml 3-4 times daily. Children: 6-12 yrs: 5ml 3-4 times daily. 3-6 yrs: 2.5-5ml 3-4 times daily. 2-3 yrs:

1.25-2.5ml 3-4 times daily.

❗Use with caution in patients with heart disease or who are receiving digitalis therapy.

Pharmacy only: Yes

CLEARWAY INHALANT OIL
E J Bodkin & Co Ltd

PA No: N/A

▣10ml glass bottle dispenser of blended natural aromatic plant oils.

☑Menthol BP (5% w/w), eucalyptus oil BP (35% w/w), wintergreen oil BPC (7% w/w), fractionated coconut oil (.53% w/w).

▣To relieve symptoms of catarrh, blocked sinuses, coughs and colds.

▣Adults: Fill cup to ⅔ level with very hot water and add 2-5 drops of inhalant oil. Inhale deeply up to 4 or 5 times.

Children: For children over 2 yrs, use no more than 2 drops of inhalant added to hot rather than very hot water, under close adult supervision.

❗Not for use by asthmatics or children under 2 yrs.

Pharmacy only: Yes

Always Read The Label

CLEARWAY STEAM INHALER & INHALANT OIL
E J Bodkin & Co Ltd

PA No: N/A

Green, two-handled, plastic steam inhaler cup with soft transparent PVC nose/mouth mask. Sold in conjunction with natural decongestant inhalant oil.

Inhalant oil: Menthol BP (5% w/w), eucalyptus oil BP (35% w/w), wintergreen oil BPC (7% w/w), fractionated coconut oil

(53% w/w).

To relieve symptoms of catarrh, blocked sinuses, coughs and colds. Steam inhalation traditionally used to relieve croup. Speech therapists use to hydrate vocal chords.

Adults: Fill cup to ⅔ level with very hot water and add 2-5 drops of inhalant oil. Inhale deeply up to 4 or 5 times.

Children: For children over 2 yrs, use no more than 2 drops of inhalant added to hot rather than very hot water, under close

adult supervision.

Inhalant oil not for use by asthmatics or children under 2 yrs. To avoid scalding, do not tilt the inhaler during use.

Pharmacy only: Yes

CODINEX
Pinewood Healthcare

PA No: 281/5/1

100ml, 200ml or 500ml bottles of dark yellow/orange flavoured syrup.

Codeine phosphate Ph Eur 15mg/5ml.

An antitussive for dry cough.

Adults: 5-7.5ml, 3-4 times daily. Dosage should be reduced in the elderly or debilitated patients.

Children: 5-12 yrs: 2.5ml (7.5mg) repeated if necessary 3-4 times daily.

Contraindicated in cases of hypersensitivity to codeine and liver dysfunction, ventilary

failure.

May cause constipation, dizziness and respiratory depression at high doses. Drowsiness may occur.

Pharmacy only: Yes

DAY NURSE CAPSULES
GlaxoSmithKline

PA No: 678/13/1

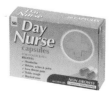

Packs of 20 capsules.

Paracetamol Ph Eur 500mg, phenylpropanolamine hydrochloride Ph Eur 12.5mg, dextromethorphan hydrobromide Ph Eur 7.5mg.

For the relief of tickly cough, sore throat pain, blocked nose and aches associated with colds and flu. Does not cause drowsiness.

Adults: 2 capsules every 4 hrs. Maximum 8 capsules in 24 hrs.

Adults/children over 16 yrs who take Night Nurse before bed should take no more than 6 capsules in 24 hrs.

Children: 6-12 yrs: 1 capsule every 4 hrs. Maximum 4 capsules in 24 hrs.

Not suitable for children under 6 yrs.

Do not exceed the stated dose.

Do not take with any other paracetamol-containing product.

Pharmacy only: Yes

Always Consult Your Pharmacist

DELSYM
Roche Consumer Health

PA No: 72/6/1

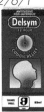

■89ml bottle containing an antitussive.

☑Dextromethorphan.

⚠For treatment of dry cough.

✒Adults: 5ml every 12 hrs. Maximum 15ml in 24 hrs.

Children: 6-12 yrs: 5ml every 12 hrs. Maximum 10ml in 24 hrs. 2-5 yrs: 2.5ml every 12 hrs. Maximum 5ml in 24 hrs.

Pharmacy only: Yes

DIMOTANE CO
Whitehall Laboratories Ltd

PA No: 86/13/5

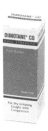

■100ml bottle containing a clear, dark pink, raspberry-scented liquid.

☑Brompheniramine maleate 2mg, pseudoephedrine hydrochloride 30mg, codeine phosphate 10mg.

⚠For the treatment of cough associated with colds and similar conditions of the upper respiratory tract.

✒Adults: 10ml 3 times daily.

Children: 6-12 yrs: 7.5ml 3 times daily. 4-6 yrs: 5ml 3 times daily. 2-4 yrs: 2.5ml 3 times daily.

⚠Not recommended for children under 2 yrs.

May cause drowsiness and patients receiving it should not drive or operate machinery unless it has been shown that their physical and mental capacity remains unaffected.

Do not use this product for persistent or chronic cough such as occurs with smoking, asthma or emphysema, or if cough is accompanied by phlegm unless directed by a doctor.

Pharmacy only: Yes

DIMOTANE CO PAEDIATRIC
Whitehall Laboratories Ltd

PA No: 86/13/6

■100ml bottle containing a clear, dark pink liquid with raspberry odour.

☑Brompheniramine maleate 2mg, pseudoephedrine hydrochloride 15mg, codeine phosphate 3mg.

⚠For the treatment of cough associated with colds and other similar conditions of the upper respiratory tract.

✒Children: 6-12 yrs: 15ml 3 times daily. 4-6 yrs: 10ml 3 times daily. 2-4 yrs: 5ml 3 times daily.

⚠Not recommended for children under 2 yrs.

May cause drowsiness.

Not recommended for use during pregnancy or breastfeeding unless under medical supervision.

Do not use this product for persistent or chronic cough such as occurs with smoking, asthma or emphysema, or if cough is accompanied by phlegm unless directed by a doctor.

Pharmacy only: Yes

If Symptoms Persist Consult Your Doctor

EXPULIN CHILDREN'S COUGH LINCTUS
Monmouth Pharmaceuticals

PA No: 488/10/1

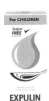

EXPULIN
Children's Cough
Linctus

100ml bottle of sugar-free linctus.

Pholcodine 2mg, chlorpheniramine maleate 1mg, menthol 1.1mg.

Relieves coughs in children by soothing the irritation.

Children: 2-5 yrs: 5ml 1-2 times daily. 6-12 yrs: 10ml 1-2 times daily.

Not recommended for children under 2 yrs.

May cause drowsiness.

Pharmacy only: Yes

EXPULIN COUGH LINCTUS
Monmouth Pharmaceuticals

PA No: 488/13/1

100ml bottle of sugar-free cough linctus.

Pholcodine 5mg, chlorpheniramine maleate 2mg, pseudoephedrine 15mg, menthol 1.1mg.

For the relief of coughs and congestion associated with colds, flu and allergy.

Adults: 10ml 3-4 times daily.

Children: 6-12 yrs: 2.5-5ml 3 times daily.

2-6 yrs: 2.5ml 3 times daily.

Not recommended for children under 2 yrs.

May cause drowsiness.

Pharmacy only: Yes

EXPULIN DRY COUGH STRONG LINCTUS
Monmouth Pharmaceuticals

PA No: 488/11/1

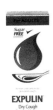

EXPULIN
Dry Cough
Strong Linctus

10ml bottle of sugar-free linctus.

Pholcodine 10mg, menthol 1.1mg.

Relieves and controls dry, persistent coughs.

Adults: 5ml (10mg) 3-4 times daily.

Not recommended for children.

Pharmacy only: Yes

Always Read The Label

EXPUTEX
Monmouth Pharmaceuticals

PA No: 488/14/1

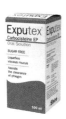

◼100ml, 200ml or 300ml bottles of mucolytic, sugar-free syrup.

◼Carbocisteine 250mg, menthol 1.1mg.

◼For the treatment of excessive or viscous mucus.

◼Adults: 15ml 3 times daily initially, reducing to 10ml 3 times daily when a satisfactory response has been obtained.

Children: 6-12 yrs: 5ml (250mg) 2-3 times daily. 2-5 yrs: 2.5ml (125mg) 2-3 times daily.

◼Under 2 yrs: Not recommended.

Consult doctor before use if pregnant or if there is a history of peptic ulcer.

Pharmacy only: Yes

MEGGEZONES PASTILLES
Schering-Plough Ltd

PA No: 277/54/1

◼Pastilles.

◼Menthol 16mg.

◼For the symptomatic relief of sore throats, coughs, catarrh and nasal congestion.

◼Adults: Allow 1 pastille to

dissolve slowly in the mouth as required. Maximum 15 pastilles in 24 hrs.

◼Children: Not recommended.

Pharmacy only: Yes

MELTUS COUGH LINCTUS HONEY AND LEMON
SSL Healthcare Ireland Ltd

PA No: 258/38/1

◼100ml bottle of syrup.

◼Guaiphenesin 50mg.

◼Symptomatic relief of deep, chesty coughs and to soothe the throat.

◼Adults: 10-20ml 3-4 times daily.

Children: 6-12 yrs: 10ml 3-4 times daily. 2-6 yrs: 5ml 3-4 times daily.

◼Not recommended for children under 2 yrs except on medical advice.

Pharmacy only: No

MELTUS EXPECTORANT (ADULT)
SSL Healthcare Ireland Ltd

PA No: 258/26/1

◼10ml or 200ml bottles of

linctus.

◼Guaiphenesin 100mg, purified honey 500mg, cetylpyridinium chloride 2.5mg, sucrose 1.75g.

◼Symptomatic relief of coughs

and catarrh associated with flu, colds and mild throat infections.

◼Adults: 5-10ml every 3-4 hrs.

◼Children: Not recommended for children under 12 yrs.

Pharmacy only: No

MELTUS JUNIOR EXPECTORANT LINCTUS
SSL Healthcare Ireland Ltd

PA No: 258/26/2

◼100ml bottle of linctus.

◼Guaiphenesin 50mg, cetylpyridinium chloride 2.5mg.

◼Symptomatic relief of coughs and catarrh associated with flu, colds and mild throat infections.

◼Children: Over 6 yrs: 10ml

3-4 times daily. 2-6 yrs: 5ml 3-4 times daily.

◼Not recommended for children under 2 yrs except on medical advice.

Pharmacy only: No

Always Consult Your Pharmacist

MUCOGEN SYRUP
Antigen

PA No: 73/92/1

100ml or 250ml bottles of clear, red, mobile syrup with the odour and taste of raspberry.

250mg carbocisteine per 5ml of syrup.

For use in the management of lower respiratory tract disorders characterised by excessive viscous mucus.

Adults: 3 tsp 2-3 times daily, reducing to 2 tsp 2-3 times daily when a satisfactory response has been obtained. In acute exacerbation a treatment period of 5-10 days is usually sufficient.

Children 6-12 yrs: 5ml 2-3 times daily.

Children 2-5 yrs: 2.5ml 2-3 times daily.

Children under 2 yrs: Not recommended.

Not recommended in cases of hypersensitivity to carbocisteine, or in active peptic ulceration.

Should not be used during pregnancy unless considered essential by the physician.

When oral antibiotics or other drugs are required, they should be administered 1-2 hrs apart from carbocisteine. The addition of other drugs to the carbocisteine solution should be avoided.

Pharmacy only: Yes

NIGHT NURSE CAPSULES
GlaxoSmithKline

PA No: 678/21/2

Cartons of 10 capsules.

Paracetamol Ph Eur 500mg, promethazine hydrochloride Ph Eur 10mg, dextromethorphan hydrobromide Ph Eur 7.5mg per capsule.

For the relief of tickly cough, sore throat pain, runny nose and aches associated with colds and flu.

Adults: 2 capsules before bedtime.

Not suitable for children under 16 yrs.

Do not exceed the stated dose.

Do not take with any other paracetamol-containing product. May cause drowsiness.

Pharmacy only: Yes

NIGHT NURSE COLD REMEDY LIQUID
GlaxoSmithKline

PA No: 678/14/1

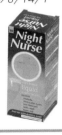

160ml bottle of green syrup.

Paracetamol BP 1,000mg, promethazine hydrochloride BP 20mg, dextromethorphan hydrobromide BP 15mg per 20ml.

For the relief of tickly cough, runny nose, sore throat pain and aches associated with colds and flu.

Adults and children 16 yrs and over: 20ml before bedtime.

Under 16 yrs: Only as directed by doctor.

Do not exceed the stated dose.

Do not take with any other paracetamol-containing product.

May cause drowsiness.

Pharmacy only: Yes

PHOLCOLIN
Antigen

PA No: 73/18/1

150ml bottle of linctus.

Pholcodine 5mg/5ml.

For the management of dry cough.

Adults: 10ml up to 3 times daily.

Children: Over 2 yrs: 5ml up to 3 times daily. 1-2 yrs: 2.5ml up to 3 times daily.

Use only for suppression of non-productive cough.

May cause drowsiness.

Pharmacy only: Yes

If Symptoms Persist Consult Your Doctor

PULMOCLASE 500
U.C.B. (Pharma) Ireland Ltd

PA No: 230/6/1

70ml or 125ml bottles of mucolytic, sugar-free syrup.

Carbocisteine 500mg per 5ml.

For treatment of excessive or viscous mucus.

Adults: 5ml 3-4 times daily.

Consult doctor before use if pregnant or if there is a history of peptic ulcer.

Pharmacy only: Yes

ROBITUSSIN CHESTY COUGH
Whitehall Laboratories Ltd

PA No: 86/19/1

100ml bottle containing a deep wine russet-coloured syrup with a raspberry odour and taste.

Guaiphenesin 100mg, ethanol (96%) 2.5% v/v.

As an adjunct in the treatment of chesty cough.

Adults: 10ml 4 times daily.

Children: 6-12 yrs: 5ml 4 times daily. 2-6 yrs: 2.5ml 4 times daily.

Not recommended for children under 2 yrs unless under medical supervision.

If symptoms persist consult your doctor. If pregnant or breastfeeding consult doctor before use.

Pharmacy only: Yes

ROBITUSSIN DRY COUGH
Whitehall Laboratories Ltd

PA No: 86/24/2

100ml bottle containing a clear, red liquid with the odour of cherry/grenadine.

Dextromethorphan hydrobromide 7.5mg, ethanol (96%) 2.5% v/v.

For the relief of dry, irritant cough.

Adults: 10ml 3-4 times daily.

Children: 6-12 yrs: 5ml 3-4 times daily.

Not recommended for children under 6 yrs.

Do not exceed the stated dose. If symptoms persist for more than 7 days or you have a recurrent cough consult your doctor. If pregnant or breastfeeding consult doctor before use.

Pharmacy only: Yes

ROBITUSSIN JUNIOR
Whitehall Laboratories Ltd

PA No: 86/24/1

100ml bottle containing a clear, red liquid with cherry odour.

Dextromethorphan hydrobromide 3.75mg, ethanol (96%) 2.5% v/v.

For the relief of dry, irritant cough.

Children: 6-12 yrs: 10ml 3-4 times daily. 2-6 yrs: 5ml 3-4 times daily.

Not recommended for children under 2 yrs.

Do not exceed the stated dose. If symptoms persist for more than 7 days or your child has a recurrent cough consult your doctor. If pregnant or breastfeeding consult doctor before use.

Pharmacy only: Yes

Always Read The Label

ROBITUSSIN PLUS
Whitehall Laboratories Ltd

PA No: 86/23/1

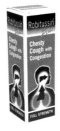

🔲100ml bottle containing a clear, pale pink, slightly viscous liquid with a raspberry odour.

☑Guaiphenesin 100mg, pseudoephedrine hydrochloride 30mg, ethanol (96%) 2.5% v/v.

❓For use as a nasal decongestant and for chesty cough.

☑Adults: 10ml 3 times daily.

Children: 6-12 yrs: 5ml 3 times daily. 2-6 yrs: 2.5ml 3 times daily. Not recommended for children under 2 yrs.

❗Do not exceed the stated dose.

If symptoms persist consult your doctor.

If pregnant or breastfeeding consult doctor before use.

Pharmacy only: Yes

TIXYLIX CHESTY COUGH
Novartis Consumer Health

PA No: 30/22/1

🔲100ml bottle containing a clear, sugar-free linctus with a blackcurrant flavour.

☑Guaiphenesin 50mg per 5ml.

❓Symptomatic relief of chesty coughs. Helps loosen mucus to make breathing easier.

☑Under 2 yrs on medical advice. 2-5 yrs: 5ml given every 4 hrs. 6-10 yrs: 5-10ml given every 4 hrs.

Pharmacy only: Yes

TRADITIONAL IRISH COUGH SWEETS
Rose Confectionery Ltd

PA No: N/A

🔲Clear cellophane 130g bag containing black, oblong lozenges with a citrus/aniseed flavour.

❓Soothing properties and pleasant taste. Glucose based.

Pharmacy only: Yes

VICKS ORIGINAL COUGH SYRUP CHESTY
Procter & Gamble (Health & Beauty Care) Limited

PA No: 441/7/2

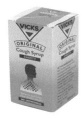

🔲Bottle of clear, reddish-pink syrup.

☑Guaiphenesin 50mg BP, cetylpyridinium chloride 1.25mg BP, sodium citrate 200mg BP.

❓For the treatment of nasal and throat irritation and relief of chesty cough.

☑Adults: 10ml (2 tsps), to be repeated every 3 hours as needed.

Children 6-12 yrs: 5ml (1 tsp), to be repeated every 3 hours as needed.

❗If symptoms persist, consult your doctor.

Pharmacy only: No

Always Consult Your Pharmacist

VISCOLEX
Pinewood Healthcare

PA No: 281/70/1

◨100ml or 250ml bottles of clear yellow syrup, with an orange flavour. Mucolytic agent.

☑Carbocisteine 250mg/5ml.

▣Used for adjunctive therapy in lower respiratory tract disorders characterised by viscous mucus.

☑Adults: 15ml 3 times daily reducing to 10ml 3 times daily when satisfactory response is achieved.

Children: 6-12 yrs: 5ml 2 or 3 times daily.

2-5 yrs: 2.5ml 3 times daily.

❗Under 2 yrs: Not recommended.

Use with caution in patients with a history of peptic ulcers or during pregnancy or breastfeeding.

Pharmacy only: Yes

DECONGESTANTS
See **Colds and Flu** for information on decongestants.

ACTIFED CHESTY NON-DROWSY
Pfizer/Warner Lambert Consumer Healthcare

PA No: 823/2/1

◨100ml bottle of clear, orange-red, cherry-flavoured syrup.

☑Pseudoephedrine

hydrochloride BP 30mg, guaiphenesin BP 100mg.

▣Contains a decongestant to provide relief from nasal congestion and blocked sinuses. Also contains an expectorant to relieve a chesty cough without causing drowsiness.

☑Adults: 10ml 3 times daily.

Children over 12 yrs: 10ml 3 times daily.

Children 6-12 yrs: 5ml 3 times daily.

Children 2-5 yrs: 2.5ml 3 times daily.

❗Children under 2 yrs: Not recommended.

Pharmacy only: Yes

ACTIFED SYRUP
Pfizer/Warner Lambert Consumer Healthcare

PA No: 823/6/2

◨100ml bottle of clear, yellow syrup.

☑Triprolidine hydrochloride 1.25mg, pseudoephedrine hydrochloride 30mg, syrup base

per 5ml.

▣Contains a decongestant to provide relief from nasal congestion and blocked sinuses. Also contains an antihistamine to relieve the symptoms of allergies such as sneezing and a runny nose. Suitable for children 2 yrs and upwards.

☑Adults: 10ml 3 times daily.

Children: Over 12 yrs: 10ml 3 times daily. 6-12 yrs: 5ml 3 times daily. 2-5 yrs: 2.5ml 3 times daily.

❗Not recommended for children under 2 yrs.

Pharmacy only: Yes

ACTIFED TABLETS
Pfizer/Warner Lambert Consumer Healthcare

PA No: 823/6/3

◨12 white, uncoated, biconvex tablets.

☑Pseudoephedrine

hydrochloride 60.0mg, triprolidine hydrochloride 2.5mg.

▣Contains a decongestant to provide relief from nasal congestion and blocked sinuses. Also contains an antihistamine to relieve the symptoms of allergies such as sneezing and a runny

nose.

☑Adults: 1 tablet 3 times daily.

Children: Over 12 yrs: 1 tablet 3 times daily.

❗Not recommended for children under 12 yrs.

Pharmacy only: Yes

If Symptoms Persist Consult Your Doctor

ADVIL COLD AND FLU
Whitehall Laboratories Ltd

PA No: 172/24/1

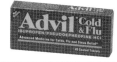

Blister packs containing 10 or 20 oval-shaped, butterscotch-coloured, sugar-coated tablets imprinted 'Advil cold and flu'.

Ibuprofen 200mg and pseudoephedrine HCl 30mg.

For relief of the symptoms associated with the common cold and influenza including blocked sinuses.

Adults and children over 12 yrs: 1 or 2 tablets should be taken every 4-6 hrs. No more than 6 tablets to be taken in 24 hrs.

Not recommended for children under 12 yrs.

Not to be taken by patients with stomach ulcers or those allergic to aspirin or other similar medicines. Patients who are pregnant, breastfeeding, elderly, have asthma or are receiving regular treatment should consult the doctor before taking Advil Cold and Flu.

Pharmacy only: Yes

CLEARWAY INHALANT OIL
E J Bodkin & Co Ltd

PA No: N/A

10ml glass bottle dispenser of blended natural aromatic plant oils.

Menthol BP (5% w/w), eucalyptus oil BP (35% w/w), wintergreen oil BPC (7% w/w), fractionated coconut oil (53% w/w).

To relieve symptoms of catarrh, blocked sinuses, coughs and colds.

Adults: Fill cup to ⅔ level with very hot water and add 2-5 drops of inhalant oil. Inhale deeply up to 4 or 5 times.

Children: For children over 2 yrs, use no more than 2 drops of inhalant added to hot rather than very hot water, under close adult supervision.

Not for use by asthmatics or children under 2 yrs.

Pharmacy only: Yes

CLEARWAY STEAM INHALER & INHALANT OIL
E J Bodkin & Co Ltd

PA No: N/A

Green, two-handled, plastic steam inhaler cup with soft transparent PVC nose/mouth mask. Sold in conjunction with natural decongestant inhalant oil.

Inhalant Oil: Menthol BP (5% w/w), eucalyptus oil BP (35% w/w), wintergreen oil BPC (7% w/w), fractionated coconut oil (53% w/w).

To relieve symptoms of catarrh, blocked sinuses, coughs and colds. Steam inhalation traditionally used to relieve croup. Speech therapists use to hydrate vocal chords.

Adults: Fill cup to ⅔ level with very hot water and add 2-5 drops of inhalant oil. Inhale deeply up to 4 or 5 times.

Children: For children over 2 yrs, use no more than 2 drops of inhalant added to hot rather than very hot water, under close adult supervision.

Inhalant oil not for use by asthmatics or children under 2 yrs. To avoid scalding, do not tilt the inhaler during use.

Pharmacy only: Yes

Always Read The Label

DRISTAN NASAL SPRAY
Whitehall Laboratories Ltd

PA No: 172/07/1

▭15ml bottle of colourless, aqueous solution with a characteristic odour.

☑Oxymetazoline hydrochloride

0.05% w/w.

❓Nasal decongestant for relief of the symptoms of acute rhinitis in head cold, hayfever, catarrh and nasal congestion.

☑Adults: 1-2 sprays up each nostril every 8-10 hrs. Maximum 4 sprays per nostril in 24 hrs.

Children: 6-16 yrs: Spray once lightly in each nostril every 8-10 hrs. Maximum of 2 sprays per nostril in 24 hrs.

❗Do not use for more than 7 days. Consult doctor before use if receiving medication, if pregnant or breastfeeding.

Pharmacy only: Yes

KARVOL
Boots Healthcare Ltd

PA No: 43/4/1

▭Pack of 10 capsules.

☑Chlorbutol 2.25mg, menthol 35.55mg, pine oil sylvestris 9mg, pumilio pine oil 103.05mg, terpineol 66.6mg, thymol 3.15mg.

❓For the relief of symptoms of nasal congestion and head colds.

☑Adults: Snip tip off capsule. Dab contents onto bedding or handkerchief secured nearby and inhale the vapour freely. Or squeeze contents into hot water and inhale the vapours freely.

Children: Dab contents onto handkerchief in the vicinity but out of reach of the child.

❗Not recommended for children under 3 months.

Avoid contact with eyes and skin.

Pharmacy only: Yes

NOSOR MENTHOL VAPOUR RUB STICK
Intrapharma/J Pickles Healthcare

PA No: N/A

▭Stick.

☑Blend of menthol and camphor with eucalyptus oils.

❓Used in vapour inhalation to

relieve breathing.

Pharmacy only: Yes

NOSOR NASAL BALM
Intrapharma/J Pickles Healthcare

PA No: N/A

▭Ointment.

☑Menthol, eucalyptus and geranium oils.

☑Apply around the nostrils.

Pharmacy only: Yes

NOSOR NASAL INHALER
Intrapharma/J Pickles Healthcare

PA No: N/A

▭Inhaler.

☑Contains a blend of eucalyptus and pine oils with menthol and methyl salicylate.

❓Relieves blocked stuffy noses and helps breathing.

Pharmacy only: Yes

NOSOR NOSE BALM
Intrapharma/J Pickles Healthcare

PA No: N/A

▭Blend of oils and waxes based on a lip balm formulation.

☑Contains dibromopropamidine,

eucalyptus, menthol and pine oil.

Pharmacy only: Yes

Always Consult Your Pharmacist

NOSOR VAPOUR RUB
Intrapharma/J Pickles Healthcare
PA No: N/A

🔲Vapour rub.

☑Camphor, turpentine menthol, eucalyptus oil, nutmeg oil, cedarwood oil and thymol.

Pharmacy only: Yes

NUROFEN COLD & FLU
Boots Healthcare Ltd
PA No: 43/12/1

🔲Packs of 12 or 24 round, biconvex, yellow, film-coated tablets; embossed 'N'.

☑Ibuprofen 200mg, pseudoephedrine hydrochloride 30mg.

❓For fast, effective relief of symptoms of colds and flu

including aches and pains, headache, fever. Eases the pain of sore throat, plus a decongestant for blocked nose and sinuses.

☑Adults and children 12 yrs and over: Swallow 2 tablets with water, then, if necessary, take 1-2 tablets every 4 hrs. Do not exceed 6 tablets in 24 hrs.

❗Do not take Nurofen Cold & Flu if you have or ever had a stomach ulcer or other digestive system disorder, if you are

allergic to any of the ingredients, to aspirin or to any other NSAIDs.

Consult your doctor before use if you are pregnant, breastfeeding, elderly, asthmatic, on any regular medication or treatment, if you have heart problems, high blood pressure, diabetes, glaucoma, thyroid or prostate problems.

Pharmacy only: Yes

OTRIVINE ADULT MENTHOL NASAL SPRAY
Novartis Consumer Health
PA No: 30/26/5

🔲10ml bottle of nasal spray/solution.

🔲0.1% w/v xylometazoline hydrochloride BP.

❓For the symptomatic relief of nasal congestion, perennial and allergic rhinitis (including hayfever), and sinusitis.

☑One application in each nostril 2-3 times daily.

❗Not suitable for children under 12 yrs.

Do not use for more than 7 consecutive days.

Pharmacy only: Yes

ROBITUSSIN PLUS
Whitehall Laboratories Ltd
PA No: 86/23/1

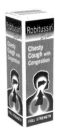

🔲100ml bottle of clear, pale pink, slightly viscous liquid with a raspberry odour.

☑Guaiphenesin 100mg, pseudoephedrine hydrochloride 30mg, ethanol (96%) 2.5% v/v.

❓For use as a nasal decongestant and for chesty cough.

☑Adults: 10ml 3 times daily.

Children: 6-12 yrs: 5ml 3 times daily. 2-6 yrs: 2.5ml 3 times

daily.

❗Not recommended for children under 2 yrs.

Do not exceed the stated dose. If symptoms persist consult your doctor. If pregnant or breastfeeding consult doctor before use.

Pharmacy only: Yes

If Symptoms Persist Consult Your Doctor

SINUTAB
Pfizer/Warner Lambert Consumer Healthcare

PA No: 823/28/1

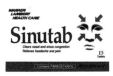

Packs of 15 smooth, circular, yellow, biconvex, film-coated tablets.

Paracetamol 500mg, phenylpropanolamine hydrochloride 12.5mg.

For the relief of symptoms of headache, sinusitis, allergic or vasomotor rhinitis, common cold and flu.

Adults and children over 12 yrs: 2 tablets 3 times daily. Maximum 6 tablets in 24 hrs.

Children: 6-12 yrs: 1 tablet 3 times daily. Maximum 3 tablets in 24 hrs.

Not recommended for children under 6 yrs.

Pharmacy only: Yes

SUDAFED ELIXIR
Pfizer/Warner Lambert Consumer Healthcare

PA No: 823/9/1

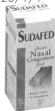

100ml bottle of clear, red syrup with raspberry odour and taste.

Pseudoephedrine hydrochloride 30mg.

Decongestant of mucous membranes of the upper respiratory tract, especially the nasal mucosa and sinuses. It is indicated for the symptomatic relief of allergic rhinitis, vasomotor rhinitis, common cold and flu.

Adults: 10ml 3 times daily.

Children: Over 12 yrs: 10ml 3 times daily. 6-12 yrs: 5ml 3 times daily. 2-5 yrs: 2.5ml 3 times daily.

Pharmacy only: Yes

SUDAFED TABLETS
Pfizer/Warner Lambert Consumer Healthcare

PA No: 823/9/3

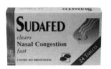

Packs of 12 or 24 brownish-red, round, biconvex, film-coated tablets.

Pseudoephedrine hydrochloride 60mg.

Decongestion of mucous membranes of the upper respiratory tract, especially the nasal mucosa and sinuses. It is indicated for the symptomatic relief of conditions such as allergic rhinitis, vasomotor rhinitis, the common cold and flu.

Adults and children over 12 yrs: 1 tablet 3 times daily.

Children under 12 yrs: Not recommended.

Pharmacy only: Yes

VICKS INHALER
Procter & Gamble (Health & Beauty Care) Limited

PA No: 441/27/1

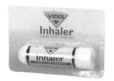

Nasal stick inhaler, for nasal use.

Menthol 125mg EP, camphor 50mg EP, Siberian pine needle oil 10mg FP.

For the relief of symptoms of nasal congestion such as are associated with allergic and infectious upper respiratory tract disorders.

Adults and children over 6 yrs: Insert the inhaler into each nostril, holding the other nostril closed and inhaling deeply. Can be used as frequently as needed.

Not recommended for children under 6 yrs.

If there is no improvement of this disorder, a doctor should be consulted.

Pharmacy only: No

Always Read The Label

VICKS SINEX NASAL PUMP SPRAY
Procter & Gamble (Health & Beauty Care) Limited

PA No: 441/24/3

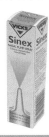

■Non-pressurised, metered dose spray containing nasal spray solution.

■Oxymetazoline hydrochloride 0.05% w/w EP.

■For the symptomatic relief of congestion of the upper respiratory tract due to the common cold, hayfever or sinusitis.

■Adults and children over 6 yrs: 1-2 sprays per nostril every 6-8 hours unless otherwise advised by your doctor. Topical application as a nasal spray.

■Not recommended for children under 6 yrs.

See your doctor if you feel worse, do not feel better after 7 days, or if you develop new symptoms.

Pharmacy only: No

VICKS VAPORUB
Procter & Gamble (Health & Beauty Care) Limited

PA No: 441/2/2

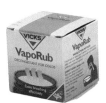

■Jar of ointment.

■Levomenthol 2.75% w/w EP, camphor 5% w/w EP, eucalyptus oil 1.5% w/w EP, turpentine oil 5% w/w FP.

■For the symptomatic relief of nasal catarrh and congestion, sore throat and cough due to colds.

■Adults: Rub VapoRub liberally on the chest, throat and back. Rub in well over the whole area and leave night-clothes loose for easy inhalation. Alternatively,

melt 2 tsps of VapoRub in very hot water and inhale the vapours.

Children over 2 yrs: Apply lightly to chest and back. Rub gently and leave clothes loose for easy inhalation.

■In case of fever consult your doctor. Do not swallow or place in nostrils. As with all medicines, keep out of the reach of children. If symptoms persist, consult your doctor.

Pharmacy only: No

DEVICES - ASTHMA

AEROCHAMBER VHC
Intrapharma/Dugdale

PA No: N/A

■Range of spacer devices to suit all ages. Adult/infant/child. Peak flow meter.

Pharmacy only: Yes

Always Consult Your Pharmacist

SORE THROATS

A sore throat may accompany a cold or cough or it may be caused by either a bacterial or a viral infection. If you suffer repeatedly from sore throat, it may be a sign that your immune system is not working properly and you should see your doctor.

Many of the medicines available for sore throat include **antibacterial agents** (**dequalinium, cetylpyridinium, domiphen bromide, amyl metacresol, dichlorobenzyl alcohol, phemol, thymol, tyrothricin**). Antibacterial agents are, of course, of no use if the infection is caused by a virus, but other ingredients can help in this case. These include **local anaesthetics**, which will help to reduce pain. Examples of local anaesthetics included in medicines for sore throat include **benzocaine** and **lignocaine**. The sugary nature of a lozenge also has a helpful soothing action. Lozenges should be allowed to dissolve slowly in the mouth so that the throat is exposed to the active ingredients for as long as possible.

BRADOSOL PLUS SUGAR FREE
Novartis Consumer Health

PA No: 30/37/1

❑Packs of 24 bright green, cylindrical, sugar- free lozenges.

❚Domiphen bromide 0.5mg, lignocaine hydrochloride 5.0mg.

❓For the symptomatic relief of sore throats.

✍Adults: 1 lozenge to be sucked every 2-3 hrs up to 8 lozenges per day.

❚Children: Not recommended for children under 12 yrs.

If symptoms persist consult a doctor.

Pharmacy only: Yes

DAY NURSE CAPSULES
GlaxoSmithKline

PA No: 678/13/1

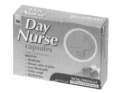

❑Packs of 20 capsules.

❚Paracetamol Ph Eur 500mg, phenylpropanolamine hydrochloride Ph Eur 12.5mg, dextromethorphan hydrobromide Ph Eur 7.5mg.

❓For the relief of tickly cough, sore throat pain, blocked nose and aches associated with colds and flu. Does not cause drowsiness.

✍Adults: 2 capsules every 4 hrs. Maximum 8 capsules in 24 hrs.

Adults/children over 16 yrs who take Night Nurse before bed should take no more than 6 capsules in 24 hrs.

Children: 6-12 yrs: 1 capsule every 4 hrs. Maximum 4 capsules in 24 hrs.

❚Not suitable for children under 6 yrs.

Do not exceed the stated dose. Do not take with any other paracetamol-containing product.

Pharmacy only: Yes

DEQUACAINE
Boots Healthcare Ltd

PA No: 43/19/1

❑Packs of 24 amber-coloured lozenges.

❚Dequalinium chloride 0.25mg, benzocaine 10mg.

❓For the relief of pain and discomfort associated with sore throat, minor mouth infections or with dental procedures.

✍Adults: 1 lozenge to be sucked every 2 hrs or as needed. Maximum 8 lozenges in 24 hrs.

❚Children: Not suitable for children under 12 yrs.

Pharmacy only: Yes

If Symptoms Persist Consult Your Doctor

DEQUADIN
Boots Healthcare Ltd

PA No: 43/20/1

Packs of 20 orange lozenges.

Dequalinium chloride 0.25mg.

For the symptomatic relief of common mouth and throat infections.

Adults and children over 10 yrs: 1 lozenge every 2-3 hrs. Maximum 8 lozenges in 24 hrs.

Pharmacy only: Yes

DIFFLAM ORAL RINSE
3M Healthcare

PA No: 57/59/2

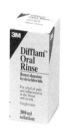

300ml oral rinse.

Benzydamine hydrochloride 0.15% w/v.

For relief of pain and inflammation in the throat and mouth.

Rinse or gargle with 15ml (approx. 1 tbsp) every 1 $\frac{1}{2}$-3 hours, as required for pain relief.

Not suitable for children under 12 yrs.

Avoid contact with eyes. Not to be swallowed.

Pharmacy only: Yes

DIFFLAM SPRAY
3M Healthcare

PA No: 357/59/3

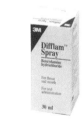

30ml spray.

Benzydamine hydrochloride 0.15% w/v, sodium bicarbonate, menthyl hydroxybenzoate, ethanol.

For relief of pain and inflammation in the throat and mouth.

Adults and children over 12 yrs: 4-8 puffs, 1 $\frac{1}{2}$-3 hourly.

Children: 6-12 yrs: 4 puffs 1 $\frac{1}{2}$-3 hourly. Under 6 yrs: 1 puff to be administered per 4kg body weight up to a maximum of 4 puffs 1 $\frac{1}{2}$-3 hourly. 6-12 yrs: 4 puffs, 1 $\frac{1}{2}$-3 hourly.

Avoid contact with eyes. Not to be swallowed.

Pharmacy only: Yes

MEROCAINE LOZENGES
SSL Healthcare Ireland Ltd

PA No: 618/37/1

Packs of 24 lozenges.

Benzocaine 10mg, cetylpyridinium chloride 1.4mg.

For the relief of pain and discomfort in the mouth.

Adults and children over 12 yrs: Allow to dissolve slowly in the mouth. 1 lozenge every 2 hrs or as needed. Maximum 8 lozenges in 24 hrs.

Not recommended for children under 12 yrs.

Pharmacy only: Yes

Always Read The Label

MEROCETS LOZENGES
SSL Healthcare Ireland Ltd

PA No: 618/27/1

Packs of 24 lozenges.

Cetylpyridinium chloride 1.4mg.

For the symptomatic treatment of sore throat and minor irritations of the mouth and throat.

Adults: Dissolve 1 lozenge slowly in the mouth every 3 hrs.

Children: Over 6 yrs: Dissolve 1 lozenge slowly in the mouth

every 3 hrs.

Not recommended for children under 6 yrs.

Pharmacy only: No

MEROCETS PLUS
SSL Healthcare Ireland Ltd

PA No: 618/28/1

Packs of 24 lozenges.

Cetylpyridinium chloride 1.4mg, cineole (eucalyptol)

3mg, menthol 5mg.

For the symptomatic relief of sore throat and nasal congestion.

Adults and children over 6 yrs: Dissolve 1 lozenge slowly in the mouth every 3 hrs.

Not recommended for children under 6 yrs.

Pharmacy only: No

NIGHT NURSE CAPSULES
GlaxoSmithKline

PA No: 678/21/2

Cartons of 10 capsules.

Paracetamol Ph Eur 500mg, promethazine hydrochloride Ph Eur 10mg, dextromethorphan

hydrobromide Ph Eur 7.5mg per capsule.

For the relief of tickly cough, sore throat pain, runny nose and aches associated with colds and flu.

Adults: 2 capsules before bedtime.

Not suitable for children under 16 yrs.

Do not exceed the stated dose.

Do not take with any other paracetamol-containing product.

May cause drowsiness.

Pharmacy only: Yes

NIGHT NURSE COLD REMEDY LIQUID
GlaxoSmithKline

PA No: 678/14/1

160ml botle of green syrup.

Paracetamol BP 1,000mg, promethazine hydrochloride BP 20mg, dextromethorphan hydrobromide BP 15mg per 20ml.

For the relief of tickly cough, runny nose, sore throat pain and aches associated with colds and flu.

Adults and children 16 yrs and over: 20ml before bedtime.

Under 16 yrs: Only as directed by doctor.

Do not exceed the stated dose.

Do not take with any other paracetamol-containing product.

May cause drowsiness.

Pharmacy only: Yes

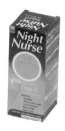

Always Consult Your Pharmacist

Takes the sting out of cystitis

fast.

If you've ever had cystitis, you'll remember how painful it can be. That stinging, burning feeling just can't be ignored. That's why it's essential to use an effective remedy straightaway. Cystopurin® with natural cranberry juice extract is a complete low sodium treatment which relieves the pain – fast.

Cystopurin contains potassium citrate which helps to counteract the symptoms and take away that stinging sensation.

Ask your pharmacist for Cystopurin today and keep a pack handy, just in case. Cystopurin - the fast way to take the sting out of cystitis.

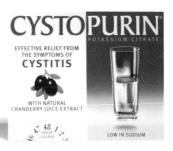

Available from your pharmacist. Always read the label.

In most cases, using Cystopurin at the first signs of cystitis is all the treatment you need. But remember, if you develop other symptoms such as blood in the urine, abdominal pain or fever, then it's important to see your doctor at once, as you might need an antibiotic. See your doctor if symptoms persist after 48 hours treatment.

Cystopurin is a registered trademark.

Takes the sting out of cystitis

fast.

If you've ever had cystitis, you'll remember how painful it can be. That stinging, burning feeling just can't be ignored. That's why it's essential to use an effective remedy straightaway. Cystopurin® with natural cranberry juice extract is a complete low sodium treatment which relieves the pain – fast.

Cystopurin contains potassium citrate which helps to counteract the symptoms and take away that stinging sensation.

Ask your pharmacist for Cystopurin today and keep a pack handy, just in case. Cystopurin - the fast way to take the sting out of cystitis.

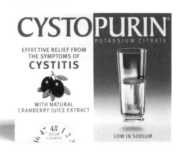

Available from your pharmacist. Always read the label.

In most cases, using Cystopurin at the first signs of cystitis is all the treatment you need. But remember, if you develop other symptoms such as blood in the urine, abdominal pain or fever, then it's important to see your doctor at once, as you might need an antibiotic. See your doctor if symptoms persist after 48 hours treatment.

Cystopurin is a registered trademark.

STREPSILS DUAL ACTION LOZENGES
Boots Healthcare Ltd

PA No: 43/22/1

🔲Packs of 24 pale blue/green lozenges.

🔲Lignocaine 10mg, dichlorobenzyl alcohol 1.2mg and amylmetacresol 0.6mg.

🔲For the relief of severe sore throat, pain and infection.

🔲Adults: 1 lozenge sucked every 2 hrs as required.

Maximum 8 lozenges in 24 hrs.

🔲Children: Not recommended for children under 12 yrs.

Pharmacy only: Yes

STREPSILS DUAL ACTION THROAT SPRAY
Boots Healthcare Ltd

PA No: 43/22/2

🔲20ml spray.

🔲Lignocaine, dichlorobenzyl alcohol and amylmetacresol.

🔲For the symptomatic relief of severe sore throat and infection.

🔲Adults and children over 12 yrs: Spray affected area twice and swallow gently. Repeat every 2 hrs, as required. Maximum 8 times in 24 hrs.

🔲Not recommended for children under 12 yrs.

Contraindications: Hypersensitivity to any of the ingredients.

Safety for use during pregnancy and breastfeeding has not yet been established. The product is therefore not recommended during pregnancy and breastfeeding except under medical supervision.

Asthmatics should consult their doctor before first using this product.

Pharmacy only: Yes

STREPSILS LOZENGES
Boots Healthcare Ltd

PA No:43/3/2

🔲Packs of 24 lozenges.

🔲Original: Amylmetacresol 0.6mg, 2, 4-dichlorobenzyl alcohol 1.2mg.

Vitamin C: Amylmetacresol 0.6mg, 2, 4-dichlorobenzyl alcohol 1.2mg, vitamin C 100mg.

Honey & Lemon: Amylmetacresol 0.6mg, 2, 4-dichlorobenzyl alcohol 1.2mg.

Sugar-free lemon and herb: Amylmetacresol 0.6mg, 2, 4 dichlorbenzyl alcohol 1.2 mg.

🔲For the symptomatic relief of mouth and throat infections.

🔲Adults and children: Dissolve 1 lozenge slowly in the mouth every 2-3 hrs.

Pharmacy only: No

If Symptoms Persist Consult Your Doctor

TCP LIQUID ANTISEPTIC
Pfizer/Warner Lambert Consumer Healthcare

PA No: 823/37/2

📋50ml, 100ml or 200ml bottles of aqueous liquid antiseptic.

☑Phenol 0.175% w/v, halogenated phenols 0.68% w/v.

❓For the symptomatic relief of common mouth ulcers, cuts, grazes, bites and stings, boils, spots and pimples, and sore throat including those associated with colds and flu.

📑Adults: Gargle: Twice daily diluted 1:5 with water. Mouth ulcer: Apply undiluted 3 times daily. Spots: Apply undiluted every 4 hrs. Cuts: Apply diluted 1:1.

Pharmacy only: No

TYROZETS
Janssen Pharmacy Healthcare

PA No: 755/2/1

📋Packs of 24 lozenges in 2 tubes of 12.

☑Tyrothricin 1mg, benzocaine 5mg.

❓For the relief of mild sore throat and minor mouth irritations.

📑Adults: 1 lozenge every 3 hrs. Maximum 8 lozenges in 24 hrs.

Children: As per adult dose.

Pharmacy only: Yes

VALDA PASTILLES
GlaxoSmithKline

PA No: 678/46/1

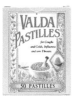

📋Packs of 50 pastilles.

☑Menthol BP 3.280mg, eucalyptol Fr P 0.451mg, thymol Ph Eur 0.016mg, compound extract of pinewood 0.016mg, guaiacol 0.016mg per pastille.

❓For the symptomatic relief of congestion with coughs, colds and flu, and for soothing sore throats.

📑Adults: Dissolve 1 pastille in the mouth as required. Maximum 10 pastilles in 24 hrs.

Children: Over 5 yrs: Dissolve 1 pastille in the mouth as required. Maximum 10 pastilles in 24 hrs.

⚠Not recommended for children under 5 yrs.

Pharmacy only: Yes

Always Read The Label

CYSTITIS

Cystitis affects about one-third of women at some time or other. Symptoms include a sensation of wanting to pass water which produces an increased frequency of urination. There is usually a burning sensation while water is passed. Sometimes there is pain over the pubic area during and after passing water.

Cystitis occurs as a consequence of a bacterial infection. In about three-quarters of cases, the bacterium involved is one that normally colonises the intestine – *E. coli*. This is not to be confused with the strain of *E. coli* that causes food poisoning. Sexual intercourse may assist in transferring the bacterium.

While the initial infection occurs externally, the distance between the external opening at the vagina and the bladder is short and the bladder may therefore quite easily become infected. Ultimately, the infection may pass upwards to the kidneys, producing back pain. Drinking plenty of water is helpful in flushing the infection out of the urinary system so you are advised to do this.

Treatment
Over the counter treatment for cystitis is limited to the use of **citrate** which turns the urine alkaline. *E. coli* does not like alkaline conditions and if the infection is minor it may be cleared. However, if symptoms persist, you should see your doctor so that appropriate antibiotic treatment can be given before the kidneys become infected.

Precautions and Warnings
- Seek medical advice if symptoms persist, if you experience back pain, if there is blood in the urine or if you get cystitis repeatedly.

To help prevent recurrence if you suffer from repeated infections:
- Drink at least two litres of water per day
- Empty the bladder every three hours and before going to bed, and ensure that it is fully emptied
- Apply a cream containing **cetrimide** (see **Skin Care**) before intercourse
- Empty the bladder before and after intercourse and wash afterwards.

CYMALON
SSL Healthcare Ireland Ltd

PA No: 618/23/1

▢ Packs of 6 sachets of granules.

▢ Sodium citrate 2.8g, citric acid (anhydrous) 1g, sodium bicarbonate 1.2g, sodium carbonate 0.1g.

▢ For relief of the symptoms of cystitis in women.

▢ Adults: 1 sachet dissolved in water 3 times daily over 2 days. Take all 6 sachets to complete the course.

▢ Not recommended for children.

Do not exceed the stated dose.

Pharmacy only: No

CYSTOPURIN
Roche Consumer Health

PA No: 50/105/1

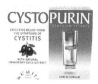

▢ Packs of 6 x 3g sachets of cranberry-flavoured, effervescent granules.

▢ Potassium citrate 3g.

▢ To relieve the symptoms of cystitis.

▢ Adults, elderly and children over 6 yrs: 1 sachet dissolved in 200ml cold water taken 3 times daily for 2 days.

▢ Do not exceed the stated dose.

Not to be given to children under 6 yrs.

Pharmacy only: Yes

Always Consult Your Pharmacist

DIABETES CARE

BLOOD GLUCOSE METERS

If you have diabetes you will know that there is very good evidence that the better you are able to control your blood glucose levels, the less likely it is that you will suffer from the long term complications of diabetes. The dietary measures that you will have been informed about, as well as strict compliance with the use of your medication, are the key to this, but you need to know how well these measures are working.

Modern technology has ensured that nowadays laboratory tests are kept to a minimum, since meters that give very accurate estimates of blood glucose are available for home or outdoor use. Only a very small amount of blood is needed and modern sampling devices are discreet, hygienic and very simple to use. They can even keep a record of your tests so that treatment can be optimised.

ACCU-CHEK ADVANTAGE
Roche Diagnostics

PA No: N/A

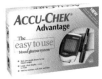

Blood glucose system.

The Accu-Check Advantage makes diabetes control extremely easy. No buttons to press, a large, clear display and requires only a tiny blood sample (4µL). The touchable, comfort curve test strip is shaped to the finger for added comfort and ease of use. Capillary action gently draws in blood.

The pen-like finger pricker is small and discreet, with easy loading and priming. 11 variable depth settings give virtually pain-free testing.

100 test memory with date and time. Computer download facility for reviewing results.

Pharmacy only: No

GLUCOMETER ELITE®
Bayer Diagnostics

PA No: N/A

Glucometer Elite is an easy to use blood glucose meter.

Quick and simple, with sip in sampling – the sample test is automatically drawn into the test strip upon contact with fluid. Tiny

2µL drop of blood reduces patient discomfort. No buttons, no wiping, no timing, no mess and no hanging drops. Test memory.

Pharmacy only: Yes

GLUCOMETER ESPRIT
Bayer Diagnostics

PA No: N/A

Glucometer Esprit has been specially designed for people on the go who want a meter that

gives them the freedom to test wherever and whenever they like, in or out of the home.

The 10-test sensor disc preloads quickly and easily, so less to carry around. Sips in blood sample through unique capillary action. Small blood sample (3-4µl). 100

test memory with time, date and averages. Lab-comparable results in three easy stages. PC download facility with WinGlucofacts for easy to use diabetes management.

Pharmacy only: Yes

GLUCOTREND PREMIUM
Roche Diagnostics

PA No: N/A

For home monitoring and management of diabetes. Product line extension of the

Glucotrend meter, featuring extra benefits to allow greater control of diabetes management.

Features a 300 reading memory allowing patients an accurate time and day record, a large display screen and a PC download function to help

patients keep an accurate, long-term record of their diabetes management.

This is particularly important for children and pregnant women with diabetes.

Pharmacy only: No

If Symptoms Persist Consult Your Doctor

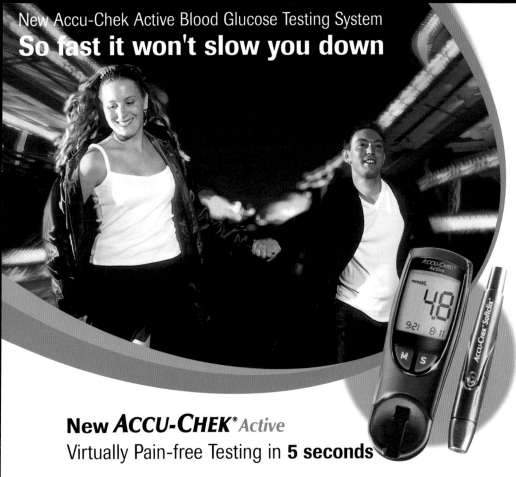
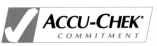

GLUCOTREND SOFT TEST SYSTEM
Roche Diagnostics

PA No: N/A

◻Complete home monitoring system enabling people with diabetes to monitor their blood glucose levels.

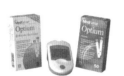To produce a near laboratory accurate measurement of blood glucose levels in seconds, the meter requires minimal blood (just 3-4µl), which removes the need to prick deeper or even to prick again to supply sample a sufficient quantity of blood.

Designed for virtually pain-free testing, the easy-to-use kit comprises the Glucotrend meter and test strips, and the Softclix II finger pricker and lancets, in a soft carry case.

Pharmacy only: No

MEDISENSE OPTIUM METER
Abbott Diagnostics

PA No: N/A

◻Blood glucose meter.

The Optium meter is a unique sensor in that it allows measurement of both blood glucose and ketone levels. Measurement of ketones is of particular relevance to type 1 diabetics who are at risk of developing ketosis. The glucose test takes 20 seconds; the ketone test takes 30 seconds.

450 test memory with date and time, plus computer download facility enables optimal control.

Pharmacy only: No. Please attend diabetes clinic

MEDISENSE Q.I.D. METER
Abbott Diagnostics

PA No: N/A

◻Blood glucose meter.

The Medisense Q.I.D. meter provides an accurate, efficient 20 second test, with a discreet, hand held meter.

The Q.I.D. has a computer download facility to enable optimal control.

Pharmacy only: No. Please attend diabetes clinic

POCKETSCAN BLOOD GLUCOSE MONITORING SYSTEM
LifeScan

PA No: N/A

◻Easy to use, accurate and convenient, blood glucose monitoring system.

Requiring a tiny amount of blood (2.5 microlitres), PocketScan combines a large, easy to read display with clear usage prompts and a fast, accurate 15 second test time. 150 test memory with date and time plus computer download facility helps people to achieve good diabetes control.

The PocketScan pack contains everything needed to start testing straight away, including the Penlet Plus adjustable finger pricker for maximum comfort. Any type A lancet can be used with the Penlet Plus Sampler.

Pharmacy only: No

Always Read The Label

EAR CARE

Ear Infection

Earache is caused by an infection that is usually bacterial. It is common in children and often follows an infection of the nose or throat. It occurs because inflammation causes an accumulation of fluid that blocks the inner part of the ear.

In about 80% of cases, the problem will get better within about three days without treatment. However, if it progresses, the pressure caused by the fluid may distort or burst the ear-drum leading to temporary deafness. There may also be interference with balance. Worse still, if the infection is left untreated for several days, it may spread to other areas within or close to the ear and rarely, it can cause meningitis.

'Glue ear' is the name given to the persistent presence of fluid within the ear, with or without infection. It affects about 20% of children around the age of two years with another peak at around age five. The immature ear is not as well drained as the adult ear. Although about half the cases of glue ear will improve within three months without treatment, it should be managed medically since it can result in some hearing loss.

Treatment

Over the counter remedies for earache contain **analgesics (salicylate** or **phenazone)** and you can also take **paracetamol** (see **Pain Relief** section). **Glycerine** – which softens wax – or **antibacterial agents (methylhydroxybenzoate)** may also be found in ear drops. These products give some relief but if the earache or deafness continues beyond 48-72 hours, or if it is accompanied by a discharge or dizziness, it is advisable to see your doctor. You should also see your doctor if ear infection recurs frequently.

Ear Wax

Preparations for removing ear wax usually contain oils (**arachis oil, almond oil**) or **glycerol**. They also sometimes include an antibacterial agent (e.g. **chlorbutol, paradichlorobenzene**). Although syringing is the most effective way to remove wax, these preparations are useful to soften the wax and should be used daily for a few days before syringing. If you experience earache or a discharge followed by deafness, the ear should be examined by a doctor to ensure that the ear-drum is intact before these preparations are used.

Precautions and Warnings
- Avoid aspirin in children under 12 (see **Pain Relief**)
- You should seek medical advice if the earache does not disappear within 48-72 hours, if there is discharge or dizziness or if recurrent earache is a problem
- Avoid poking any object into the ear in an attempt to remove wax.

AUDAX EAR DROPS
SSL Healthcare Ireland Ltd

PA No: 618/9/1

◻ 10ml bottle of ear drops.

◪ Choline salicylate 20%, glycerol 12.6%.

◪ Pain in acute earache and as an aid to earwax removal.

◪ Adults and children: For pain: Fill ear and plug with cotton wool every 3-4 hrs.

◪ Contraindications: Hypersensitivity to salicylates, perforated ear-drum.

Pharmacy only: Yes

Always Consult Your Pharmacist

CERUMOL
LAB Ltd

PA No: 300/4/1

⬛11ml bottle of drops.

☑Paradichlorobenzene 2%, chlorbutal 5%, arachis oil 57%.

◻Removal of ear wax.

☑Adults: 5 drops twice daily for 3 days.

Children: As adult dose.

⬛Do not use if ear canal is sore or inflamed (e.g. as a result of eczema).

Pharmacy only: Yes

EARCALM ASCETIC ACID SPRAY
Intrapharma/Stafford-Miller Ltd.

PA No: 69/22/1

⬛5ml bottle with special nozzle.

☑Ascetic acid (glacial) Ph Eur

2.0% w/w.

◻Helps prevent the recurrence of irritation and itching of the ear in susceptible individuals.

☑Adults and children over 6 yrs: One metered dose in each affected ear three times daily

(morning, evening and after swimming, showering or bathing).

⬛Not recommended for children under 6 yrs without medical advice.

Pharmacy only: Yes

EAREX EAR DROPS
SSL Healthcare Ireland Ltd

PA No: 547/1/1

⬛10ml bottle of oily liquid.

☑Almond oil 33.33% v/v, arachis oil 33.33% v/v,

camphor oil rectified 33.33% v/v.

◻For removal of ear wax.

☑Adults and children: Insert 4 drops with applicator, closing ear with cotton wool. Repeat

every night and morning for up to 4 days.

⬛Do not use if the ear is inflamed, infected or the ear-drum is perforated.

Pharmacy only: No

EXTEROL EAR DROPS
Dermal Laboratories

PA No: 278/9/1

⬛8ml easy squeeze plastic dropper bottle containing clear, straw-coloured, viscous ear drops.

☑Urea hydrogen peroxide

5.0%.

◻For the removal of hardened ear wax.

☑Adults: Up to 5 drops into the ear. Retain drops in ear for several minutes by keeping the head tilted and then wipe away any surplus. Repeat once or twice daily for 3-4 days, or as required.

Children: As per adult dose.

⬛Do not use if the ear-drum is known or suspected to be damaged, in cases of dizziness, or if there is, or has been, any other ear disorder (such as pain, discharge, inflammation, infection or tinnitus).

Pharmacy only: Yes

TROPEX EAR DROPS
Rowa® Pharmaceuticals Ltd

PA No: 74/2/1

Tropex
EAR DROPS
10 ml
SOFTENS WAX
& EASES PAIN

⬛10ml dropper bottle of ear drops.

☑Phenazonc 5%, methylhydroxybenzoate Ph Eur 0.1% w/v, glycerol Ph Eur 94.9%.

◻For the treatment of earache and the softening and removal of ear wax.

☑Adults: 4-6 drops 3-4 times daily.

Children: As adult dose.

⬛If infection is present consult the doctor.

Pharmacy only: Yes

If Symptoms Persist Consult Your Doctor

EYE CARE

REDNESS

The simplest cause of redness in the eye is a burst blood vessel. This will be visible on the white part of the eye as a red spot or a clot. This is often caused by objects coming into contact with the eye. It often looks worse than it is and usually heals within a couple of weeks like a bruise under the skin. However, if this keeps happening it may indicate high blood pressure and you should see your doctor.

If there is a more generalised redness on the white of the eye accompanied by soreness or itching — it may feel like there is a piece of grit in the eye — then the problem is inflammation of the eye (**conjunctivitis**). This may be allergic in origin but is more often infectious. Infectious conjunctivitis usually worsens rapidly within a day or two. The inside of the eyelids may also be reddened and yellow flecks of pus may be present. The eyelids will often be stuck together first thing in the morning.

Allergic conjunctivitis is slower in onset with no pus but often with a watery discharge and sometimes swelling of the eyelids. Pollen or cosmetics may produce the allergic response. Chlorine in swimming pools or tobacco smoke are also common causes of 'allergic' conjunctivitis, although these substances are really irritants.

Treatment

OTC preparations for infectious conjunctivitis contain **antibacterials (propamidine, dibromopropamidine)**. **Eye ointment** is generally more effective than **eye drops** because the ointment stays in the eye longer. However, it is more difficult to apply and will cloud your vision for a while. These preparations should be used for a maximum of two days. If the infection does not improve by that time, see your doctor.

Allergic conjunctivitis may be treated with preparations that suppress the allergic response (**sodium chromoglycate**). Eye irritation caused by exposure to smoke, chlorine or pollen may be reduced by an agent which constricts the blood vessels (**naphazoline**). Mild eye irritation may respond to the traditionally used **witch hazel (hamamelis)**.

Precautions and Warnings

- Do not attempt self-treatment if there is any cloudiness in the pupil, any disturbance of vision, if there is sensitivity to light or if any deep-seated pain is apparent.
- Contact lenses may interfere with treatment and should not be worn
- Try not to touch the eye directly with the container when applying eye drops or ointment
- Seek medical advice if your condition does not improve after two days of self-treatment
- Discard any remaining medication within one month of opening.

BROLENE EYE DROPS

Aventis Pharma

PA No: 40/66/1

10ml dropper bottle containing clear, colourless, sterile, aqueous solution.

Propamidine isethionate 0.1% w/v.

For the treatment of local infections of the superficial structures of the eye.

Adults: 1-2 drops up to 4 times daily. Use for a maximum of 2 days.

Children: As adult dose.

Discontinue use if increased inflammation occurs.

Pharmacy only: Yes

Always Read The Label

BROLENE EYE OINTMENT
Aventis Pharma

PA No: 40/66/2

■5g tube of yellow, smooth, sterile ointment.

■Dibromopropamidine

isethionate 0.15% w/w in eye ointment base.

?For the treatment of local infections of the superficial structure of the eye.

☒Adults: Cleanse affected eye with warm water. Apply

ointment to the eyelids or conjunctival sacs 2-3 times daily for not more than 2 days.

Children: As adult dose.

■Discontinue use if increased inflammation occurs.

Pharmacy only: Yes

GOLDEN EYE DROPS
Typharm

PA No: 219/2/1

■10ml bottle of eye drops.

■Propamidine isethionate 0.1%.

?For the treatment of minor eye infections such as sticky eyes and mild cases of conjunctivitis.

☒Adults: 1-2 drops 4 times daily.

Children: As adult dose.

■Do not wear hard or soft contact lenses while using eye drops.

Pharmacy only: Yes

GOLDEN EYE OINTMENT
Typharm

PA No: 219/2/2

■5g tube of ointment.

■Dibromopropamidine

isethionate 0.15%.

?For treatment of minor eye infections, sticky eyes, inflammation and mild conjunctivitis.

☒Adults: Apply once or twice daily.

Children: As adult dose.

Pharmacy only: Yes

MURINE EYE DROPS
Abbott Laboratories

PA No: 38/32/1

■10ml bottle of eye drops.

■Naphazoline hydrochloride BP 19680.0 12% w/v.

?To remove redness, and soothe away the irritation caused by dust, pollen, swimmimg, smoking etc.

☒Adults: 1-2 drops 2-3 times daily.

■Do not use if suffering from glaucoma or while wearing

contact lenses.

Pharmacy only: Yes

OPTREX CLEAR EYES EYE DROPS
Boots Healthcare Ltd

PA No: 275/2/1

■10ml bottle of eye drops.

■Distilled witch hazel (hamamelis) 12.5% w/v, naphalozine hydrochloride 0.01% w/v.

?For the temporary relief of redness of the eye due to minor eye irritations.

☒Adults and children over 12 yrs: 1-2 drops into each eye. Repeat as necessary. Maximum 4 doses in 24 hrs.

■Do not use whilst, or 30 mins before, wearing contact lenses. Do not use if you suffer from eye

disease or have had eye surgery.

Do not use if sensitive to any of the ingredients.

Pharmacy only: Yes

Always Consult Your Pharmacist

OPTREX EYE DROPS
Boots Healthcare Ltd

PA No: 275/6/1

▢ 18ml bottle of eye drops.

☑ Distilled witch hazel (hamamelis) 13% w/v.

▢ For the relief of minor eye irritations.

☑ Adults and children: Squeeze 1-2 drops into each eye as often as required.

❚ Do not use while wearing contact lenses or if suffering from ulceration or infection of the eyes.

Do not use if sensitive to any of the ingredients.

Pharmacy only: No

OPTREX EYE LOTION
Boots Healthcare Ltd

PA No: 275/5/1

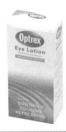

▢ 110ml bottle of eye lotion.

☑ Distilled witch hazel (hamamelis) 13% w/v, borax, boric acid, benzalkonium chloride.

▢ For the relief of minor eye irritations.

☑ Adults and children: Clean eye bath before use. Gently pour lotion into eye bath until it is one-third full. Bend head slightly forward and, holding the eye bath by its base, apply it to the eye. Slowly raise head slightly with the eye open, so that the lotion flows freely over it. Gently rock the head from side to side for at least 30 seconds.

❚ Do not use whilst, or 30 mins before, wearing contact lenses.

Do not use if suffering from ulceration or infection of the eyes.

Do not use if sensitive to any of the ingredients.

Pharmacy only: No

VIVIDRIN (EYE DROPS)
Pharma Global Ltd

PA No: 141/24/2

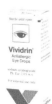

▢ 13.5ml bottle containing mast cell stabiliser.

☑ Disodium chromoglycate 2%; sterile eye drops.

▢ Prevention and treatment of acute allergic conjunctivitis (hayfever), chronic allergic conjunctivitis (inflammation of the eyelids) and vernal kerato-conjunctivitis (vernal or spring catarrh).

☑ Adults and children: 1 drop into each eye 4 times daily.

❚ Not suitable for soft contact lens users. Discard any remaining contents 4 weeks after opening.

Pharmacy only: Yes

If Symptoms Persist Consult Your Doctor

FOOT CARE

ATHLETE'S FOOT

Athlete's foot is caused by a fungus that lives on skin. Fungi thrive in damp conditions and the moist conditions surrounding the foot provide the ideal environment, making athlete's foot the most common fungal infection we experience. The infection is picked up by contact with bits of shed skin containing the fungus and changing rooms are the most common source of infection. The infection usually starts in the space between the toes and it causes intense itching.

It is important that athlete's foot is effectively and promptly treated because if it is left untreated it can infect the nails. Once this happens, it is difficult to eradicate and requires medical attention. Simple hygiene precautions such as taking care not to walk barefoot and making sure that socks are not swapped from one foot to the other can help to prevent the spread of infection.

Treatment

There are many effective antifungal treatments available for athlete's foot including some medicines that were, until recently, only available on prescription (**clotrimazole** and **miconazole**). Other antifungal agents include **zinc undecenoate** and **tolnaftate**. Treatment with these preparations should be continued for two weeks after symptoms disappear to ensure that no new infection erupts.

CORNS AND CALLOUSES

Callouses are areas of thickened skin. They usually occur over bony projections and are caused by repeated friction or pressure. Corns are small thickened areas of skin with a central core, usually found on the upper surface of the toes (hard corns) or between the toes (soft corns). They are usually caused by badly fitting shoes and are painful if pressed.

Treatment

Treatment of corns and callouses is by the application of a substance which gradually dissolves the hardened skin (a **keratolytic**). **Salicylic acid** is the most frequently used keratolytic.

Keratolytics are more effective if they are covered with a plaster and products generally contain self-adhesive pads which help to relieve the pain associated with pressure. Washing the feet in warm water to soften the skin, then rubbing the affected skin with a pumice stone, helps penetration of the keratolytic and speeds up treatment. Since keratolytics will also dissolve and burn normal skin it is important that they are only applied to the surface which is being treated.

VERRUCAE

Verrucae are warts that are found on the feet. They are caused by infection with a virus that is picked up by contact with the floor, usually in a changing room or swimming pool. They generally occur in clusters on the sole of the foot at points of contact with the floor. If you look carefully at them you may see tiny black dots. These are damaged capillaries.

Treatment

Keratolytic agents are also used to treat verrucae and preparations based on **formaldehyde** or salicylic acid are available. The advice given above concerning use of keratolytics for treatment of corns and callouses applies also to treatment of verrucae. In addition, because of the infectious nature of verrucae, some simple hygiene rules are appropriate including the use of a separate towel and care not to swap socks from one foot to the other.

Always Read The Label

Treatment with keratolytics, though effective, is a slow process and medical treatment of verrucae consists of freezing (**cryotherapy**). A home-based form of cryotherapy, using a single application of a freezing aerosol, is available.

Precautions and Warnings

- All products used to dissolve or freeze skin should only be applied to the affected area since they may damage normal skin
- If you are diabetic do not self-treat corns, callouses or verrucae because poor circulation in your feet may make you much more susceptible to the possible harmful effects of the treatments.

CANESTEN POWDER
Bayer Ltd

PA No: 21/4/6

⬜ Powder 30g.

☑ Clotrimazole 1% w/w.

⬜ Treatment and prevention of athlete's foot infections.

☑ Adults, the elderly and children: Sprinkle onto the affected areas 2-3 times daily.

Also dust inside articles of clothing and footwear in contact with the infected area.

Pharmacy only: Yes

DAKTARIN CREAM
Janssen Pharmacy Healthcare

PA No: 748/16/1

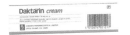

⬜ 30g tube of white cream.

☑ Miconazole nitrate 20mg per gram.

⬜ For the treatment of fungal and associated bacterial infections of the skin, such as athlete's foot, sweat rash, ringworm and

infected nappy rash.

☑ Adults: Apply once or twice daily to affected areas. Continue treatment for 10 days after lesions have disappeared.

Children: As adult dose.

Pharmacy only: Yes

DAKTARIN POWDER
Janssen Pharmacy Healthcare

PA No: 748/16/3

⬜ 20g pack of white powder.

☑ Miconazole nitrate 20mg per gram colloidal silicon dioxide,

zinc oxide and talc.

⬜ For the treatment of fungal and associated bacterial infections of the skin, such as athlete's foot, sweat rash, ringworm and infected nappy rash.

☑ Adults: Apply once or twice daily to affected area. Continue treatment until lesions have disappeared.

Children: As adult dose.

Pharmacy only: Yes

DESENEX
Roche Consumer Health

PA No: 72/8/2

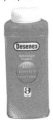

⬜ 55g tin of powder or 30g tube of ointment.

☑ Zinc undecenoate 20%, undecenoic acid 2%.

⬜ For the treatment of athlete's foot.

Pharmacy only: Yes

Always Consult Your Pharmacist

MYCIL OINTMENT
Boots Healthcare Ltd

PA No: 43/17/1

◻️25g of ointment.

◻️Benzalkonium chloride 0.1% w/w, tolnaftate 1% w/w, polyethylene glycol, cetostearyl alcohol, dimethicone 20, glycerol, liquid paraffin.

◻️For the treatment and prevention of athlete's foot.

◻️Adults and children: Apply to the affected area morning and night. Continue treatment for at least a week after the infection has cleared up.

◻️Do not use if sensitive to any of the ingredients.

Pharmacy only: Yes

MYCIL POWDER
Boots Healthcare Ltd

PA No: 43/16/1

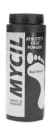

◻️55g of powder.

◻️Chlorhexidine hydrochloride 0.25% w/w, tolnaftate 1% w/w, silica, maize, starch, purified talc.

◻️For the treatment and prevention of athlete's foot.

◻️Adults and children: Apply to affected area morning and night. Continue treatment for at least a week after the infection has cleared up.

◻️Do not use if sensitive to any of the ingredients.

Pharmacy only: Yes

MYCIL PUFFER PACK
Boots Healthcare Ltd

PA No: 43/16/1

◻️55g powder puffer pack.

◻️Chlorhexidine hydrochloride 0.25% w/w, tolnaftate 1% w/w, silica, maize, starch, purified talc.

◻️For the treatment and prevention of athlete's foot.

◻️Adults and children: Apply to affected area morning and night. Continue treatment for at least a week after infection has cleared up.

◻️Do not use if sensitive to any of the ingredients.

Pharmacy only: Yes

MYCIL SPRAY
Boots Healthcare Ltd

PA No: 43/21/1

◻️150ml spray.

◻️Tolnaftate 1% w/w, butylated hydroxytoluene, dichlorodifluoromethane, polyethylene glycol, talc, trichlorofluoromethane.

◻️For the treatment and prevention of athlete's foot.

◻️Adults and children: Spray the affected area morning and night. Continue treatment for at least a week after the infection has cleared up.

◻️Do not use if sensitive to any of the ingredients.

Pharmacy only: Yes

PEDAMED CREAM
Ricesteele Manufacturing

PA No: 95/12/1

◻️30g tube of white cream.

◻️Zinc undecenoate 10% w/w.

◻️For the prevention of athlete's foot and other fungal skin infections. For the elimination of foot odours and antiperspirant effect.

◻️Adults: Cleanse and dry affected area; apply cream twice daily.

◻️If symptoms persist or worsen consult doctor.

Pharmacy only: Yes

If Symptoms Persist Consult Your Doctor

PEDAMED POWDER
Ricesteele Manufacturing

PA No: 95/12/2

☐65g shaker pack of white powder.

☑Zinc undecenoate 10% w/w.

For the prevention of athlete's foot and other fungal skin infections. For the elimination of foot odours and antiperspirant effect.

☑Adults: Cleanse and dry affected area; apply powder twice daily.

❗If symptoms persist or worsen consult doctor.

Pharmacy only: Yes

SCHOLL ATHLETE'S FOOT CREAM
SSL Healthcare Ireland Ltd

PA No: 455/1/1

☐25g tube of antifungal cream.

☑Tolnaftate 1% w/w.

For the treatment of athlete's foot.

☑Adults and children: Wash and dry infected area. Apply cream twice daily, or as directed by a doctor. Spread 2-3cms cream evenly onto affected area. Wear clean socks or hosiery every day. Continue treatment for 2 weeks after symptoms disappear.

❗If condition does not improve within 10 days, discontinue use and consult a doctor.

Pharmacy only: No

SCHOLL ATHLETE'S FOOT POWDER
SSL Healthcare Ireland Ltd

PA No: 455/1/2

☐75g plastic container of antifungal powder.

☑Tolnaftate 1% w/w.

For the treatment of athlete's foot.

☑Adults and children: Wash and dry infected area. Apply powder twice daily, or as directed by a doctor. Dust feet liberally, especially between toes. For added protection dust on socks, hosiery and inside shoes. Continue treatment for 2 weeks after symptoms disappear.

❗If condition does not improve within 10 days, discontinue use and consult a doctor.

Pharmacy only: No

SCHOLL ATHLETE'S FOOT SPRAY
SSL Healthcare Ireland Ltd

PA No: 455/1/4

☐150ml of antifungal spray.

☑Tolnaftate (to deliver a 1% w/v solution).

For the treatment of athlete's foot.

☑Adults and children: Wash and dry infected area and apply twice daily, or as directed by a doctor. Shake can well before use, point nozzle towards affected area, holding 10-15cm away. Spray liberally over area. Wear clean socks or hosiery every day. Allow to dry before wearing shoes. Continue treatment for 2 weeks after symptoms disappear.

❗Do not apply to broken or sensitive skin, discontinue use if irritation develops.

Pharmacy only: No

SCHOLL CALLOUS REMOVERS
SSL Healthcare Ireland Ltd

PA No: 455/6/3

☐Packs of 2 pads and 2 medicated discs.

☑Salicylic acid 40% w/w.

For the removal of callouses.

☑Adults: Ensure feet are clean and dry. Remove medicated disc from backing paper. Place firmly over centre of callous, adhesive next to skin. Cover with pad. Repeat treatment daily until callous can be removed.

❗Not recommended for diabetics or children under 16 yrs.

Discontinue use if excessive discomfort or irritation is experienced or if sensitivity develops.

Pharmacy only: No

Always Read The Label

SCHOLL CORN AND CALLOUS REMOVAL LIQUID
SSL Healthcare Ireland Ltd

PA No: 455/3/1

10ml bottle of medicated liquid.

Salicylic acid 11.25% w/v, camphor 2.8% w/v.

For the removal of corns and callouses.

Adults and children over 12 yrs: Ensure feet are clean and dry. Apply a thin film of liquid over the corn or callous using the applicator provided and allow to dry. When using pads to relieve shoe pressure and friction, confine the application of the liquid to the area of the skin covered by the central part of the pad. Repeat the treatment twice daily until the corn or callous can be removed.

Not recommended for diabetics or children under 12 yrs.

Discontinue use if excessive discomfort or irritation is experienced or if sensitivity develops.

Pharmacy only: No

SCHOLL CORN REMOVERS FABRIC
SSL Healthcare Ireland Ltd

PA No: 455/7/1

Packs of 4 plasters and 4 medicated discs.

Salicylic acid 40% w/w.

For the removal of corns.

Adults: Ensure feet are clean and dry. Remove medicated disc from backing paper. Place firmly over centre of corn, adhesive next to skin. Cover with pad, fix with strap. Repeat treatment daily until corn can be removed.

Not recommended for diabetics or children under 16 yrs.

Discontinue use if excessive discomfort or irritation is experienced or if sensitivity develops.

Pharmacy only: No

SCHOLL CORN REMOVERS ORIGINAL
SSL Healthcare Ireland Ltd

PA No: 455/6/1

Packs of 4 plasters and 4 medicated discs.

Salicylic acid 40% w/w.

For the removal of corns.

Adults: Ensure feet are clean and dry. Remove medicated disc from backing paper. Place firmly over centre of corn, adhesive next to skin. Cover with pad, repeat treatment daily until corn can be removed.

Not recommended for diabetics or children under 16 yrs.

Discontinue use if excessive discomfort or irritation is experienced or if sensitivity develops.

Pharmacy only: No

SCHOLL CORN REMOVERS WASHPROOF
SSL Healthcare Ireland Ltd

PA No: 455///1

Packs of 4 plasters and 4 medicated discs with washproof fixing strap.

Salicylic acid 40% w/w.

For the removal of corns.

Adults: Ensure feet are clean and dry. Remove medicated disc from backing paper. Place firmly over centre of corn, adhesive next to skin. Cover with pad, fix with strap. Repeat treatment daily until corn can be removed.

Not recommended for diabetics or children under 16 yrs. Discontinue use if excessive discomfort or irritation is experienced or if sensitivity develops.

Pharmacy only: No

Always Consult Your Pharmacist

VERACUR GEL
Typpharm

PA No: 219/1/1

▭ 15g tube of gel.

☑ Formaldehyde 0.75%.

▨ For the treatment of warts

and verrucae.

◪ Adults: Apply twice daily and cover with plaster. Rub with pumice between applications.

Children: As adult dose.

▮ Not to be used on facial or

genital warts.

Pharmacy only: Yes

VERRUGON COMPLETE
Intrapharma/Dugdale/J Pickles Healthcare

PA No: N/A

▭ 1 tube of ointment, 9 rings, 9 plaster discs and 1 emery

board.

☑ Salicylic acid in a specially formulated base containing lanesta S, an ingredient which enhances the penetration of the salicylic acid.

▨ A complete treatment to

eradicate verrucae.

Pharmacy only: Yes

WARTNER
Shield Health

PA No: N/A

▭ Home-based freezing kit for removal of warts and verrucas. Consists of a 35ml aerosol container, 10 foam applicators and a holder.

☑ Dimethylether and propane.

▨ For the treatment of warts and verrucas by freezing.

◪ Should require only 1 application per wart or verruca.

Adults and children over 4 yrs: Fit a foam applicator onto the holder. Place the holder (with applicator) into the opening on

top of the aerosol. Press down firmly for 3 seconds. Place the tip of the foam applicator onto the wart or verruca for 20 seconds.

In persistent cases, repeat treatment after 10 days.

▮ Not suitable for children under 4 yrs.

Not suitable for areas of tender skin or for patients with diabetes.

If no improvement after 3 treatments, consult your doctor.

Pharmacy only: Yes

ZEASORB
Stiefel Laboratories (Ireland) Ltd

PA No: 144/26/1

▭ 50g sifter pack of medicated dusting powder for topical application.

☑ Aluminium dihydroxy allantoinate 0.2%.

▨ For the treatment of intertrigo, hyperhidrosis, bromhidrosis and

other conditions where the absorption of skin surface moisture is required. It is useful in the prevention of athlete's foot and related conditions.

◪ Adults: Dry the area as thoroughly as possible before application; smooth the powder over the surface of the skin and between the joints and folds. Powder should be used as often as necessary.

▮ Avoid inhalation.

Pharmacy only: Yes

If Symptoms Persist Consult Your Doctor

HAEMORRHOIDS

Haemorrhoids are swellings of the network of veins that surround the anus. They are caused by straining during a bowel movement, possibly as a result of constipation. Women often get haemorrhoids after childbirth.

Haemorrhoids often rupture and bleed during or after a bowel movement and the shed blood is bright red. This is often painful and there may also be itching around the anus. Haemorrhoids may be either external swellings around the anus (which can be easily felt) or they may be internal.

Treatment

In order to prevent and treat haemorrhoids, it is important to avoid straining during bowel movements. The best way to achieve this is by increasing the **fibre** content of your diet so that a softer, more easily passed stool is produced. If this is not possible, then a suitable fibre-like product may be appropriate (see **Constipation**).

OTC treatment for piles consists of **astringents** which strengthen the wall of the vein (e.g. **bismuth oxide, balsam of Peru, bismuth subgallate, zinc oxide**), **local anaesthetics** which dull the pain (**lignocaine**) and **antiseptics**. The greasy nature of the products also helps to soothe the itching. It is also important to wash frequently. Suppositories are the best treatment for internal haemorrhoids and creams or ointments are best for external haemorrhoids.

Precautions and Warnings

- Bleeding can be a symptom of a serious disease. If you are not certain that haemorrhoids are the cause of bleeding, seek medical advice
- If there is blood mixed in with the stool, if the blood is dark or the stool has a tarry appearance, seek medical advice
- If the haemorrhoids protrude on straining or if there is a large mass protruding all the time, seek medical advice

ANUSOL CREAM
Pfizer/Warner Lambert Consumer Healthcare

PA No: 823/23/1

23g aluminium tube containing a buff-coloured cream with an odour of balsam Peru.

Bismuth oxide 2.14g, zinc oxide 10.75g, balsam Peru 1.80g per 100g.

For the symptomatic relief of uncomplicated internal and external haemorrhoids, pruritus ani, proctitis and fissures. Also indicated postoperatively in anorectal surgical procedures.

Adults: Apply to the affected area at night, in the morning and after each bowel movement until the condition is controlled. Thoroughly cleanse the affected area, dry and apply cream. For internal conditions, use rectal nozzle provided and clean it after each use.

Not recommended for children.

Not to be taken orally.

Pharmacy only: Yes

Always Read The Label

ANUSOL HC OINTMENT
Pfizer/Warner Lambert Consumer Healthcare

PA No: 856/16/1

▣15g aluminium tube containing a buff-coloured ointment.

▧Hydrocortisone acetate Ph Eur 250mg, bismuth oxide 875mg, zinc oxide Ph Eur 10.75g, bismuth subgallate FP 2.25g, balsam Peru Ph Eur 1.875g, benzyl benzoate Ph Eur 1.25g.

▧Anusol HC Ointment is used to treat the pain and discomfort associated with internal and external haemorrhoids (piles) and pruritus ani (itching around the anus).

▧Apply to the affected area at night, in the morning and after each bowel movement. Thoroughly cleanse the affected area, dry and apply cream. For internal conditions, use rectal nozzle provided and clean after each use.

▯Not recommended for children.

Not to be taken orally.

Pharmacy only: Yes

ANUSOL OINTMENT
Pfizer/Warner Lambert Consumer Healthcare

PA No: 823/23/2

▣25g aluminium tube containing a cream-coloured ointment.

▧Bismuth oxide 0.875g, zinc oxide 10.75g, balsam Peru 1.875g, bismuth subgallate 2.25g.

▧For the relief of uncomplicated internal and external haemorrhoids, pruritus ani, proctitis and fissures. Also indicated postoperatively in anorectal surgical procedures.

▧Adults: Apply to the affected area at night, in the morning and after each bowel movement until the condition is controlled. Thoroughly cleanse the area, dry, and apply ointment on a gauze dressing. For internal conditions, use rectal nozzle provided and clean it after each use.

▯Children: Not recommended for children.

Not to be taken orally.

Pharmacy only: Yes

ANUSOL SUPPOSITORIES
Pfizer/Warner Lambert Consumer Healthcare

PA No: 823/23/3

▣Packs of 12 or 24 white or off-white suppositories with a characteristic odour of balsam Peru.

▧Bismuth oxide anhydrous 24mg, zinc oxide 296mg, balsam Peru 49mg, bismuth subgallate 59mg.

▧For the relief of internal haemorrhoids and other related anorectal conditions.

▧Adults: Remove wrapper and insert suppository into the anus at night, in the morning and after each bowel movement.

▯Children: Not recommended for children.

Not to be taken orally.

Pharmacy only: Yes

ANUSOL SUPPOSITORIES HC
Pfizer/Warner Lambert Consumer Healthcare

PA No: 856/16/2

▣Packs of 12 olive green suppositories, packaged in a plastic strip.

▧Hydrocortisone acetate Ph Eur 10mg, bismuth oxide 24mg, bismuth subgallate 1980 BP 59mg, balsam Peru Ph Eur 49mg, zinc oxide Ph Eur 296mg, benzyl benzoate Ph Eur 33mg.

▧For the relief of internal haemorrhoids and other related anorectal conditions.

▧Remove wrapper and insert suppository into the anus at night, in the morning and after each bowel movement.

▯Not recommended for children.

Not to be taken orally.

Pharmacy only: Yes

Always Consult Your Pharmacist

HEMOCANE
Eastern Pharmaceuticals/ Intra Pharma Ltd

PA No: 739/2/1

■25g tube of cream and applicator.

■Lignocaine hydrochloride Ph Eur 0.65%, zinc oxide Ph Eur 10.0%, bismuth oxide 2.0%, cinnamic acid 0.45%, benzoic acid Ph Eur 0.4%.

■For treatment of the symptoms of haemorrhoids and allied anorectal conditions.

■Adults: Apply morning and night after bowel movements until the condition is controlled. Cream is inserted into the rectum (via an applicator) and/or externally in the anal region.

■Live yeast cell derivative 1.00% w/w, shark liver oil 3.00% w/w.

■As an adjunct for the topical relief of the symptoms associated with uncomplicated external haemorrhoids.

■Adults: Apply morning and evening and after defecation.

■Not recommended for children.

If symptoms persist or worsen, or if an allergic reaction occurs, discontinue use immediately and consult your doctor. Persons who suffer from haemorrhoids are advised to consult their doctor. Keep out of reach of children.

Pharmacy only: Yes

PREPARATION H OINTMENT
Whitehall Laboratories Ltd

PA No: 172/11/1

■25g or 50g collapsible aluminium tubes with detachable polythene cannula containing a soft yellow ointment with an odour of thyme oil.

■In the case of bleeding, if there is no improvement or if the condition is aggravated discontinue treatment and consult the doctor.

Patients with haemorrhoids should consult the doctor to determine the cause.

Pharmacy only: Yes

PREPARATION H SUPPOSITORIES
Whitehall Laboratories Ltd

PA No: 172/11/2

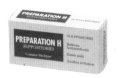

■Blister packs of 6, 12 or 24 pale yellow, bomb-shaped suppositories with one hemispherical end.

■Live yeast cell derivative 1.00% w/w, shark liver oil 3.00% w/w.

■As an adjunct for the topical relief of the symptoms associated with uncomplicated external haemorrhoids.

■Adults: Insert one suppository morning and evening and after each bowel movement.

■In the case of bleeding, if there is no improvement or if the condition is aggravated discontinue treatment and consult the doctor. Patients with haemorrhoids should consult the doctor to determine the cause.

Pharmacy only: Yes

ROWATANAL CREAM
Rowa® Pharmaceuticals Ltd

PA No: 74/16/1

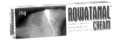

■26g tube of soothing, antiseptic, astringent cream.

■Bismuth subgallate 2%, zinc oxide 8%, menthol 1%.

■For the treatment of haemorrhoids and anal irritation.

■Adults: Apply 3 times daily and after each bowel movement. For internal haemorrhoids, use cannula nozzle provided.

■Not recommended for children.

Pharmacy only: Yes

If Symptoms Persist Consult Your Doctor

HAIR AND SCALP

DANDRUFF

It is now recognised that dandruff occurs as a result of infection with a common yeast organism (*Pityrosporum*). Also, some authorities regard dandruff as a mild form of the more serious scalp condition, **seborrhoiec dermatitis**.

Nevertheless, it is a common complaint, usually only of a cosmetic nature. We usually get dandruff at adolescence, which is a sensitive time, and it is at its worst between young adulthood and middle age, but is rare in the elderly.

Treatment

Traditional treatment of dandruff consists of the use of shampoos containing **coal tar**. More recently, **zinc pyrithione** and **selenium sulphide** have been used. Most recently of all, a potent anti-yeast preparation (**ketoconazole**) – formerly available only on prescription – has become available for OTC use.

Twice weekly use of the above products for two to four weeks should clear dandruff. After that, twice weekly use of an ordinary shampoo, with use of an anti-dandruff shampoo once a fortnight, should keep the scalp clear. It is important when using an anti-dandruff shampoo to allow sufficient time for it to work (up to five minutes) before rinsing.

ALPHOSYL CONDITIONING SHAMPOO
Stafford-Miller/Intra Pharma

PA No: 69/18/1

☐ Green, pearlescent shampoo.

☑ Alcoholic extract of coal tar 5%; conditioning agent: Guar, hydroxypropyl-trimonium chloride.

☐ For the treatment of scalp psoriasis, dandruff and seborrhoeic dermatitis.

☑ Adults: For dandruff: Once or twice a week. For dermatitis: Every 2-3 days.

❗ Discontinue if irritation occurs.

Pharmacy only: Yes

CAPASAL HERBAL SHAMPOO
Dermal Laboratories Ltd

PA No: N/A

☐ 100ml bottle of shampoo.

☑ Tea tree oil, coconut oil, water, triethanolamine lauryl sulphate, coco amido propyl dimethyl betaine, lauric acid diethanolamide, croquat L, salicylic acid, phenoxyethanol, Hexaspray Brilliant Blue 91100 (E133).

☐ To treat dandruff and soothe an itchy scalp. Suitable for all hair types.

☑ Use as a shampoo, daily if necessary. Wet hair thoroughly. Massage a small amount of the shampoo into the scalp, ideally leaving on for a few minutes before washing out. Repeat, producing a rich lather. Rinse hair well, and dry.

❗ Do not use if sensitive to any of the ingredients, or if irritation occurs. Keep undiluted shampoo away from the eyes. For external use only.

Pharmacy only: Yes

CAPASAL THERAPEUTIC SHAMPOO
Dermal Laboratories

PA No: 278/16/1

⬛ 100ml or 250ml bottles of golden-brown therapeutic shampoo.

🔻 Salicylic acid 0.5% w/w, coconut oil 1.0% w/w, distilled coal tar 1.0% w/w.

🔲 For the treatment of dry, scaly scalp conditions such as seborrhoeic eczema, seborrhoeic dermatitis, dandruff, psoriasis and cradle cap in children. It may also be used to remove previous scalp applications.

☑ Adults: Use as a shampoo, daily if necessary. Wet hair thoroughly. Massage a small amount of the shampoo into the scalp, leaving on for a few minutes before washing out. Repeat, producing a rich lather. Rinse hair well and dry.

Children: As per adult dose.

Pharmacy only: Yes

CEANEL CONCENTRATE
Quinoderm Ltd

PA No: 308/5/1

⬛ 50ml, 150ml or 500ml bottles of liquid.

🔻 Phenylethyl alcohol 7.5%, cetrimide 10%, undecenoic acid 1%.

🔲 For the treatment of psoriasis, dandruff, seborrhoeic dermatitis.

☑ Adults: Use as shampoo, initially 3 times weekly, then twice weekly.

Children: As adult dose.

❗ Protect eyes.

Pharmacy only: Yes

COCOIS
Celltech

PA No: 365/77/1

⬛ 40g or 100g tubes of scalp ointment plus applicator.

🔻 Coal tar solution BP 12%, sulphur BP 4%, salicylic acid Ph Eur 2%, coconut oil.

🔲 For the treatment of common scaly scalp disorders such as psoriasis, eczema, seborrhoeic dermatitis and dandruff.

☑ Adults and children over 6 yrs: Rub in to scalp. Leave in contact for 1 hr, wash out with mild shampoo. Use for 3-7 days.

❗ Avoid contact with eyes.

Pharmacy only: Yes

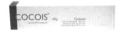

DENOREX SHAMPOO
Whitehall Laboratories Ltd

PA No: 172/23/1

⬛ 125ml bottle containing an amber-brown liquid shampoo with a pleasant menthol fragrance masking the penetrant coal tar smell.

🔻 Coal tar solution 7.5% w/w, menthol 1.5% w/w.

🔲 For the treatment of dandruff, seborrhoeic dermatitis and psoriasis of the scalp. Relieves scaling, itching, flaking of dandruff, seborrhoeic dermatitis and psoriasis.

☑ Adults: Apply liberally to wet hair, massage thoroughly and briskly until a rich lather is obtained. The lather should be allowed to remain on the scalp for 3 mins. Rinse thoroughly and repeat. Shampoo every other day for the first 10 days then 2-3 times weekly thereafter.

❗ Avoid contact with eyes, inflamed or broken skin. If no improvement consult doctor.

Pharmacy only: Yes

Always Consult Your Pharmacist

GELCOTAR LIQUID
Quinoderm Ltd

PA No: 308/12/1

📦150ml or 350ml bottles of liquid shampoo.

⚠Strong coal tar solution 1%, cade oil 0.5%.

ℹPsoriasis of the scalp, dandruff and seborrhoeic dermatitis.

✏Adults: Use as shampoo twice weekly or as required.

Children: As adult dose.

⚠Avoid contact with eyes.

Pharmacy only: Yes

NIZORAL DANDRUFF SHAMPOO
Janssen Pharmacy Healthcare

PA No: 748/15/2

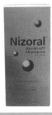

📦100ml bottle of pink unperfumed shampoo.

⚠Ketoconazole 20mg/g.

ℹPrevention and treatment of dandruff, seborrhoeic dermatitis.

✏Adults, the elderly and children: Wash hair and leave for 3-5 mins before rinsing. For the first 2-4 wks, use every 3-4 days to clear dandruff. Thereafter, use once every 1-2 wks to prevent dandruff from coming back.

⚠If you have had an allergic reaction to Nizoral Dandruff Shampoo or any of the ingredients in the past, then do not continue to use this shampoo.

To prevent a rebound effect, withdraw topical scalp steroids gradually over 2-3 weeks, or as directed by doctor or pharmacist. Local burning, itching, irritation, dry/oily hair, rash, periorbital oedema or increased hair shedding may occur, but are rare. Rarely, in patients with chemically damaged or grey hair, hair discoloration has been seen. Can be used during pregnancy and breastfeeding.

Pharmacy only: Yes

OILATUM SCALP TREATMENT SHAMPOO
Stiefel Laboratories (Ireland) Ltd

PA No: N/A

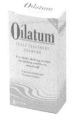

📦50ml or 100ml bottles of shampoo.

⚠Ciclopirox olamine 1.5%.

ℹFor the treatment of itchy, flaking scalps including stubborn dandruff.

✏Adults/children: Apply a small amount to wet hair. Gently massage into scalp to produce a lather. For best results it should be left on for 3-5 mins. Rinse thoroughly and repeat if necessary. Use twice weekly.

⚠For external use only. As with most shampoos avoid contact with eyes. If contact occurs, rinse thoroughly with water. If irritation persists, consult a doctor. Do not use if you have a known sensitivity to any of the ingredients in this shampoo.

Pharmacy only: Yes

If Symptoms Persist Consult Your Doctor

POLYTAR LIQUID
Stiefel Laboratories (Ireland) Ltd

PA No: 144/20/2

150ml or 250ml bottles of medicated scalp cleanser.

1% blend of tars (cold tar, pine tar, cade oil, coal tar solution and arachis oil extract).

For the treatment of scalp disorders such as itchy, flaky scalp, eczema, seborrhoea, psoriasis, and problem dandruff. Also for the removal of ointments and the pastes used in the treatment of psoriasis. Helps to clear and soothe the scalp and relieve irritation.

Adults and children: Wet the hair and apply sufficient liquid to produce an abundant lather. Massage into the scalp and adjacent areas with the fingertips. Rinse thoroughly.

If rash develops consult a doctor. Contains arachis oil.

Pharmacy only: Yes

SELSUN
Abbott Laboratories

PA No: 38/33/1

50ml or 100ml bottles of shampoo.

Selenium sulphide as a 2.5% w/v suspension.

For the treatment of dandruff.

Adults: Use as ordinary shampoo twice weekly.

Children: Over 5 yrs: Twice weekly. Not recommended for children under 5 yrs.

Avoid using during first 3 months of pregnancy.

Pharmacy only: Yes

HAIR LOSS
Recently, it was discovered that some prescribed medicines will lead to hair growth. Among these is **minoxidil** which is now available on an OTC basis. Early use is helpful and dedicated long term use is necessary. The hair which re-grows may be finer and softer than that which has been lost.

PREGAINE SHAMPOO
Pharmacia Consumer Healthcare

PA No: N/A

200ml plastic bottle of clear gel. Only shampoo specifically formulated and recommended for use with Regaine.

Cleans thin delicate hair and new hair growth.

Pharmacy only: Yes

REGAINE
Pharmacia Consumer Healthcare

PA No: 936/3/1,3

Regaine Regular Strength: 60ml bottle. Regaine Extra Strength: 60ml bottle and packs of 3 x 60ml bottles. Colourless, fragrance-free, topical solution.

Regaine Regular Strength: Minoxidil 2%, Regaine Extra Strength: Minoxidil 5%.

For the treatment of hereditary hair loss (alopecia androgenetica) in both men and women.

Adults: Apply 1ml twice daily directly on to the scalp. Massage in and allow to dry naturally.

Not to be used while pregnant or breastfeeding.

Pharmacy only: Yes

Always Read The Label

HEAD LICE

There is still an unnecessary stigma attached to head lice in the public mind. The presence of head lice does not indicate poor hygiene or dirty hair. Children of primary school age are most susceptible and most primary schools experience episodes of infestation among pupils. These are transmitted by head to head contact among the children. Lice do not jump from head to head or live on clothing.

Infestation is indicated by the child complaining of intense itching and by scratching his or her scalp, especially behind the ears. A fine tooth comb can be used to comb out the lice which can most easily be seen on a background of white paper. The small flecks (nits) that are glued to the hair strand are the eggs of the lice. If they are white and easy to see they have probably already hatched. The presence of nits after treatment does not necessarily indicate active infection. It is more important to observe how close they are to the scalp, because the egg or its shell moves up the hair shaft as the hair grows.

There is no doubt that head lice are becoming more difficult to treat since they are developing resistance to the established forms of treatment. It is therefore important to follow directions carefully, particularly concerning the method of application and the length of time for which the product should be left in the hair. It is a good thing to examine all susceptible members of the family and treat where infestation is found. A second treatment may be appropriate after a week or so to ensure that any eggs which have hatched are dealt with. However, head lice treatments should not be used as a precautionary measure so do not treat unless you are sure that lice are present.

Treatment

Preparations for head lice contain insecticides which fall into three categories. The first is **lindane**, the second is **malathion** and **carbaryl**, and the third is **permethrin** and **phenothrin**. If the initial treatment is unsuccessful, switch to a product from a different category.

In order to reduce the development of resistance, some regions in the UK have a policy to stick with a particular category of product for a while and then switch to another. However, there are no such policies in Ireland as yet.

Precautions and Warnings

- Use a fine tooth comb to detect the lice
- Do not assume that 'nits' indicate active infestation
- Do not use head lice preparations as a precaution against infestation
- Strictly observe the directions for application and duration of treatment
- Switch to a different class of product if treatment is unsuccessful
- Avoid using dry heat with some lotions as they may be inflammable – see product for details.

DERBAC-M LIQUID
SSL Healthcare Ireland Ltd

PA No: 618/14/1

◼ 50ml or 200ml bottles containing white, creamy, liquid emulsion.

◪ Malathion 0.5% w/v.

◪ For the eradication of head and pubic lice and their eggs. For treatment of scabies.

◪ Adults and children over 6 months: Head lice: Apply liberally and leave to dry naturally, shampoo hair after 12 hrs. Use nit comb while hair is still wet. Pubic lice: Apply to all areas including beard and moustache, leave for 1-12 hrs before washing off. Scabies: Apply liberally after thorough cleansing and leave for 24 hrs before washing off.

▮ In adults it may not be necessary to apply above the neck, but children under 2 yrs should have a thin film applied to the scalp, face and ears, avoiding the eyes and mouth.

Avoid contact with eyes. Not recommended for children under 6 months.

Pharmacy only: Yes

Always Consult Your Pharmacist

HEADMASTER LOTION
SSL Healthcare Ireland Ltd

PA No: 618/15/1

55ml or 160ml bottles of aqueous, alcoholic lotion.

Phenothrin 0.2%.

For treatment of head and pubic lice.

Adults and children: For head lice: Apply lotion to dry hair and rub gently until the entire scalp is moistened, especially back of neck and behind ears. Allow hair to dry naturally. Wash hair after 2 hrs and comb while wet.

For pubic lice: As above, but apply lotion to the pubic hair and hair between the legs and around the anus.

Avoid contact with eyes and broken skin. Do not use artificial heat.

Pharmacy only: Yes

LYCLEAR CREME RINSE
Pfizer/Warner Lambert Consumer Healthcare

PA No: 823/8/1

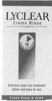

59ml bottle containing orange, cream rinse. Available in single and twin packs.

Permethrin 1% w/w.

For the treatment of pediculosis capitis (head lice).

Adults: Apply to hair and scalp as conditioner. Allow solution to remain on for 10 mins, then rinse thoroughly.

Children: As adult dose.

Pharmacy only: Yes

PRIODERM CREAM SHAMPOO
SSL Healthcare Ireland Ltd

PA No: 618/16/1

40g tube of cream shampoo.

Malathion 1% w/w.

For eradication of head and pubic lice.

Adults and children: Wet hair, rub in well, leave for 5 mins before rinsing off. Repeat procedure, comb through before drying. Repeat twice at 3 day

intervals.

Avoid contact with eyes.

Pharmacy only: Yes

PRIODERM LOTION
SSL Healthcare Ireland Ltd

PA No: 618/32/1

55ml or 160ml bottles of alcohol lotion.

Malathion 0.5% w/v.

Treatment of infestation of head lice.

Adults and children: Lice: Rub into hair, leave to dry naturally then shampoo after 12 hrs.

Comb hair while wet.

May be repeated after 7 days.

Avoid contact with eyes.

Pharmacy only: Yes

QUELLADA PC
Stafford-Miller/Intra Pharma

PA No: N/A

100ml bottle of shampoo.

Lindane 1%.

For the treatment of head and pubic lice.

Adults and children: Apply to dry infested areas. Rub in well and leave for 4 mins, shampoo and comb through before drying.

Pharmacy only: Yes

If Symptoms Persist Consult Your Doctor

RAPPELL
Pfizer/Warner Lambert Consumer Healthcare

PA No: N/A

☐90ml pump action spray.

☑Piperonal.

☐Head lice repellent.

☑Use daily during periods when lice infections are likely.

Children under 2 yrs: Refer to doctor.

☑Avoid spraying in eyes. Use with caution if you are asthmatic, or have sensitive skin.

Pharmacy only: Yes

PSORIASIS OF THE SCALP

Psoriasis (see **Skin Care**) takes the form of raised and reddened areas of skin (plaques) with dry silvery scales. These are the result of an increased rate of skin production in the affected area. Psoriasis should be medically rather than self-diagnosed and should be kept under medical supervision.

Mild forms of psoriasis affecting the scalp can be effectively treated with shampoos containing **coal tar**. This reduces inflammation, decreases the rate of skin production and has a mild **keratolytic (skin dissolving)** action. **Salicylic acid** is included in some products as an additional keratolytic.

ALPHOSYL CONDITIONING SHAMPOO
Stafford-Miller/Intra Pharma

PA No: 69/18/1

☐Green, pearlescent shampoo.

☑Alcoholic extract of coal tar 5%, conditioning agent: Guar, hydroxypropyl-trimonium chloride.

☐For the treatment of scalp psoriasis, dandruff and seborrhoeic dermatitis.

☑Adults: For dandruff: Once or twice a week. For dermatitis: Every 2-3 days.

☑Discontinue if irritation occurs.

Pharmacy only: Yes

ALPHOSYL CREAM
Stafford-Miller/Intra Pharma

PA No: 69/15/1

☐100g of tan-coloured cream.

☑Alcoholic extract of coal tar 5%, allantoin 2%.

☐For the treatment of psoriasis and psoriasis of the scalp.

☑Adults: Apply to affected area 2-4 times daily.

Pharmacy only: Yes

ALPHOSYL LOTION
Stafford-Miller/Intra Pharma

PA No: 69/15/2

☐250ml bottle containing light, free-flowing emulsion.

☑Coal tar.

☐For the treatment of psoriasis.

☑Adults: Apply to affected area 2-4 times daily.

Pharmacy only: Yes

CAPASAL THERAPEUTIC SHAMPOO
Dermal Laboratories

PA No: 278/16/1

☐100ml or 250ml bottles of golden-brown therapeutic shampoo.

☑Salicylic acid 0.5% w/w, coconut oil 1.0% w/w, distilled coal tar 1.0% w/w.

☐For the treatment of dry, scaly scalp conditions such as seborrhoeic eczema, seborrhoeic dermatitis, dandruff, psoriasis and cradle cap in children. It may also be used to remove previous scalp applications.

☑Adults: Use as a shampoo, daily if necessary. Wet hair thoroughly. Massage a small amount of the shampoo into the scalp, leaving on for a few minutes before washing out. Repeat, producing a rich lather. Rinse hair well and dry.

Children: As per adult dose.

Pharmacy only: Yes

Always Read The Label

COCOIS
Celltech

PA No: 365/77/1

40g or 100g tubes of scalp ointment with applicator.

Coal tar solution BP 12%, sulphur BP 4%, salicylic acid Ph Eur 2%, coconut oil.

For the treatment of common scaly scalp disorders such as psoriasis, eczema, seborrhoeic dermatitis and dandruff.

Adults and children over 6 yrs: Rub in to scalp. Leave in contact for 1 hr, wash out with mild shampoo. Use for 3-7 days.

Avoid contact with eyes.

Pharmacy only: Yes

DENOREX SHAMPOO
Whitehall Laboratories Ltd

PA No: 172/23/1

125ml bottle containing an amber-brown, liquid shampoo with a pleasant menthol fragrance masking the penetrant coal tar smell.

Coal tar solution 7.5% w/w, menthol 1.5% w/w.

For relief of scaling, itching, flaking of dandruff, seborrhoeic dermatitis and psoriasis of the scalp.

Adults: Apply liberally to wet hair, massage thoroughly and briskly until a rich lather is obtained. The lather should be allowed to remain on the scalp for 3 mins. Rinse thoroughly and repeat. Shampoo every other day for the first 10 days then 2-3 times weekly thereafter.

Avoid contact with eyes, and inflamed or broken skin. If no improvement consult doctor.

Pharmacy only: Yes

GELCOTAR
Quinoderm Ltd

PA No: 308/9/1

50g tube or 500g tub of gel.

Strong coal tar solution 5%, tar (pine tar) 5%.

For the treatment of psoriasis, chronic dermatitis.

Adults: Massage into affected area twice daily.

Children: As adult dose.

Avoid contact with eyes.

Pharmacy only: Yes

IONIL T
Galderma/IntraPharma Ltd

PA No: 590/3/1

Shampoo.

Salicylic acid Ph Eur 2.0% w/w, benzalkonium chloride solution Ph Eur 0.4% w/w, coal tar solution 4.25% w/w, polyethylene glycol (4) lauryl ether 7.2% w/w, polyethylene glycol (23) lauryl ether 14.4% w/w.

For the treatment of psoriasis and seborrhoeic dermatitis of the scalp.

Adults, the elderly and children: Apply to wet hair, rinse off and apply again, working into a lather, which should be left for 5 mins. Rinse thoroughly. Use once or twice weekly or as directed by the doctor. For best results do not use soap, detergent or other shampoo on the hair immediately before or after using Ionil T.

Do not apply to broken or inflamed skin. Should only be used in pregnancy when considered essential by the doctor.

Pharmacy only: Yes

Always Consult Your Pharmacist

OILATUM SCALP TREATMENT SHAMPOO
Stiefel Laboratories (Ireland) Ltd

PA No: N/A

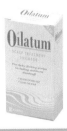

50ml or 100ml bottles of scalp treatment shampoo.

Ciclopirox olamine 1.5%.

For the treatment of itchy, flaking scalps including stubborn dandruff.

Adults/children: Apply a small amount to wet hair. Gently massage into scalp to produce a lather. For best results it should be left on for 3-5 mins. Rinse thoroughly and repeat if necessary. Use twice weekly.

For external use only. As with most shampoos avoid contact with eyes. If contact occurs, rinse thoroughly with water. If irritation persists, consult a doctor. Do not use if you have a known sensitivity to any of the ingredients in this shampoo.

Pharmacy only: Yes

POLYTAR LIQUID
Stiefel Laboratories (Ireland) Ltd

PA No: 144/20/2

150ml or 250ml bottles of medicated scalp cleanser.

1% blend of tars (cold tar, pine tar, cade oil, coal tar solution and arachis oil extract).

For the treatment of scalp disorders such as itchy, flaky scalp, eczema, seborrhoea, psoriasis, and problem dandruff; also for the removal of ointments and the pastes used in the treatment of psoriasis. Helps to clear and soothe the scalp and relieve irritation.

Adults and children: Wet the hair and apply sufficient liquid to produce an abundant lather. Massage into the scalp and adjacent areas with the fingertips. Rinse thoroughly.

If rash develops, consult a doctor. Contains arachis oil.

Pharmacy only: Yes

PROCAM HAIR SHAMPOO
Perrans Distributors Ltd

PA No: N/A

200ml bottle of shampoo.

A unique blend of Eastern and Western herbs.

Provides relief and effectively helps control dry and itchy scalp conditions. Conditions hair, should be used in conjunction with Procam Scalp Lotion. Suitable for all hair types.

Apply to wet hair and gently massage over scalp to produce a rich lather. For best results leave shampoo on the hair for five minutes. Rinse thoroughly and repeat if necessary. Procam should be used daily if possible. If not, it should be used at least twice a week.

For external use only. Avoid contact with eyes. If shampoo enters the eye area bathe immediately with cold water. Not recommended for children under 3 yrs. Keep out of the reach of children. Local irritation may occur in rare cases. If this continues, cease product use. Do not use if there is a known sensitivity to any ingredients.

Pharmacy only: No

If Symptoms Persist Consult Your Doctor

HAYFEVER

HAYFEVER

Hayfever usually starts in children at around ten years of age. It is generally easy to recognise because it occurs at the same time each year due to a specific allergy to grass or conifer pollen. The peak of the hayfever season in Ireland runs from late May until the end of July.

The symptoms are the familiar snuffling, nasal congestion and sneezing. A night time cough may arise as a consequence of secretions from the nose dripping into the throat and causing infection. The internal ear may also be involved leading to increased fluid secretion and deafness (see **Ear Care**).

General measures to cut down on exposure to pollen are useful. These include avoiding high pollen count areas including open grassy spaces or woodland (especially in the evening when pollen counts are highest) keeping windows closed and using a pollen filter in the car.

Treatment

For mild hayfever, **antihistamines (brompheniramine, clemastine, chlorpheniramine)** are the traditional form of treatment, but these cause drowsiness. If you drive or your work involves complex tasks such as operating machinery, the newer, relatively non-sedating antihistamines (**loratadine, cetirizine**) are now available over the counter.

Decongestants are also helpful in reducing nasal stuffiness and are available either alone or together with an antihistamine (see **Coughs and Colds** for further information and for **Precautions and Warnings**).

The allergic reaction is very effectively suppressed by steroids and recently one such steroid, **beclomethasone**, became available for OTC use as a nasal spray. Although some steroids can produce side effects if taken by mouth, the risk of any such effects is minimised with the nasal spray form. The most common problems are nasal irritation and occasional nose bleeds. Nevertheless, it is wise to avoid excessive or long term use of any steroid preparation.

The allergic response can also be suppressed by **sodium chromoglycate** which is available as a nasal spray and as eye drops (see **Eye Care**). Treatment with this substance is most effective if it starts before the hayfever season begins. It must be continued even if symptoms are not present since sodium chromoglycate is preventive rather than curative. It may occasionally cause nosebleeds or wheezing in the early stages of use.

Early treatment is also important if you are using a nasal spray because a stuffy nose may reduce the absorption of the active ingredients from this type of product.

Precautions and Warnings

- See **Coughs and Colds** for precautions with antihistamines and decongestants
- Ask your pharmacist for advice before taking any antihistamine if you are taking a prescribed medicine
- Avoid non-sedating antihistamines if you have a heart complaint
- If you experience nose bleeds, wheezing or tight chest, discontinue treatment and seek medical advice
- If you are unsure as to how to use them, ask your pharmacist for advice on how to use nose drops or sprays correctly
- Do not use a steroid long-term except under medical supervision
- If using a steroid, observe the dosage instructions carefully
- If symptoms are not relieved seek medical advice
- Seek medical advice if you are pregnant.

Always Read The Label

BECONASE ALLERGY RELIEF NASAL SPRAY
GlaxoSmithKline

PA No: 24/12/3

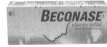

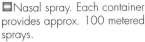Nasal spray. Each container provides approx. 100 metered sprays.

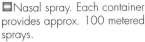Each 100mg spray contains beclomethasone dipropionate monohydrate equivalent to 50µg of beclomethasone dipropionate BP.

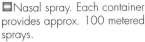Prevents and relieves nasal congestion, sneezing and a runny, itchy nose due to hayfever and other seasonal allergic conditions. Once nasal congestion is cleared the pressure and pain around the eyes is also reduced.

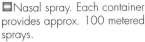Adults 18 yrs and over: 2 applications into each nostril twice daily. If symptoms persist after 14 days of treatment, consult with doctor.

Pharmacy only: Yes

CLARITYN
Schering-Plough Ltd

PA No: 277/53/1

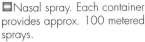Blister packs of 7 small, oval, white tablets.

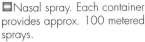Loratadine 10mg.

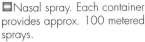For the relief of hayfever and allergic skin conditions such as rash, itching and urticaria (hives).

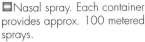Adults and children over 12 yrs: 1 tablet daily.

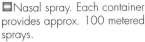Not recommended for children under 12 yrs.

Pharmacy only: Yes

DRISTAN NASAL SPRAY
Whitehall Laboratories Ltd

PA No: 172/07/1

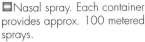15ml bottle of colourless, aqueous solution with a characteristic odour.

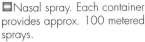Oxymetazoline hydrochloride 0.05% w/w.

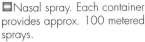Nasal decongestant for relief of the symptoms of acute rhinitis in head colds, hay fever, catarrh and nasal congestion.

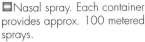Adults: 1-2 sprays up each nostril every 8-10 hrs. Maximum 4 sprays per nostril in 24 hrs.

Children: 6-16 yrs: Spray once lightly in each nostril every 8-10 hrs. Maximum 2 sprays per nostril in 24 hrs.

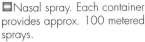Do not use for more than 7 days. Consult doctor before use if receiving medication, if pregnant or breastfeeding.

Pharmacy only: Yes

OPTICROM EYE DROPS
Aventis Pharma

PA No: 18/2/1

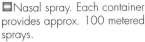5ml bottle of eye drops.

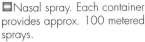Sodium cromoglycate 2%.

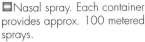For the relief of seasonal allergic conjunctivitis.

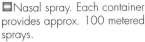Adults: 1-2 drops in each eye 4 times daily.

Children: As adult dose.

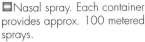Do not use while wearing soft contact lenses.

Pharmacy only: Yes

Always Consult Your Pharmacist

PHENERGAN ELIXIR
Aventis Pharma Ltd

PA No: 40/42/3

100ml bottles or tablets.

5mg phenothiazine HCL for 5ml syrup for oral use.

Long-acting antihistamine with additional sedative and anti-emetic effect. For symptomatic relief of allergic conditions of the respiratory tract and skin. For sedation, hypnosis and insomnia as a tranquilliser. For sensitisation reactions to drugs or foreign proteins; anaphylactic reactions.

Adults: Use tablets x 25mgs.

Children 2 yrs and over: 2-5 yrs: 1-3 x 5ml spoonfuls (15mg) once daily at bedtime. 5-10 yrs: 2-5 x 5ml spoonfuls (25mg) once daily at bedtime.

Protect from light and store below 30° centigrade.

Solutions of Phenergan are incompatible with alkaline substances which precipitate the insoluble promethazine base.

Pharmacy only: Yes

PIRITON
Intrapharma/Dugdale/ Stafford Miller GSK

PA No: 69/21/2

Blister card of 30 tablets.

Piriton 4mg containing 4mg chlorphenamine maleate.

Symptomatic relief of allergic conditions.

Adults: 1 tablet every 4-6 hrs. Maximum 6 tablets in 24 hrs.

Children 6-12 yrs: ½ a tablet (0.1mg/kg) every 4-6 hrs. Maximum 6 x ½ tablets in 24 hrs.

Hypersensitivity. Pre-coma states, concurrent or recent treatment with MAOIs. May increase effects of alcohol.

Pharmacy only: Yes

RYNACROM NASAL SPRAY
Aventis Pharma

PA No: 18/3/4

13ml bottle of metered dose aerosol spray.

Sodium cromoglycate.

For the relief of seasonal allergic rhinitis.

Adults and children: 1 spray into each nostril 4-6 times daily.

Pharmacy only: Yes

VIVIDRIN (NASAL SPRAY)
Pharma Global Ltd

PA No: 141/24/1

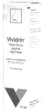

15ml nasal spray. Mast cell stabiliser.

Disodium cromoglycate 2%, aqueous nasal spray.

For the treatment of allergic rhinitis (perennial), seasonal allergic rhinitis and hay fever.

Adults and children: Prophylactic and therapeutic: 1 spray into each nostril 4 times daily.

Transient nasal irritation, rarely bronchospasm.

Pharmacy only: Yes

ZIRTEK
U.C.B. (Pharma) Ireland Ltd

PA No: 230/3/1

Packs of 7 small, white, oblong tablets.

Cetirizine dihydrochloride 10mg.

For the symptomatic relief of hayfever, allergic rhinitis, urticaria and senile pruritus.

Adults and children over 12 yrs: 1 daily.

Not recommended for children under 12 yrs.

Pharmacy only: Yes

If Symptoms Persist Consult Your Doctor

MATERNITY DEVICES

Nowadays it is taken for granted that, where possible, when feeding a newborn baby, 'breast is best'. The benefits to both mother and baby have been extensively researched and recorded. A number of devices are now available to help new mothers to breastfeed as easily and conveniently as possible, whether they are at home, or returning to work outside the home. These are classified not as medicines, but as devices, and therefore do not require a product authorisation (PA) number (see **Introduction**). If you are not sure which products will best suit your needs, your pharmacist, midwife or public health nurse will be able to offer assistance.

AQUAFLEX PELVIC FLOOR EXERCISE SYSTEM
Intrapharma/SSL International

PA No: N/A

Cones/weights/personal container.

Designed to help women who suffer from stress incontinence (accidentally leak urine when they laugh, cough, sneeze or exercise).

Use as per instructions.

Pharmacy only: Yes

AVENT DISPOSABLE
EJ Bodkin & Co Ltd

PA No: N/A

Breast-shaped teat, combined with pre-sterilised disposable bottle bags.

As the baby feeds, the bag collapses, ensuring that air swallowing is prevented and the risk of colic reduced.

Can fit onto the AVENT ISIS Breast Pump, allowing milk to be expressed directly into the bottle bags for storage in the fridge freezer.

Pharmacy only: No

AVENT FEEDING BOTTLE
EJ Bodkin & Co Ltd

PA No: N/A

Feeding bottle.

Patented teat designed to mimic the form and function of the breast, allowing the baby to suckle continuously and reducing the risk of air swallowing. To reduce colic in the newborn.

Pharmacy only: No

AVENT FUTURE MOTHER RELAXING BATH & SHOWER ESSENCE
E J Bodkin & Co Ltd

PA No: N/A

250ml plastic tube of blue gel, naturally perfumed. Citrus-based fragrance (lemon and grapefruit) with hint of lavender oil.

Undaria Pinnatifida seaweed extract, vitamin E and provitamin B5.

Marine extracts are used to cleanse, moisturise and soften skin, and improve elasticity. Fragrance to help relax.

Adults: As required, especially when tired. Pre- and post birth.

Children: Not applicable.

Pharmacy only: Yes

AVENT TEAT
EJ Bodkin & Co Ltd

PA No: N/A

▭ Bottlefeeding teat.

▨ Soft wide shape encourages baby to open the mouth wide when feeding and to literally 'latch on' to the teat. He or she can then suckle, using the same movements of tongue and jaw as when breastfeeding. Helps mother to easily combine breast- and bottlefeeding.

Unique patented skirt system at the base of the teat flexes to allow air into the bottle, replacing the milk at the baby's own suckling rhythm and eliminating the vacuum.

Pharmacy only: No

BEBE CONFORT UMBILICAL CORD BAND/NET
EJ Bodkin & Co Ltd

PA No: N/A

▭ Elasticated waistband to cover a baby's umbilical stump.

▨ Helps to prevent the cord or its clamp from accidental stress or damage, providing peace of mind for parents.

Pharmacy only: No

BEBE NURSING WIPES
EJ Bodkin & Co Ltd

PA No: N/A

▭ Specially designed wipes for breastfeeding mothers.

▨ Wipes contain an antiseptic and cleaning agent that helps to prevent skin from cracking when used regularly. Moisturised to ensure maximum comfort and hygiene. Neutral to the baby.

▨ Should be used from birth onwards to clean the delicate skin of the breast before and after each feed.

Pharmacy only: No

ISIS BREAST PUMP
EJ Bodkin & Co Ltd

PA No: N/A

▭ Breast pump. Works without electricity or batteries.

▨ Soft silicone petals massage the breast, imitating the baby's suckling to stimulate fast 'let down'.

Can also help to overcome early common problems such as engorgement or cracked nipples.

Pharmacy only: No

ISIS COMFORT BREAST SHELL SET
EJ Bodkin & Co Ltd

PA No: N/A

▭ Pack of breast shells containing 2 Ventilated Shells, 2 Breast Milk Saver Shells and 2 Ultrasoft Silicone Backing Cushions.

▨ Ventilated Shells protect sore or cracked nipples to help them heal more quickly. Gentle pressure helps relieve engorgement. Holes allow air to circulate. Breast Milk Saver Shells (no holes) collect leaking breast milk.

▨ Worn inside the bra to protect nipples from chafing and to collect leaking breast milk.

Pharmacy only: No

NATURE'S MOTHER STRETCH MARK CREAM
Power Health Products Ltd

PA No: N/A

▭ White opaque cream. No animal ingredients.

▨ Macadamia nut oil, vitamin E oil, jasmine oil, aqua, decyloleate, glyceryl stearate, macadamia ternifolia, ceteareth 20, cetearyl alcohol, D-alpha tocopheryl acetate, methylparaben, ethylparaben, propylparaben, butyparaben, phenoxyethanol, imidazolidiny, urea, jasminum officinale.

▨ To prevent stretch marks.

▨ For use prior to and during the full term of pregnancy. Warm a generous amount in the hand, then gently massage onto all areas susceptible to stretch marks such as the stomach and thighs.

Pharmacy only: Yes

Always Consult Your Pharmacist

NATURE'S MOTHER STRETCH MARK MASSAGE OIL
Power Health Products Ltd

PA No: N/A

❑Pale yellow oil. No animal ingredients.

❑Macadamia nut oil, jasmine oil, vitamin E oil, wheatgerm oil & jojoba oil, decyl oleate, octyl dodecanol, capric/caprylic triglyceride, macadamia ternifolia simmondsia chimenses, triticum vulgare, D-alpha tocopheryl acetate, polysorbate-20, jasminum officinale.

❓To prevent stretch marks.

❓For use prior to and during the full term of pregnancy. Gently massage the oil onto all areas susceptible to stretch marks such as the stomach and thighs.

Pharmacy only: Yes

NIPPLE PROTECTORS
EJ Bodkin & Co Ltd

PA No: N/A

❑Packs of 2 silicone nipple protectors.

❓Butterfly shaped to allow baby more contact with the breast. Baby can still feed and smell the mother's skin and continue to stimulate the milk supply whilst suckling, and will return easily to the breast once nipples are healed.

Pharmacy only: Yes

NIPLETTE
EJ Bodkin & Co Ltd

PA No: N/A

❑Pack of 2 Niplettes and 2 disposable breast pads.

❓To overcome the problem of flat or inverted nipples.

Through gentle suction the Niplette pulls the nipple out into a small plastic thimble-like cup.

Can also be used for the first few days after delivery for a few minutes only before each feed to pull the nipple out so that the baby can latch on more easily and breastfeeding can be established.

Pharmacy only: Yes

NUK BABY RANGE
IntraPharma Healthcare/Dugdale Trading/MAPA GMBH

PA No: N/A

❑Blister packs. Individually packed accessories. Breastfeeding equipment. Information leaflet.

❓A range of orthodontically designed teats and soothers that mimic the shape and function of a mother's nipple during breastfeeding. Includes a range of accessories and breastfeeding equipment.

Pharmacy Only: Yes

NUK BREAST PADS 30S
Intrapharma/Dugdale/MAPA GMBH

PA No: N/A

❑Box of 30 NUK Breast Pads.

❓Highly absorbant pads.

Pharmacy only: Yes

NUK CLEFT LIP/CLEFT PALATE TEATS
Intrapharma/Dugdale/MAPA GMBH

PA No: N/A

❑Box containing 1 teat.

❓Teats specially designed for babies who are born with a cleft lip or palate. These babies cannot breastfeed and NUK teats allow them to obtain nourishment from expressed breast milk.

Pharmacy only: Yes

If Symptoms Persist Consult Your Doctor

NUK ELECTRIC BREAST
Intrapharma/Dugdale/MAPA GMBH

PA No: N/A

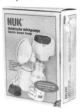

🔲Battery operated dual electric breast pump.

Pharmacy only: Yes

NUK NASAL DECONGESTOR
Intrapharma/Dugdale/MAPA GMBH

PA No: N/A

🔲Blister pack containing 1 decongestor.

❓Device used to clear baby's nose of mucus.

Pharmacy only: Yes

NUK NIPPLE SHIELDS
Intrapharma/Dugdale/MAPA GMBH

PA No: N/A

🔲Blister card containing 2 latex or silicone orthodontic shaped nipple shields.

Pharmacy only: Yes

STERZAC POWDER
Intrapharma/Seton

PA No: N/A

🔲30g in easy to apply powder dispenser.

🔳0.33% hexachlorophene powder.

❓Protection from neonatal infection.

Cord care effective against *Staph. aureus* and other pathogens.

Pharmacy only: Yes

Always Read The Label

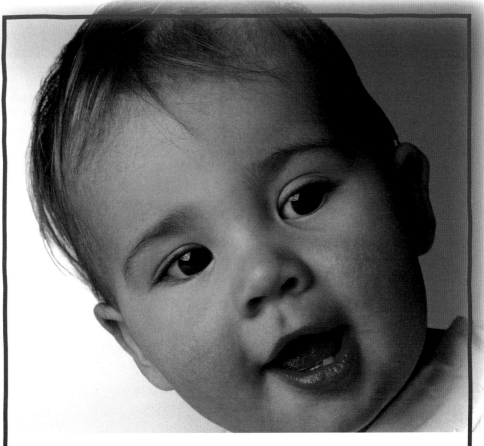

Which Soother?

**The NUK orthodontic soother is probably the best.
The difference is in the 'size' and the 'shape'.**

Feeding isn't always enough to satisfy a baby's natural sucking desire. Many derive considerable enjoyment from a soother and, unlike a baby's thumb, soothers are easily cleaned and sterilised.

To ensure that the soother fits your baby's mouth correctly, and to give the best support to your baby's growing oral cavity, NUK® soothers are available in three different sizes (Size 1 to 3) depending on age of baby.

The special NUK orthodontic shape ensures the correct positioning of the soother against the lips and palate, while allowing the lower jaw to move freely forwards and backwards naturally.

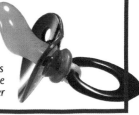

NUK®
Aus Liebe und Verantwortung

NUK is available throughout retail pharmacies.
For further information please contact: Intra Pharma / Dugdale Trading,
86 Broomhill Road, Tallaght, Dublin 24. Telephone : (01) 4520388

MOUTH CARE

COLD SORES

Cold sores are caused by the Herpes simplex virus. The usual cause of infection is direct contact, by kissing someone with a cold sore. The initial infection takes the form of sores inside the mouth. After a while, the virus travels up the nerve that serves the facial area and lies dormant until it is reactivated. Exposure to sunlight, stress or hormonal changes are just a few of the factors which can reactivate the virus. It then travels back down the nerve and the familiar cold sore breaks out on the lip area. Subsequently, each time the virus reactivates a cold sore reappears.

Treatment

Local anaesthetics (lignocaine) are useful to dull the pain of a cold sore. Traditional treatments for cold sores included **alcohol** or **antibacterial agents (povidone iodine, cetrimide)**. These agents might help to prevent secondary bacterial infection but they do not kill the virus. More recently a specific antiviral agent, **aciclovir**, has become available. This stops the virus reproducing and has some anaesthetic action of its own. It is very important that acyclovir is used as early as possible in the development of the cold sore – as soon as the first tingling sensation is felt – or it may not be fully effective. Used early, it may prevent the sore from developing.

Precautions and Warnings

- Do not kiss babies or other people if you have a cold sore
- Wash your hands thoroughly after applying medication
- Wash your eyes and face separately and dry your lips with tissue rather than a towel
- Do not touch your eyes as the infection can be transferred to them causing serious damage
- Avoid orogenital contact
- Use a lip sunscreen if your cold sores tend to be activated by sunlight.

MOUTH ULCERS – SEE PAIN RELIEF

ORAL THRUSH

About half of us carry a yeast called *Candida albicans* as part of the normal bacteria and other organisms within the mouth. In normal circumstances, Candida is invisible and harmless and it lives quietly in balance with the other organisms (do not be persuaded into believing otherwise or be frightened by being told by a non-expert that you have 'Candida').

In some circumstances this normal balance can be upset. This can happen, for example, if antibiotics are taken, since antibiotics are not selective for harmful bacteria but also kill friendly ones. If the bacterial population of the mouth is reduced then Candida, which is not killed by the antibiotic, will overgrow and thrush will develop. We call Candida an 'opportunistic' organism because it takes advantage of this situation.

Candida is also kept in balance by the normal immune system and if this is suppressed, for example by steroid treatment, overgrowth can occur. Since their immune system may not be fully developed, babies may be particularly susceptible to thrush but this will diminish as the immune system develops.

Oral thrush manifests as creamy-white raised patches on the tongue or cheeks. This can be scraped off revealing an underlying inflamed area which may bleed. Thrush may occur in denture users who do not remove and sterilise dentures at night (especially poorly fitted dentures) because trapped food particles may nourish Candida and encourage its growth. This type of thrush leads to

You have standards.
So do we.

CORSODYL

THE GOLD STANDARD TREATMENT FOR GINGIVITIS

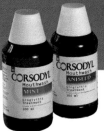

Chlorhexidine gluconate

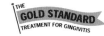

CORSODYL
Chlorhexidine gluconate

A dental practice is no place for compromise, especially when it comes to chlorhexidine mouthwashes.

For over 21 years Corsodyl has been 'The Gold Standard'™ treatment for gingivitis. Also used for the management of aphthous ulceration, dental stomatitis, oral thrush and the promotion of gingival healing after oral surgery. No wonder Corsodyl is recommended by 78% of all dentists in the treatment of gingivitis.*

Corsodyl. Tried, tested and trusted. Why settle for anything less?

Presentation: Corsodyl Mouthwash, Mint and Aniseed flavours containing 0.2% w/w chlorhexidine gluconate (ROI:PA678/2/2,4) (UK: PL0079/312,313) **Uses:** For the prevention of formation of dental plaque, in the prevention and treatment of gingivitis, to promote gingival healing post-periodontal surgery, in the management of recurrent oral ulceration and recurrent oral candidal infections. **Dosage:** Thoroughly rinse the mouth with 10 ml. twice daily. For the treatment of gingivitis a course of about one month is advisable, although some variation in response is to be expected. In the case of oral ulceration or candidal infections, treatment should be continued for 48 hours following clinical resolution. For the treatment of denture stomatitis, the dentures should be cleaned and soaked in the mouthwash for 15 minutes twice daily. Corsodyl mouthwashes should be used after conventional dentifrices or at a different time of the day as they are incompatible with anionic agents normally present in these dentifrices. **Contra-indications:** In patients who have previously shown hypersensitivity to chlorhexidine. **Precautions:** For external use only. Keep out of the eyes and ears. If Corsodyl comes into contact with the eyes, wash out promptly and thoroughly with water. **Adverse reactions:** Superficial discolouration of the tongue which disappears upon discontinuation of treatment may occur. Discolourations of the teeth or tooth-coloured restorations may also occur. This stain is not permanent and can largely be removed by brushing with a conventional toothpaste daily before using Corsodyl. Transient disturbances of taste and a burning sensation of the tongue may occur on initial use, usually disappearing with continued use. Occasional oral desquamation. Very occasionally, transient swelling of the parotid glands. Occasional irritative skin reactions. Extremely rarely generalised allergic reactions. **Product authorisation holder:** SmithKline Beecham (Ireland) Ltd., Corrig Avenue, Dun Laoghaire, Co. Dublin. Further information is available from: GlaxoSmithKline Consumer Healthcare, Dun Laoghaire, Co. Dublin, Tel: 01-2147777 or GlaxoSmithKline Consumer Healthcare, Wallis House, Great West Road, Brentford, Middlesex TW8 9BD, Tel: 020 8975 3792. August 1999. 'Corsodyl' and 'Corsodyl the Gold Standard' are registered trademarks. *Source: TMS survey 1996.

gsk GlaxoSmithKline

bright red inflammation between the dental plate and the palate and usually involves the upper dentures. If untreated, the infection can cause cracking at the corners of the mouth (angular stomatitis).

Treatment

Some of the antibacterials are also effective against Candida, especially **chlorhexidine**.

Miconazole is a specific agent that kills yeast. It was previously only available on prescription, but is now available over the counter in a gel form to treat oral thrush. Because saliva tends to wash away medicines from inside the mouth, repeated application (up to four times per day) is necessary. It helps if you do not eat or drink for an hour or so after the application.

Precautions and Warnings

- If you suffer repeatedly from thrush, see your doctor as your immune system may not be fully functional
- If you are using a steroid inhaler, rinsing your mouth out with water after using the inhaler will reduce the chances of thrush developing
- If you wear dentures, take them out at night and sterilise them with a hypochlorite-based product
- Chlorhexidine may temporarily stain the teeth.

CARBOSAN GEL
Rowa® Pharmaceuticals Ltd

PA No: 74/11/1

▢ 5g tube of cytoprotectant gel.

Carbenoxolone sodium 2%.

For the relief of lip sores and mouth ulcers.

Adults and children over 3 yrs: Apply thickly to lesions 4 times daily, preferably after meals and before bedtime.

Not recommended for children under 4 yrs.

Pharmacy only: Yes

CORSODYL ANISEED MOUTHWASH
GlaxoSmithKline

PA No: 678/2/4

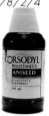

300ml bottle of aniseed-flavoured mouthwash.

Chlorhexidine gluconate Ph Eur 0.2% w/v.

For the treatment of gingivitis, oral thrush, denture stomatitis, mouth ulcers and general oral hygiene. Also inhibits the formation of plaque. Promotes gum healing following surgery.

Wash mouth with 10ml twice daily.

Can cause temporary discolouration of teeth.

Pharmacy only: Yes

CORSODYL DENTAL GEL
GlaxoSmithKline

PA No: 678/2/1

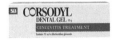

50g tube of gel.

Chlorhexidine gluconate Ph Eur 1% w/w.

For the treatment of gingivitis, mouth ulcers, oral thrush, denture stomatitis and general oral hygiene. Inhibits formation of dental plaque. Promotes gum healing following surgery.

Brush teeth with gel twice daily for 1 month.

Can cause temporary discolouration of teeth.

Pharmacy only: Yes

If Symptoms Persist Consult Your Doctor

CORSODYL MINT MOUTHWASH
GlaxoSmithKline

PA No: 678/2/2

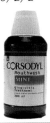

300ml bottle of mint-flavoured mouthwash.

Chlorhexidine gluconate Ph Eur 0.2% w/v.

For the treatment of gingivitis, oral thrush, denture stomatitis, mouth ulcers and general oral hygiene. Also inhibits the formation of plaque. Promotes gum healing following surgery.

Wash mouth with 10ml twice daily.

Can cause temporary discolouration of teeth.

Pharmacy only: Yes

DAKTARIN ORAL GEL
Janssen Pharmacy Healthcare

PA No: 545/8/3

40g tube of orange-flavoured, sugar-free gel.

Miconazole 20mg.

For the treatment of oral thrush and cracked corners of the mouth secondary to thrush.

Adults: 2.5ml 4 times daily.

Children: Over 1 yr: 2.5ml 4 times daily. Infants: $\frac{1}{4}$ tsp 4 times daily.

Pharmacy only: Yes

LISTERINE COOLMINT
Pfizer/Warner Lambert Consumer Healthcare

PA No: N/A

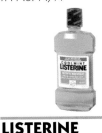

250ml or 500ml bottle of antiseptic mouthwash.

Aqua, alcohol, sorbitol, poloxamer 407, benzoic acid, eucalyptol, menthol, thymol, methyl salicylate, aroma, sodium saccharin, sodium benzoate, CI 42053.

Prevents and reduces plaque, a major cause of gum disease. Freshens breath.

Adults: Especially effective when used morning and evening after brushing. Pour 20ml (4 x 5ml tsp) into a glass, rinse around the teeth and gums, gargle, then spit out after 30 seconds.

Store below 30°C. Not suitable for children under 12 yrs. Do not use if bottle seal is broken when purchased. Do not dilute, swallow or swig from the bottle. If problems in the mouth persist for more than a few days, see your dentist.

Pharmacy only: No

LISTERINE FRESHBURST
Pfizer/Warner Lambert Consumer Healthcare

PA No: N/A

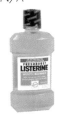

250ml or 500ml bottle of antiseptic mouthwash.

Aqua, alcohol, sorbitol, poloxamer 407, benzoic acid, eucalyptol, menthol, thymol, methyl salicylate, aroma, sodium saccharin, sodium benzoate, CI 42053, CI 47005.

Prevents and reduces plaque, a major cause of gum disease. Freshens breath.

Adults: Especially effective when used morning and evening after brushing. Pour 20ml (4 x 5ml tsp) into a glass, rinse around the teeth and gums, gargle, then spit out after 30 seconds.

Store below 30°C. Not suitable for children under 12 yrs. Do not use if bottle seal is broken when purchased. Do not dilute, swallow or swig from the bottle. If problems in the mouth persist for more than a few days, see your dentist.

Pharmacy only: No

Always Read The Label

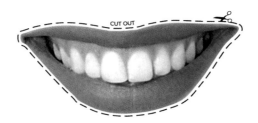

CUT OUT

What to use when you don't use Tartar Control Listerine.

Unsightly deposits of tartar on your teeth can take the sparkle out of any smile. But with Tartar Control Listerine, you've got nothing to hide.

By getting to places toothbrushes find hard to reach, its the only mouthwash that prevents tartar build-up. Thats what makes it unique.

So make it part of your daily routine. And make your smile your own.

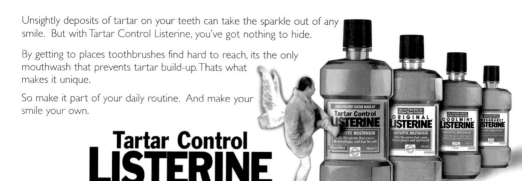

Tartar Control
LISTERINE
What brushing starts, Listerine finishes.

LISTERINE ORIGINAL
Pfizer/Warner Lambert Consumer Healthcare

PA No: N/A

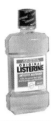

📁250ml or 500ml bottle of antiseptic mouthwash.

☑Aqua, alcohol, benzoic acid, poloxamer 407, eucalyptol, methyl salicylate, thymol, menthol, sodium benzoate, caramel.

❓Prevents and reduces plaque, a major cause of gum disease. Freshens breath.

☑Adults: Especially effective when used morning and evening after brushing. Pour 20ml (4 x 5ml tsp) into a glass, rinse around the teeth and gums, gargle, then spit out after 30 seconds.

❗Store below 30°C. Not suitable for children under 12 yrs. Do not use if bottle seal is broken when purchased. Do not dilute, swallow or swig from the bottle. If problems in the mouth persist for more than a few days, see your dentist.

Pharmacy only: No

LISTERMINT
Pfizer/Warner Lambert Consumer Healthcare

PA No: N/A

📁300ml bottle of antiseptic mouthwash.

☑Aqua, alcohol, sorbitol, poloxamer 407, polysorbate 80, cetylpiridinium chloride, aroma, sodium saccharin, saccharin, zinc chloride, CI 47005, CI 42053

❓Prevents and reduces plaque, a major cause of gum disease. Freshens breath.

☑Sloosh or rinse out with half a capful every morning and evening.

❗Do not swallow. Keep away from direct sunlight. Store at a temperature not exceeding 25°C. Keep out of the reach of children. Do not use if bottle seal is broken.

Pharmacy only: No

LYPSYL COLD SORE GEL
Novartis Consumer Health

PA No: 30/30/1

📁3g tube of colourless, viscous gel with a characteristic menthol odour.

☑Lidocaine hydrochloride 2.0% w/w, zinc sulphate 1.0% w/w, cetrimide 0.5% w/w.

❓For the symptomatic relief of cold sores.

☑Adults and children over 12 yrs: Apply a small amount to the affected area with fingertip 3-4 times daily.

❗Avoid contact with eyes.

Not recommended for children under 12 yrs.

Pharmacy only: Yes

MACLEANS SENSITIVE
GlaxoSmithKline

PA No: 678/59/1

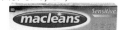

📁50ml tube of toothpaste.

☑Strontium acetate hemihydrate 8%, sodium fluoride BP 0.23% (w/w).

❓To relieve the pain of sensitive teeth.

☑Adults: Use morning and night in place of ordinary toothpaste.

❗If symptoms persist consult your dentist.

Pharmacy only: No

Always Consult Your Pharmacist

ORALDENE
Pfizer/Warner Lambert Consumer Healthcare

PA No: 823/26/1

200ml bottle containing a clear, red liquid.

Hexetidine 0.1% w/v.

Soothing antibacterial and antifungal action which relieves mouth and throat infections, including mouth ulcers, sore or bleeding gums, symptoms of sore throat and bad breath. Can be used before and after dental surgery.

Adults and children: Rinse or gargle 15ml in the mouth 3 times daily or as directed.

Pharmacy only: No

RINSTEAD ADULT GEL WITH BENZOCAINE
Schering-Plough Ltd

PA No: 277/55/1

15g tube of clear gel.

Benzocaine 2.0% w/w, chloroxylenol 0.106% w/w.

For the relief of pain due to mouth ulcers, denture sore spots and soreness of the mouth.

Adults and children over 12 yrs: Apply to the sore area with a clean finger. Maximum 6 times in 24 hrs.

Not recommended for children under 12 yrs.

Pharmacy only: Yes

RINSTEAD SUGAR FREE PASTILLES
Schering-Plough Ltd

PA No: 277/76/1

Blister packs of 24 round, red pastilles.

Menthol 0.033% w/w and cetylpyridinium chloride 0.128% w/w.

Relief of symptoms of mouth ulcers.

Adults and children over 12 yrs: Dissolve 1 pastille slowly in the mouth every 2 hrs.

Not recommended for children under 12 yrs.

Pharmacy only: Yes

SOOTHELIP
Bayer Ltd

PA No: 176/70/1

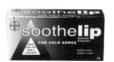

White cream 2g.

Aciclovir 5% w/w.

Treatment of cold sore infection.

Apply to cold sore or impending cold sore as early as possible after the start of an infection.

Adults and the elderly: Apply 5 times daily at approximately 4 hourly intervals. Treatment should be continued for 5 days. If, after 5 days, healing is not complete then treatment can be continued for up to an additional 5 days.

Pharmacy only: Yes

TCP LIQUID ANTISEPTIC
Pfizer/Warner Lambert Consumer Healthcare

PA No: 823/37/2

50ml, 100ml or 200ml bottles containing aqueous liquid antiseptic.

Phenol 0.175% w/v, halogenated phenols 0.68% w/v.

For the symptomatic relief of common mouth ulcers, cuts, grazes, bites and stings, boils, spots and pimples, and sore throat including those associated with colds and flu.

Adults: Gargle: Twice daily diluted 1:5 with water. Mouth ulcer: Apply undiluted 3 times daily. Spots: Apply undiluted every 4 hrs. Cuts: Apply diluted 1:1.

Pharmacy only: No

If Symptoms Persist Consult Your Doctor

the **on-target** cold sore cream...

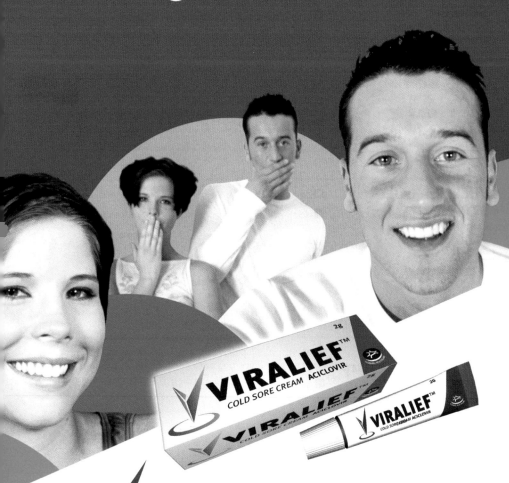

VVIRALIEF™
COLD SORE CREAM **ACICLOVIR**

FOR THE RELIEF OF COLD SORES

CLONMEL HEALTHCARE

"where quality costs less"

UVISTAT LIP SCREEN
Intrapharma/Eastern Pharmaceuticals

PA No: N/A

◻Lip screen.

☑Ethyl hexyl p-methozycinnate 3% w/w, butyl methozydibenzoylmethane 4% w/w, Novol (oleyl alcohol, Crodamol PMP (PPG myristyl proprioante).

❓Helps to prevent cold sores.

Pharmacy only: Yes

VIRALIEF COLD SORE CREAM
Clonmel Healthcare

PA No: 593/14/1

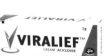

◻2g tube.

☑Aciclovir cream 2g (aciclovir 5%).

❓Enzyme inhibitor for the treatment of herpes simplex infections of the skin.

▨Adults and children: Apply 5 times daily at 4 hourly intervals for 5 days. Continue for another

5 days if healing is incomplete.

❗Not for use in eyes.

Pharmacy only: Yes

ZOVIRAX COLD SORE CREAM PUMP
Glaxo SmithKline

PA No: 17/78/10

◻2g pump dispenser.

☑Aciclovir 5% w/w.

❓For the treatment of cold

sores, herpes simplex virus infection of the lips and face.

▨Adults: Apply 5 times daily (every 4 hrs), beginning as early as possible after the start of the infection. Continue treatment for 5 days. Wash hands thoroughly before and after treatment and avoid

unnecessary rubbing or touching of the lesions to avoid aggravating or transferring the infection.

Children: As per adult dose.

Pharmacy only: Yes

ZOVIRAX COLD SORE CREAM TUBE
Glaxo SmithKline

PA No: 17/78/10

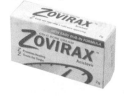

◻2g tube of white cream.

☑Aciclovir 5% w/w.

❓For the treatment of cold sores, herpes simplex virus infection of the lips and face.

▨Adults: Apply 5 times daily (every 4 hrs), beginning as early as possible after the start of the infection. Continue treatment for 5 days. Wash

hands thoroughly before and after treatment and avoid unnecessary rubbing or touching of the lesions to avoid aggravating or transferring the infection.

Children: As per adult dose.

Pharmacy only: Yes

Always Read The Label

PAIN RELIEF

GENERAL PAIN RELIEF

There are four types of painkillers (medically called **analgesics**) that you can buy over the counter without a prescription. These are **paracetamol**, **aspirin**, **ibuprofen** and **codeine**. You will find further details on the properties of each of these four under their headings below. Products containing ibuprofen or codeine can only be sold in pharmacies. Some products contain only one painkiller, while others contain a combination of them. Sometimes caffeine, which mildly enhances the analgesic effect, may also be included.

Caution

Because these substances are contained in such a wide variety of products, including prescription medicines, there is a risk that you may take more than the recommended dose without realising it.

In terms of simple pain relief there is little to choose between the various painkillers available over the counter. However, some are more suited for the treatment of particular types of pain or conditions. Aspirin and ibuprofen have anti-inflammatory as well as painkilling properties. This means that you will find them in medications for conditions such as muscle and joint pain, where inflammation may be involved.

Paracetamol, aspirin and ibuprofen reduce raised body temperature, as well as reducing pain, and so they will be found in many cold and flu remedies. The information supplied in this guide lists the active ingredients in each product. To avoid the risk of overdosing, always check the products' contents before using it.

PARACETAMOL

Used as a home medication for over 30 years, paracetamol effectively relieves pain and fever in adults and children. It can be taken by people who are sensitive to aspirin and by those with peptic ulcers. Taken in the correct dosage, paracetamol is an effective and safe analgesic with a remarkably low incidence of side effects. In overdose, however, it is dangerous.

Caution

Paracetamol overdose can lead to severe liver and kidney damage and may also damage the brain. If untreated it can lead to fatality in four to eighteen days. Fortunately, paracetamol poisoning can be effectively treated provided the treatment is given within a few hours. Tragically, although someone who has deliberately taken an overdose of paracetamol may still feel quite well next day, by then it may be too late and they will face a liver transplant at best and at worst an unpleasant lingering death. Regular alcohol intake, or a poor nutritional state, can increase a person's susceptibility to paracetamol poisoning.

In recognition of the dangers of paracetamol poisoning, some changes have recently been made to the way OTC paracetamol products are packaged. A warning that the product contains paracetamol must appear in bold type on the pack. Because of the danger of irreversible liver damage a warning that immediate medical advice should be sought in the event of overdose must also be displayed on the pack.

In order to reduce the incidence of overdose, products containing paracetamol are no longer available in bulk packs. Supply is restricted to 24 of the 500mg pack size or 120ml of the liquid product for children. Tablets must also be in a 'blister pack' – the sort that you push through a foil film. This is based on the concept that having to push tablets through one at a time will act as a deterrent to deliberate overdosing.

These measures seem to be working. One UK centre reported a 21% reduction in all overdoses and a 64% reduction in severe overdoses. Reports from Belfast also indicate a reduction in the amount consumed in overdose cases.

ASPIRIN

Among the OTC analgesics, aspirin has the longest history of use. Although the use of aspirin as a painkiller is decreasing, millions of people now take a small dose of aspirin (75mg) every day to prevent blood clotting. Accidental overdose with aspirin is much less likely than with paracetamol and deliberate overdose is less of an emergency. There are, however, significant dangers associated with aspirin use that you should be aware of.

As you may know, aspirin can cause bleeding within the stomach and intestine. This may cause nausea, vomiting and abdominal pain and sometimes, serious blood loss. If you have had an ulcer you should avoid aspirin. It is less well known that aspirin can also produce wheeze or cause an asthma attack in as many as one in five people with asthma and it is best to avoid it if you suffer from this condition.

Aspirin can interact with several types of prescription medicine. If you are prescribed one of these medicines, you should be informed of the necessary precautions. The most serious interactions occur with the anti-clotting drug, warfarin, and with methotrexate which may be used to treat arthritis or, occasionally, psoriasis.

You should also avoid aspirin during pregnancy although the chief danger is mainly associated with long term use. It should certainly not be taken in late pregnancy because of the risk of increased bleeding during the birth. About one-fifth of the dose finds its way into breast milk so it is also best avoided if you are breastfeeding.

Because of a suspected association between aspirin and a rare but serious disorder known as **Reyes syndrome**, aspirin should not be given to children under 12.

Newer uses for Aspirin

In recent times, it has been recognised that aspirin has a very potent effect in inhibiting blood clotting and, as mentioned above, it is now prescribed for this purpose for patients with angina, or for those who have had a heart attack or a certain type of stroke. This effect of aspirin, incidentally, is not produced by 'thinning the blood' but rather by preventing the clumping together of blood cells (the platelets) that start the clotting process. The effect is a very powerful one, with a single 300mg aspirin tablet having an effect for at least five days. It is not recommended that healthy people take aspirin daily to prevent heart attack or stroke.

In light of the recent publicity surrounding the risk of clotting associated with long haul flights, people are often advised to take a single aspirin tablet the evening before the journey. If there are no factors which suggest that aspirin should be avoided, it is difficult to argue against this. If you are on a long haul flight, do what you can to exercise during the flight and consume plenty of fluid (not alcohol!).

IBUPROFEN

Ibuprofen is a newer painkiller. Like aspirin, it belongs to a group of drugs known as non-

If Symptoms Persist Consult Your Doctor

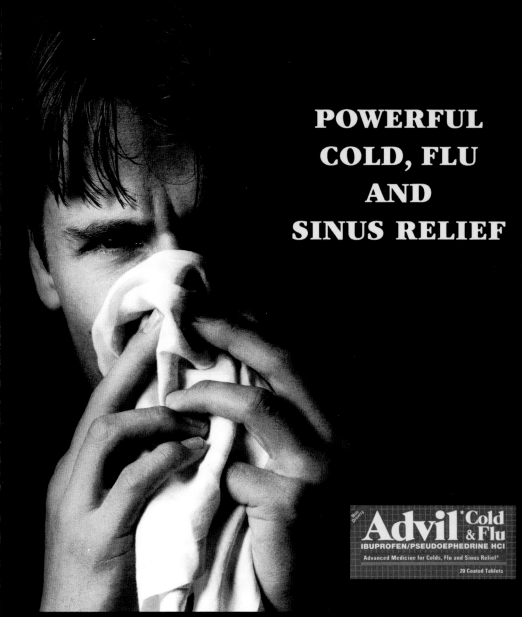

Advil* Cold & Flu

POWERFUL COLD, FLU AND SINUS RELIEF

Advil *Cold & Flu*

IBUPROFEN/PSEUDOEPHEDRINE HCl

Advanced Medicine for Colds, Flu and Sinus Relief*

20 Coated Tablets

For further information contact:
Whitehall Laboratories, 765 South Circular Road, Islandbridge, Dublin 8.
For correct use read instructions carefully.   PA 172/24/1 * Trade Mark

WHITEHALL

1 in 3 women will suffer from a significant loss in bone density

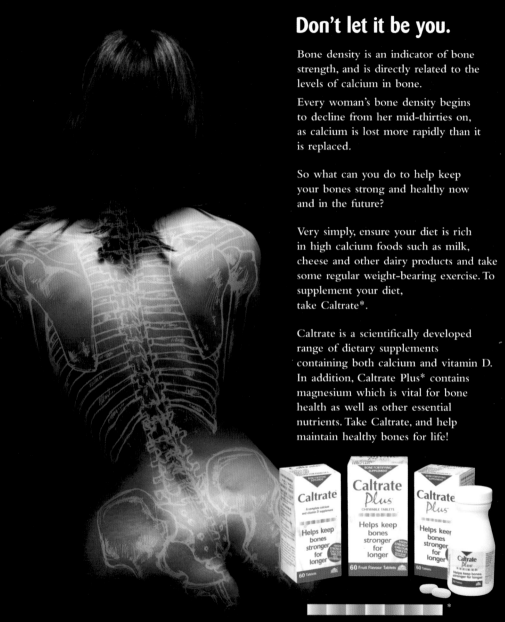

Don't let it be you.

Bone density is an indicator of bone strength, and is directly related to the levels of calcium in bone.

Every woman's bone density begins to decline from her mid-thirties on, as calcium is lost more rapidly than it is replaced.

So what can you do to help keep your bones strong and healthy now and in the future?

Very simply, ensure your diet is rich in high calcium foods such as milk, cheese and other dairy products and take some regular weight-bearing exercise. To supplement your diet, take Caltrate*.

Caltrate is a scientifically developed range of dietary supplements containing both calcium and vitamin D. In addition, Caltrate Plus* contains magnesium which is vital for bone health as well as other essential nutrients. Take Caltrate, and help maintain healthy bones for life!

Helps keep bones *stronger* for longer

*Trade Mark

steroidal anti-inflammatory drugs (NSAIDS). It therefore shares many of the properties of aspirin and some of the same precautions apply. In particular, like aspirin, it is not suitable for people with asthma. It can also produce abdominal pain, stomach and intestinal bleeding or stomach upset. Ibuprofen does not have the same effect as aspirin on blood clotting.

CODEINE

Codeine is seldom used on its own but is included in small amounts in some products to add its own analgesic action to that of the more common painkillers. It resembles morphine but is a much weaker painkiller. Nevertheless, there is a small risk of developing an addiction to codeine and this is the reason why it can only be purchased in pharmacies where sales can be professionally supervised. Do not take codeine on a continuous basis.

Like the more powerful morphine-like (**opiate**) drugs that are only available on prescription, codeine can cause constipation or drowsiness. However, these effects are seldom noticeable with short-term use. If you are taking other medicines that can cause drowsiness or constipation, you should avoid codeine. Alcohol will add to the sedative effect of codeine. Because OTC products only contain small amounts of codeine, the risks of overdose largely relate to the other ingredients.

Precautions and warnings
- Avoid aspirin and ibuprofen if you have asthma or an ulcer
- If you are pregnant, avoid aspirin, ibuprofen and codeine
- Avoid aspirin if you are about to undergo surgery or childbirth
- Do not take aspirin if you are breastfeeding
- Do not give aspirin to children under 12
- Alcohol will increase the stomach upset caused by aspirin or ibuprofen, increase the sedative action of codeine and worsen the effects of paracetamol overdose
- Avoid codeine if you suffer from bowel problems or constipation
- If you have kidney or liver disease do not take analgesics without seeking medical advice
- Do not take analgesics on a long term basis unless they have been prescribed for you. Long term consumption can lead to kidney damage.

ADVIL TABLETS
Whitehall Laboratories Ltd

PA No: 172/29/1

◻Blister packs of 10 or 20 pinkish-brown, sugar-coated tablets, printed with 'Advil'.

◻Ibuprofen 200mg.

◻For the symptomatic treatment of pain and fever conditions such as acute pain from period pain, dental pain, muscular pain, headaches, cold and flu symptoms and backache.

◻Adults, the elderly and persons over 12 yrs: 1 or 2 tablets should be taken every 4-6 hrs. Maximum 6 tablets in 24 hrs.

◻Not recommended for children under 12 yrs.

Not to be taken by patients with stomach ulcers or those allergic to aspirin or other similar medicines.

Patients who are pregnant, elderly, have asthma or are receiving regular treatment should consult the doctor before taking Advil.

Pharmacy only: Yes

Always Read The Label

ALKA-SELTZER
Bayer Ltd

PA No: 79/8/2

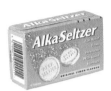

Packs of 10 or 20 white, circular, effervescent tablets with 'Alka-Seltzer' on one side.

Aspirin 324mg, sodium bicarbonate 1,625mg, citric acid 965mg.

For the relief of headache associated with upset stomach and common cold, and in the management of neuralgia or muscular aches and pains.

Adults: 1-2 tablets dissolved in water, repeated as necessary.

Maximum 8 tablets in 24 hrs.

Not recommended for children under 12 yrs except on medical advice.

Prolonged use may be harmful; if symptoms persist or if taking with other medication, consult physician.

Pharmacy only: No

ANADIN ANALGESIC TABLETS
Whitehall Laboratories Ltd

PA No:172/04/5

Packs of 6, 12 or 24 white, capsule shaped tablets embossed 'ANADIN'.

Aspirin 325mg, caffeine 15mg, quinine sulphate 1mg.

For the relief of pain such as headache, toothache etc. and for the relief of cold symptoms.

Adults: 2 tablets every 3-4 hrs if necessary. Maximum 6 doses (12 tablets) in 24 hrs.

Children (over 12 yrs): 1 tablet every 3-4 hrs.

Not to be given to children under 12 yrs except on medical advice.

Prolonged use can be harmful. If symptoms persist or if taking any other medication consult physician.

Do not exceed the stated dose.

Not to be taken by patients with stomach ulcers or those allergic to aspirin or other similar medicines.

Patients who are pregnant, breastfeeding, elderly, have asthma or are receiving regular treatment should consult the doctor before taking Anadin.

Pharmacy only: No

ANADIN EXTRA
Whitehall Laboratories Ltd

PA No: 172/18/1

Packs of 8, 12 or 24 white, film-coated, capsule-shaped cylindrical tablets with breakbar on one side and 'AE' on the other.

Aspirin 300mg, paracetamol 200mg, caffeine 45mg.

For the relief of pain such as headache, neuralgia, muscle pain, rheumatism, toothache, period pain and symptoms of the common cold and influenza.

Adults: 1-2 tablets every 4 hrs. Maximum 6 tablets in 24 hrs.

Children: Over 12 yrs: 1-2 tablets every 4 hrs. Maximum 6 tablets in 24 hrs.

Not to be given to children under 12 yrs except on medical advice.

Prolonged use can be harmful. If symptoms persist or if taking any other medication consult physician.

Do not exceed stated dose.

Do not take with any other

paracetamol-containing products.

Not to be taken by patients with stomach ulcers or those allergic to aspirin or other similar medicines.

Patients who are pregnant, breastfeeding, elderly, have asthma or are receiving regular treatment should consult the doctor before taking Anadin Extra.

Pharmacy only: No

Always Consult Your Pharmacist

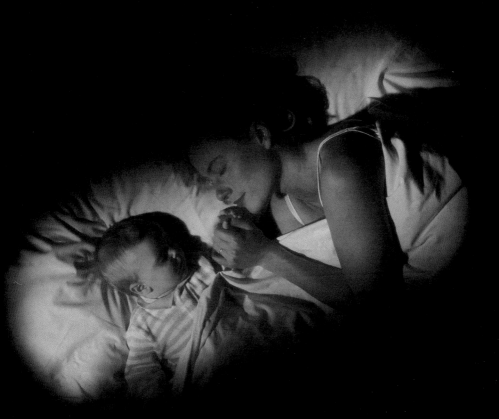

Peaceful Nights for Baby.
Peace of Mind for You.

A little one in distress can be an upsetting sound for any mother. Distress brought on by colds, flu, fever - even teething and it can happen when you feel at your most helpless.

So isn't it a great comfort to know that Calpol is close at hand. For over 25 years, mothers have trusted the soothing power of Calpol to ease pain, lower temperature - and so help a restful night.

Calpol Six Plus is perfect for the older child.

Make sure to always keep Calpol on hand. And rest easy.

Calpol is a Trademark

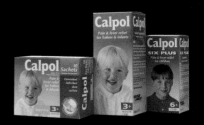

Contains Paracetamol
Always read the label

ASPRO CLEAR
Roche Consumer Health

PA No: 50/114/1

◻Blister packs of 18 or 30 round, white, bevel-edged, lemon-flavoured, soluble tablets. One side is plain, the other bisected by breakline.

✓Aspirin 300mg in an effervescent base.

For the management of pain such as that associated with headache, toothache, migraine and musculoskeletal disorders.

Adults and elderly: 2 tablets in water every 4 hrs as required.

Maximum 13 tablets in 24 hrs unless under specific direction of a physician.

Not recommended for infants, neonates or children.

Pharmacy only: No

CALPOL SACHETS
Pfizer/Warner Lambert Consumer Healthcare

PA No: 823/10/5; 823/10/2

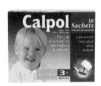

◻Packs of 10 x 5ml sachets.

✓Paracetamol 120mg per 5ml.

Children: Under 3 months: 1 x 2.5ml spoonful for fever following vaccination at 2 months, otherwise use only under medical supervision. 3 months-under 1 yr: $\frac{1}{2}$ (2.5ml) -1 x 5ml spoonful. 1yr-under 6yrs: 1-2 x 5ml spoonfuls.

Do not give with any other paracetamol-containing products.

Pharmacy only: No

CODIS
Reckitt Benckiser

PA No: 979/3/1

◻Foil packs of 24 white, circular, soluble tablets.

✓Aspirin 500mg, codeine phosphate 8mg.

Strong pain relief. For relief of pain, headaches, toothache, neuralgia, period pain, feverishness, symptoms of cold and flu.

Adults: 1 tablet dissolved in water every 3 hrs. Maximum 8 tablets in 24 hrs.

Not suitable for children.

Prolonged use without a doctor's advice can be harmful.

Pharmacy only: Yes

DISPRIN
Reckitt Benckiser

PA No: 979/6/1

◻Packs of 12, 24 or 48 white, circular soluble tablets.

✓Aspirin 300mg.

For the relief of headaches, migraine, toothache, period pain. To relieve symptoms of cold and flu, sore throat, rheumatic pain, lumbago, sciatica and neuralgia. Also lowers temperature and reduces inflammation.

Adults: Take 1-2 tablets dissolved in water. Wait 4 hrs before taking another dose. Do not take more than 12 tablets in 24 hrs.

Do not give to children, especially those under 12 yrs, except on medical advice.

Prolonged use without doctor's advice can be harmful.

Pharmacy only: No

If Symptoms Persist Consult Your Doctor

DISPRIN DIRECT
Reckitt Benckiser

PA No: 979/7/1

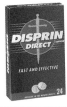

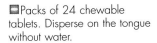Packs of 24 chewable tablets. Disperse on the tongue without water.

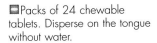Aspirin 300mg.

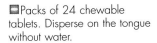For the relief of headaches, migraine, toothache, period pain. To relieve symptoms of cold and flu, sore throat, rheumatic pain, lumbago, sciatica and neuralgia. Also lowers temperature and reduces inflammation.

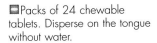Adults: 1-2 tablets dispersed on the tongue without water and then swallowed. Wait 4 hrs before taking another dose. Do not take more than 12 tablets in 24 hrs.

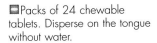Not recommended for children, except on medical advice.

Prolonged use without doctor's advice can be harmful.

Pharmacy only: No

DISPRIN EXTRA STRENGTH
Reckitt Benckiser

PA No: 979/6/2

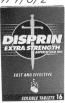

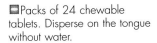Foil packs of 8 and 16 soluble white, circular tablets.

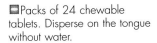Aspirin 500mg.

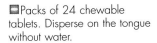Soluble pain reliever. For relief of headaches, toothache, feverishness and muscular aches and pains. To relieve symptoms of cold and flu, sore throat, neuralgia, lumbago. Also lowers temperature and reduces inflammation.

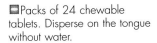Adults: 1 tablet dissolved in water every 3-4 hrs. Do not exceed 8 tablets in 24 hrs.

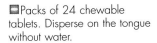Children: Not suitable for children.

Do not exceed the stated dose. Keep out of the reach of children.

Pharmacy only: No

DISPROL PARACETAMOL SUSPENSION
Reckitt Benckiser

PA No: 979/8/1

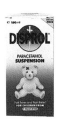

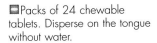100ml bottle of sugar-free, banana-flavoured suspension.

Paracetamol 120mg per 5ml.

For management of pain and fever associated with headaches, toothaches, common colds, influenza and muscular pain.

Children: 6-12 yrs: 10-20ml every 4 hrs.

1-6 yrs: 5-10ml every 4 hrs.

3-12 months: 2.5-5ml every 4 hrs.

Maximum 4 doses in 24 hrs. Do not continue dosing for more than 3 days without consulting a doctor.

Pharmacy only: Yes

Always Read The Label

DISPROL SOLUBLE PARACETAMOL TABLETS
Reckitt Benckiser

PA No: 979/8/2

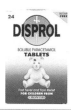

▣Foil packs of 24 sugar-free, white, circular, fruit-flavoured, soluble tablets.

▣Paracetamol 120mg.

▣For the management of pain and fever associated with headaches, toothaches, common colds, influenza and musculoskeletal pain.

▣Children: Take tablets dissolved in water or fruit juice. 6-12 yrs: 2-4 tablets every 4 hrs. Do not take more than 16 tablets in 24 hrs.

1-6 yrs: 1-2 tablets every 4 hrs.

Do not take more than 8 tablets in 24 hrs.

3-12 months: $\frac{1}{2}$ tablet every 4 hrs. Do not take more than 4 tablets in 24 hrs.

▣Do not continue dosing for more than 3 days without consulting a doctor.

Pharmacy only: Yes

HEDEX
GlaxoSmithKline

PA No: 678/28/1

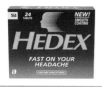

▣Packs of 12 or 24 caplets.

▣Paracetamol Ph Eur 500mg per tablet.

▣For the relief of headache, rheumatic, muscular and period pains, toothache, backache and the distress of colds and flu.

▣Adults: 2 tablets. Maximum 4 doses in 24 hrs.

Children: 6-12 yrs: 1 tablet. Maximum 4 doses in 24 hrs.

▣Do not exceed the stated dose.

Do not take with any other paracetamol-containing product.

Pharmacy only: No

HEDEX SOLUBLE
GlaxoSmithKline

PA No: 678/28/2

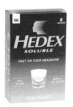

▣Packs of 6 sachets of soluble powder.

▣Paracetamol Ph Eur 1,000mg per sachet.

▣For the relief of headache, period pains, rheumatic and muscle pains, toothache, backache, colds and flu.

▣Adults: 1 sachet. Maximum 4 doses in 24 hrs.

▣Children: Not suitable for children under 12 yrs.

Do not exceed the stated dose.

Do not take with any other paracetamol-containing product.

Pharmacy only: No

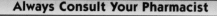

Always Consult Your Pharmacist

IBUPROFEN 200MG
Clonmel Healthcare

PA No: 126/60/1

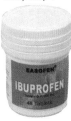

📦 Tubs of 48 round, white, coated ibuprofen tablets printed with company logo and the code '244' on one side. For oral use.

☑ Each tablet contains 200mg ibuprofen Ph Eur.

▨ For the relief of headaches, dental pain, period pain, muscle strain and cold and flu symptoms.

▨ Adults and children over 12 yrs: Initial dose of 2 tablets, then 1 or 2 tablets every 4 hrs if necessary.

❗ Consult your doctor or pharmacist before taking any other medicine.

Ibuprofen used in combination with drugs to reduce blood clotting or thiazide diuretics increases the risk of unwanted effects.

Pharmacy only: Yes

NUROFEN
Boots Healthcare Ltd

PA No: 43/6/1

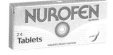

📦 Packs of 12, 24 or 48 round, white, sugar-coated tablets with 'Nurofen' printed on one side.

☑ Ibuprofen 200mg.

▨ For the relief of headaches, dental pain, period pain, backache, muscular pain, cold and flu symptoms and for reducing feverishness.

▨ Adults and children 12 yrs and over: Swallow 2 tablets with water, then if necessary, take 1-2 tablets every 4 hrs. Do not exceed 6 tablets in 24 hrs.

❗ Not suitable for children under 12 yrs (See Nurofen for Children).

Do not take Nurofen if you have or ever had a stomach ulcer or other digestive system disorder, if you are allergic to any of the ingredients, to aspirin or to any other NSAIDs.

Consult your doctor before use if you are pregnant, elderly, asthmatic or on any regular medication or treatment.

Pharmacy only: Yes

NUROFEN PLUS
Boots Healthcare Ltd

PA No: 43/24/1

📦 Packs of 12 or 24 white, capsule-shaped tablets with 'N+' printed on one side.

☑ Ibuprofen 200mg, codeine phosphate 12.8mg.

▨ For relief of migraine, cramping period pain, dental pain, sciatica, lumbago and rheumatic pain.

▨ Adults and children 12 yrs and over: Swallow 2 tablets with water, then if necessary, take 1-2 tablets every 4-6 hrs. Do not exceed 6 tablets in 24 hrs.

❗ Not suitable for children under 12 yrs (see Nurofen for Children).

Do not take Nurofen Plus if you have or ever had a stomach ulcer or other digestive system disorder, if you are allergic to any of the ingredients, to aspirin or to any other NSAIDs.

Consult your doctor before use if you are pregnant, breastfeeding, elderly, asthmatic or on any regular medication or treatment.

Pharmacy only: Yes

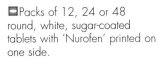

If Symptoms Persist Consult Your Doctor

PANADEINE
GlaxoSmithKline

PA No: 678/26/1

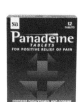

◻Packs of 12 or 24 tablets.

☑Paracetamol Ph Eur 500mg, codeine Ph Eur 8mg per tablet.

▣For the relief of headache, rheumatic and period pain, toothache, colds and flu symptoms.

▨Adults: 1-2 tablets every 4 hrs. Maximum 8 tablets in 24 hrs.

Children: 7-12 yrs: ½-1 tablet every 4 hrs. Maximum 4 tablets in 24 hrs.

▮Not recommended for children under 7 yrs.

Do not exceed the stated dose.

Do not take with any other paracetamol-containing product.

Pharmacy only: Yes

PANADOL BABY
GlaxoSmithKline

PA No: 678/39/3

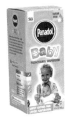

◻100ml bottle of sugar-free, strawberry-flavoured suspension.

☑Paracetamol Ph Eur 120mg per 5ml.

▣For the relief of teething pain, sore throat, toothache, and the feverishness of colds, flu, measles, whooping cough, mumps and chickenpox.

▨Children: 6-12 yrs: 10-20ml. 1-6 yrs: 5-10ml. 3 months-1 yr: 2.5-5ml. 2-3 months: 2.5ml. Repeat every 4 hrs to a maximum of 4 doses in 24 hrs.

▮Do not exceed the stated dose.

Do not take with any other paracetamol-containing product.

Not suitable for babies under 2 months.

Pharmacy only: Yes

PANADOL EXTRA
GlaxoSmithKline

PA No: 678/27/1

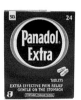

◻Packs of 12 or 24 tablets.

☑Paracetamol Ph Eur 500mg, caffeine Ph Eur 65mg per tablet.

▣Pain relief for headache, migraine, backache, period pain, rheumatic pain, toothache, neuralgia and muscle pain.

▨Adults and children over 12 yrs: take 2 tablets every 4 hrs as required. Do not take more than 8 tablets in 24 hrs.

▮Not suitable for children under 12 yrs.

Do not exceed the stated dose.

Do not take with any other paracetamol-containing product.

Pharmacy only: Yes

Always Read The Label

PANADOL NIGHT TABLETS
GlaxoSmithKline

PA No 678/39/8

🔲Packs of 10 green, film-coated, capsule-shaped tablets.

📋Per tablet: Paracetamol Ph Eur 500mg, diphenhydramine hydrochloride Ph Eur 25mg.

❓For the short-term treatment of bedtime symptoms of colds, flu and pain, for example rheumatic and muscle pain, backache, neuralgia, toothache, headache and period pain.

📃Adults and the elderly: 2 tablets to be taken 20 mins before bedtime. Other products containing paracetamol may be taken for daytime pain relief but at a reduced dose of 6 tablets in 24 hrs. The dose should not be repeated more frequently than every 4 hrs.

❗Children: Not recommended for children under 12 yrs except on medical advice.

Not to be taken by patients with closed angle glaucoma, porphyria or hypersensitivity to paracetamol or diphenhydramine. Panadol Night should be used with caution in patients suffering from epilepsy, prostatic hypertrophy, glaucoma, urinary retention or pyloroduodenal obstruction. Do not exceed the stated dose. Do not take with other products containing paracetamol. Do not take within 4 hrs of taking other paracetamol-containing products or for more than 10 consecutive nights without consulting your doctor. This product may cause drowsiness. Do not drive or operate machinery. Avoid alcoholic drink.

Pharmacy only: Yes

PANADOL SOLUBLE
GlaxoSmithKline

PA No: 678/39/4

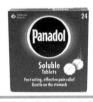

🔲Packs of 24 soluble tablets.

📋Paracetamol Ph Eur 500mg per soluble tablet.

❓For the relief of headache, neuralgia, toothache, period pain, colds, flu and rheumatic pain.

📃Adults: 1-2 tablets 3-4 times daily. Maximum 4 doses in 24 hrs.

Children: 6-12 yrs: ½ tablet. Maximum 4 doses in 24 hrs.

❗Do not exceed the stated dose. Do not take with any other paracetamol-containing product.

Not suitable for children under 6 yrs.

Pharmacy only: Yes

PANADOL TABLETS
GlaxoSmithKline

PA No: 678/39/5

🔲Packs of 12, 24 or 96 (dispense pack) tablets.

📋Paracetamol Ph Eur 500mg per tablet.

❓For the relief of headache, neuralgia, toothache, period pain, backache, rheumatic and muscular pain, colds and flu.

📃Adults: 1-2 tablets 3-4 times daily. Maximum 8 tablets in 24 hrs.

Children: 6-12 yrs: ½ tablet 3-4 times daily. Maximum 4 tablets in 24 hrs.

❗Not suitable for children under 6 yrs.

Do not exceed the stated dose.

Do not take with any other paracetamol-containing product.

Pharmacy only: No

Always Consult Your Pharmacist

PARACETAMOL TABLETS FROM THE MAKERS OF ANADIN
Whitehall Laboratories Ltd

PA No: 172/21/1

▭Packs of 8, 12 or 24 white, capsule-shaped, film-coated tablets, embossed on one side with 'Anadin-P' and a breakbar on other side.

☑Paracetamol 500mg.

❓For the treatment of pain and fever, headache, migraine, neuralgia, period pain, dental pain, symptoms of colds and flu.

☑Adults: 1-2 tablets 3-4 times daily. Maximum 8 tablets in 24 hrs.

Children: 6-12 yrs: ½ -1 tablet 3-4 times daily. Maximum 4 tablets in 24 hrs.

❗Do not exceed the stated dose.

Do not take with any other paracetamol-containing products.

Pharmacy only: No

PARACODOL
Roche Consumer Health

PA No: 18/14/2

▭Packs of 20 x 6 hard gelatin capsules, or 24 x 6 large, white, soluble, effervescent tablets.

☑Paracetamol 500mg, codeine phosphate 8mg.

❓For the relief of muscular and rheumatic pain, headache, migraine, neuralgia, toothache, sore throat, period pain and cold and flu symptoms.

☑Adults: 1-2 tablets or capsules every 4-6 hrs. Maximum 8 capsules in 24 hrs.

If symptoms persist for more than 3 days, consult a doctor.

❗Not recommended for children.

Pharmacy only: Yes

PARALIEF BLISTER PACK
Clonmel Healthcare Ltd

PA No: 126/20/1

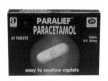

▭Blister pack of 24 white caplets.

☑Paracetamol 500mg.

❓For the treatment of pain and fever.

☑Adults: 1-2 tablets 3-4 times daily.

Children: 6-12 yrs: ½ -1 tablet 3-4 times daily.

❗Not recommended for children under 6 yrs.

Special precautions in persons with kidney or liver impairment.

Pharmacy only: Yes

PARALINK PARACETAMOL SUPPOSITORIES
Ricesteele Manufacturing

PA No: 180mg: 95/7/2; 500mg: 95/7/4

▭Packs of 10 white, tapered, cylindrical suppositories.

☑Paracetamol 180mg, 500mg.

❓For relief of pain and fever associated with common cold, flu, headaches, rheumatism, teething and postoperative pain.

☑Adults: Over 12 yrs: 1-2 suppositories (500mg) every 6 hrs.

Children: 6-12 yrs: 1 suppository (500mg) every 6 hrs.

3-6 yrs: 1 ½ suppositories (180mg) every 6 hrs.

1-3 yrs: 1 suppository (180mg) every 6 hrs.

3 months-1 yr: ½ suppository (180mg) every 6 hrs.

❗Suppositories should be administered with caution to patients with known liver or kidney impairment.

Pharmacy only: Yes

If Symptoms Persist Consult Your Doctor

PHENSIC
Merck Consumer Healthcare

PA No: 417/17/1

Packs of 12 or 24 tablets.

Aspirin 325mg, caffeine 22mg.

For the relief of headache, toothache, rheumatic pain, period pain, fibrositis, lumbago, sciatica and cold and flu symptoms.

Adults: 2 tablets every 3-4 hrs. Maximum 12 tablets in 24 hrs.

Not recommended for children under 12 yrs.

Pharmacy only: Yes

RESOLVE
SSL Healthcare Ireland Ltd

PA No: 618/34/1

Packs of 5 sachets of soluble powder.

Paracetamol 1,000mg, anhydrous citric acid 1,185mg, sodium bicarbonate 808mg, potassium bicarbonate 715mg, sodium carbonate 153mg, vitamin C 30mg.

Relieves headache and upset stomach associated with overeating and overdrinking.

Adults: 1 sachet every 4 hrs. Maximum 4 sachets in 24 hrs.

Not suitable for children under 12 yrs.

Pharmacy only: No

SOLPADEINE CAPSULES
GlaxoSmithKline

PA No: 678/40/1

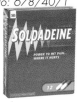

Packs of 12 or 24 capsules.

Paracetamol Ph Eur 500mg, codeine phosphate Ph Eur 8mg, caffeine Ph Eur 30mg per capsule.

For the relief of headache, rheumatic pain, toothache, period pain, neuralgia, colds, flu, sore throat and feverishness.

Adults: 2 capsules 3-4 times daily. Maximum 8 capsules in 24 hrs.

Not recommended for children under 12 yrs.

Do not exceed the stated dose.

Do not take with any other paracetamol-containing product.

Pharmacy only: Yes

SOLPADEINE SOLUBLE
GlaxoSmithKline

PA No: 678/40/2

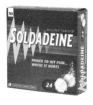

Packs of 12, 24 or 60 (dispense pack) tablets.

Paracetamol Ph Eur 500mg, codeine Ph Eur 8mg, caffeine Ph Eur 30mg per soluble tablet.

For the relief of headache, rheumatic pain, toothache, period pain, neuralgia, colds, flu, sore throat and feverishness.

Adults: 2 tablets 3-4 times daily. Maximum 8 tablets in 24 hrs.

Children: 7-12 yrs: ½ tablet 3-4 times daily. Maximum 4 tablets in 24 hrs.

Not suitable for children under 7 yrs except on medical advice.

Do not exceed the stated dose.

Do not take with any other paracetamol-containing product.

Pharmacy only: Yes

Always Read The Label

SOLPADEINE TABLETS
GlaxoSmithKline

PA No: 678/40/3

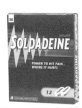

Packs of 12 or 24 tablets.

Paracetamol Ph Eur 500mg, codeine phosphate Ph Eur 8mg, caffeine Ph Eur 30mg per tablet.

For the relief of headache, rheumatic pain, period pain, toothache, neuralgia, colds, flu, sore throat and feverishness.

Adults: 2 tablets 3-4 times daily. Maximum 8 tablets in 24 hrs.

Children: Not recommended for children under 12 yrs.

Do not exceed the stated dose.

Do not take with any other paracetamol-containing product.

Pharmacy only: Yes

SYNDOL
SSL Healthcare Ireland Ltd

PA No: 618/26/1

Packs of 10 or 20 tablets.

Caffeine 30mg, codeine phosphate 10mg, doxylamine succinate 5mg, paracetamol 450mg.

For the relief of mild to moderate pain such as headache, including muscle-contraction or tension headache, migraine, neuralgia, toothache, sore throat, period pain, muscular and rheumatic aches and pains and following surgical or dental procedures.

Adults: 1-2 tablets every 4-6 hrs as required. Maximum 8 tablets in 24 hrs.

Children: Not recommended for children under 12 yrs.

Pharmacy only: Yes

TRAMIL
Whitehall Laboratories Ltd

PA No: 172/09/1

Blister packs of 12 or 24 hard, gelatin capsules with blue cap and yellow body, containing a white, free-flowing powder/granule mix. The word 'Tramil' is printed longitudinally on both cap and body.

Paracetamol 500mg, caffeine 32mg.

For the treatment of pain and fever, headache, migraine, neuralgia, colds and influenza, period and dental pain.

Adults: 1-2 capsules which may be repeated every 4 hrs as necessary. Maximum 8 capsules in 24 hrs.

Do not exceed the stated dose.

Do not take with any other paracetamol-containing products.

If pregnant or breastfeeding consult doctor before use.

Pharmacy only: No

VEGANIN TABLETS
Pfizer/Warner Lambert Consumer Healthcare

PA No: 823/27/1

Packs of 10 or 20 white, flat, circular, bevel-edged tablets with a single scoreline on one surface and a 'V' above the scoreline. The other side is unmarked.

Aspirin 250mg, paracetamol 250mg, codeine phosphate 6.80mg.

For pain and fever.

Adults: 1-2 tablets every 3-4 hrs.

Maximum 8 tablets in 24 hrs.

Pharmacy only: Yes

Always Consult Your Pharmacist

MIGRAINE

Migraine often takes the form of a series of one-sided 'throbbing' headaches. The headaches are severe enough to disrupt daily life and are often accompanied by nausea or vomiting and a sensitivity to light or noise. Sometimes visual disturbances such as flashing lights or blurred vision precede the attack by a few minutes, usually stopping within an hour. The headache, however, if untreated, may last for at least four hours and sometimes for as long as three days.

Products for treating migraine can contain any of the painkillers (**analgesics**) described under **General Pain Relief** and often include **codeine**. If your migraine is accompanied by nausea, a product containing an **anti-nauseant**, **buclizine**, may offer relief.

Precautions and Warnings
- See **General Pain Relief** for precautions concerning analgesics
- Buclizine may cause drowsiness and make driving or operating machinery dangerous.

MIGRALEVE
Pfizer/Warner Lambert Consumer Healthcare

PA No: 12s: 823/36/1,2,3; 24s: 823/36/1,3

◻Packs of 12 or 24 tablets.

◾Pink tablet: Paracetamol 500mg, codeine phosphate 8mg, buclizine hydrochloride 6.25mg. Yellow tablet: Codeine phosphate 8mg, paracetamol 500mg.

◻For the relief of migraine including headache, nausea and vomiting.

◾Adults: 2 pink tablets at onset. If required, 2 yellow tablets every 4 hrs. Maximum 2 pink and 6 yellow tablets in 24 hrs.

Children: 10-14 yrs: 1 pink tablet initially. If required 1 yellow tablet every 4 hrs. Maximum 1 pink and 3 yellow tablets in 24 hrs.

◾Not recommended for children under 10 yrs except under medical supervision.

Pharmacy only: Yes

NUROFEN PLUS
Boots Healthcare Ltd

PA No: 43/24/1

◻Packs of 12 or 24 white, capsule-shaped tablets with 'N+' printed on one side.

◾Ibuprofen 200mg, codeine phosphate 12.8mg.

◻For relief of migraine, cramping period pain, dental pain, sciatica, lumbago and rheumatic pain.

◾Adults and children 12 yrs and over: Swallow 2 tablets with water, then if necessary, take 1-2 tablets every 4-6 hrs. Do not exceed 6 tablets in 24 hrs.

◾Not suitable for children under 12 yrs (see Nurofen for Children).

Do not take Nurofen Plus if you have or ever had a stomach ulcer or other digestive system disorder, if you are allergic to any of the ingredients, to aspirin or to any other NSAIDs.

Consult your doctor before use if you are pregnant, breastfeeding, elderly, asthmatic or on any regular medication or treatment.

Pharmacy only: Yes

If Symptoms Persist Consult Your Doctor

MOUTH PAIN, ULCERS

Mouth ulcers appear as painful yellow or white shallow erosions of the cheeks, tongue or lips. They can be up to about 5 millimetres in diameter, and may be surrounded by inflammation (a red area). They may occur singly or in small groups. Although they are common there is no agreement as to their cause. The good news is that they do tend to heal spontaneously within about 7-14 days, although they may recur.

Treatment

Local anaesthetics (**benzocaine**, **lidocaine**, **lignocaine**) are useful in dulling the pain of mouth ulcers. **Choline salicylate** – related to **aspirin** – may also be used for this purpose. The ulcers are not caused by bacterial infection but **antibacterials** (**chlorhexidine**, **chloroxylenol**, **chlorocresol**, **cetylpyridinium**) are often included in OTC products to prevent any infection after the ulcer has formed.

The healing of stomach ulcers is enhanced by **carbenoxolone** and this substance is also available in gel form for treating mouth ulcers. More recently, **steroids**, which have long been used because of their powerful effect of reducing inflammation, have become available for short term OTC use to treat mouth ulcers. They are available as pellets (**hydrocortisone**) or in the form of a paste, which is specially made to stick to the inside of the mouth (**triamcinolone**).

When using products for mouth ulcers, try to keep the product in contact with the affected area for as long as possible. Pellets may be helpful in this regard for ulcers under the tongue or between the gum and cheek, whereas pastes or gels are better for other areas.

ANBESOL ANAESTHETIC ANTISEPTIC
SSL Healthcare Ireland Ltd

PA No: 618/44/1

◼6ml or 15ml bottles containing a clear, yellow, alcoholic liquid for topical application.

◼Lidocaine hydrochloride

0.90% w/w, chlorocresol 0.10% w/w, cetylpyridinium chloride 0.02% w/w, alcohol (96%) 68.24% w/w.

◼For the symptomatic relief of mouth ulcers and sore gums.

◼Adults and children 10 yrs and over: Apply to the affected area 3-4 times daily or as directed by physician or dentist.

◼If condition does not improve after 3 days, consult your doctor or dentist.

Localised allergic reactions may occur after prolonged or repeated use.

Keep away from children.

Pharmacy only: Yes

BONJELA
Reckitt Benckiser

PA No: 979/1/1

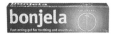

◼15g tube of aniseed-flavoured, colourless gel.

◼Choline salicylate 8.7% w/w, cetalkonium chloride 0.01% w/w.

◼For the relief of pain and discomfort of common mouth ulcers, cold sores, denture sore spots and pain due to orthodontic devices in children. It aids healing of ulcers and sore spots due to dentures in adults and orthodontic devices in children.

◼Adults: Dry affected site. Apply 1cm of gel onto sore area. The dose may be repeated every 3 hrs.

Children: Over 4 months: Dry affected site. Apply 0.5cm of gel onto sore area. The dose may be repeated every 3 hrs.

Maximum 6 doses in 24 hrs.

Pharmacy only: Yes

Always Read The Label

MEDIJEL GEL
DDD Ltd

PA No: 302/1/1

🔲 15g tube of gel.

☑ Lignocaine hydrochloride 0.66 w/w, aminacrine hydrochloride 0.05 w/w.

🔲 For pain relief of common mouth ulcers, soreness of the gums and denture rubbing.

☑ Adults: Apply to affected area with a clean finger or small pad of cotton wool. Repeat after 20 mins.

Children: Apply to affected area with a clean finger or small pad of cotton wool. Repeat after 20 mins.

❗ Do not use Medijel Gel if you are hypersensitive to lignocaine.

Pharmacy only: Yes

MUSCULAR PAIN

Salicylates (related to **aspirin**) are absorbed through the skin and are therefore suitable for the relief of localised pain such as muscle pain relating to a strain or sprain.

Similarly, some of the more powerful **NSAIDS** (see **General Pain Relief**) that combine painkilling and anti-inflammatory action (**ketoprofen** and **piroxicam**) may be used in gels for rubbing on the skin. Cooling produces a sensation of analgesia and **menthol** mimics a cooling effect whereas **nicotinates** dilate small blood vessels and produce a warming sensation.

An advantage of preparations that are applied directly to the skin is that there is relatively little absorption of the ingredients into the bloodstream, so overdose is not a problem and side effects are generally not significant. Tablets or capsules will, however, often be more effective for more severe pain because they are better absorbed. Painkillers with an anti-inflammatory action such as ibuprofen are particularly suitable for pain caused by injury.

ADVIL TABLETS
Whitehall Laboratories Ltd

PA No: 172/29/1

🔲 Blister packs of 10 or 20 pinkish-brown, sugar-coated tablets, printed with 'Advil'.

☑ Ibuprofen 200mg.

🔲 For the symptomatic treatment of pain and fever conditions such as acute pain from period pain, dental pain, muscular pain, headaches, cold and flu symptoms and backache.

☑ Adults, the elderly and persons over 12 yrs: 1 or 2 tablets should be taken every 4-6 hrs. Maximum 6 tablets in 24 hrs.

❗ Not recommended for children under 12 yrs.

Not to be taken by patients with stomach ulcers or those allergic to aspirin or other similar medicines.

Patients who are pregnant, elderly, have asthma or are receiving regular treatment should consult the doctor before taking Advil.

Pharmacy only: Yes

Always Consult Your Pharmacist

ALGIPAN RUB
Whitehall Laboratories Ltd

PA No: 22/14/1

▣ 40g of lavender-scented, smooth, homogeneous, non-greasy, pink cream for topical application.

▣ Glycol monosalicylate 10% w/w, Methyl nicotinate 1.0% w/w, Capsicin (BPC 1973) 0.1% w/w.

▣ For the management of pain of muscular, rheumatic or joint origin.

▣ Apply to the affected area and massage in thoroughly.

❗ Wash hands thoroughly after application.

Avoid contact with eyes, mucous membranes and broken skin.

Pharmacy only: Yes

CRAMPEX TABLETS
SSL Healthcare Ireland Ltd

PA No: 618/11/1

▣ Packs of 24 or 48 tablets.

▣ Nicotinic acid (niacin) 20mg, vitamin D3 (cholecalciferol) 0.02mg, calcium gluconate 200mg.

▣ For the treatment of night muscle cramp.

▣ Adults: 1-2 tablets with a drink before bedtime.

❗ Not recommended for children.

Pharmacy only: Yes

DEEP FREEZE COLD GEL
Mentholatum/Allphar

PA No: 76/5/1

▣ 35g tube of pleasant-smelling, blue gel.

▣ Racementhol 2% w/w.

▣ For the symptomatic relief of pain in muscles, tendons and joints.

▣ Adults and the elderly: Gently massage into the affected area 3-4 times daily.

❗ Not recommended for children under 5 yrs.

Pharmacy only: No

DEEP FREEZE SPRAY
Mentholatum/Allphar

PA No: 76/1/1

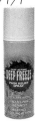

▣ 135g (200ml) aerosol spray.

▣ Levomenthol 2.00% w/w and n-Pentane 40.00% w/w.

▣ For the symptomatic relief of muscular pain.

▣ Adults and children over 6 yrs: Spray for 3-5 seconds from 6 inches onto affected area up to 2-3 times. Maximum 3 treatments in 24 hrs.

❗ Not recommended for children under 6 yrs.

Pharmacy only: No

DEEP HEAT RUB
Mentholatum/Allphar

PA No: 76/2/1

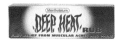

▣ Standard, medium and large tubes of emulsion cream.

▣ Turpentine oil 1.47% w/w, eucalyptus oil 1.97% w/w, racementhol 5.91% w/w, methyl salicylate 12.8% w/w.

▣ For the symptomatic relief of muscular pain, including sciatica, lumbago, fibrositis, rheumatic pain, bruises and chilblains.

▣ Adults: Massage into affected area 2-3 times daily.

❗ Children: Not recommended for children under 5 yrs.

Pharmacy only: No

If Symptoms Persist Consult Your Doctor

DEEP HEAT SPRAY
Mentholatum/Allphar

PA No: 76/3/1

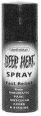

☐ 150ml aerosol spray.

🗹 Methyl salicylate 1% w/w, methyl nicotinate 1.6% w/w, ethyl salicylate 5% w/w, 2-hydroxyethyl salicylate 5% w/w.

⍰ For the symptomatic relief of muscular pain, bursitis and tendinitis including rheumatic pain, strains, fibrositis, lumbago and sciatica.

🗹 Adults and children over 5 yrs: Spray 2-3 short bursts from 6 inches above affected area.

❗ Children: Not recommended for children under 5 yrs.

Pharmacy only: No

FELDENE TOPIGEL
Pfizer/Warner Lambert Consumer Healthcare

PA No: 823/38/1

☐ 30g tube of topical NSAID

gel.

🗹 Piroxicam 0.5%.

⍰ For relief of pain from rheumatism, sprains, strains and backache.

🗹 Adults: Rub 3cm (about a fingertip) onto affected site 3-4 times daily.

❗ Children: Not recommended.

Pharmacy only: Yes

IBUPROFEN 200MG
Clonmel Healthcare

PA No: 126/60/1

☐ Tubs of 48 round, white, coated ibuprofen tablets printed with company logo and the code '244' on one side. For oral use.

🗹 Each tablet contains 200mg ibuprofen Ph Eur.

⍰ For the relief of headaches, dental pain, period pain, muscle strain and cold and flu symptoms.

🗹 Adults and children over 12 yrs: Initial dose of 2 tablets, then 1 or 2 tablets every 4 hrs if necessary.

❗ Consult your doctor or pharmacist before taking any other medicine.

Ibuprofen used in combination with drugs to reduce blood clotting or thiazide diuretics increases the risk of unwanted effects.

Pharmacy only: Yes

NUROFEN
Boots Healthcare Ltd

PA No: 43/6/1

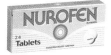

☐ Packs of 12, 24 or 48 round, white, sugar-coated tablets with 'Nurofen' printed on one side.

🗹 Ibuprofen 200mg.

⍰ For the relief of headaches, dental pain, period pain, backache, muscular pain, cold and flu symptoms, and for reducing fever.

🗹 Adults and children 12 yrs and over: Swallow 2 tablets with water, then if necessary, take 1-2 tablets every 4 hrs. Do not exceed 6 tablets in 24 hrs.

❗ Not recommended for children under 12 yrs (see Nurofen for Children).

Do not take Nurofen if you have or ever had a stomach ulcer or other digestive system disorder, if you are allergic to any of the ingredients, to aspirin or to any other NSAIDs.

Consult your doctor before use if you are pregnant, elderly, asthmatic or on any regular medication or treatment.

Pharmacy only: Yes

Always Read The Label

ORUVAIL GEL
Aventis Pharma

PA No: 40/70/5

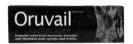

■30g tube of colourless, transparent gel with lavender fragrance.

☑Ketoprofen 2.5% w/w.

▣For the topical management of rheumatic or inflammatory conditions and soft tissue injury due to sports injuries, sprains, tendinitis, bruising and oedema.

◩Adults: To be applied by gentle massage to the affected

area 3 times daily for up to 7 days. After application the affected area should be well massaged to ensure local absorption of ketoprofen.

▪Children: Not recommended.

Not for use on broken skin, or conditions such as eczema or infected skin lesions.

Pharmacy only: Yes

PROFLEX PAIN RELIEF CREAM
Novartis Consumer Health

PA No: 30/20/1

■30g of white/cream-coloured cream.

☑Ibuprofen 5% w/w.

▣Relief of symptoms of rheumatic and muscular pain, backache, sprains, lumbago, fibrositis and tendinitis.

◩Adults and children over 12

yrs: Massage into affected area 3-4 times daily.

▪Not recommended for children.

Pharmacy only: Yes

RADIAN-B
Roche Consumer Health

PA No: 50/106/1

■Muscle spray (100ml); rub (40g, 100g); Lotion (125ml, 250ml, 500ml).

☑Rub: Menthol, camphor, methyl salicylate, capsicum. Spray: Menthol, camphor, ammonium salicylate, salicylic acid. Lotion: Menthol, camphor and ammonium salicylate.

▣Rub: For the symptomatic relief of muscular stiffness, sprains, fibrositis and similar

rheumatic conditions. Lotion and spray: For temporary relief of minor arthritic and muscular pain.

◩Rub: Adults and children over 6 yrs: Massage well into affected area.

Muscle lotion: Adults: Apply to affected area 2-3 times daily. Children: Not recommended for children under 12 yrs.

Spray: Adults: Spray as required onto the affected area, followed by a second application after 10-15 mins.

Repeat if necessary up to 3 times daily. Children: Not recommended for children under 12 yrs.

▪Not recommended for use in those with hypersensitivity to aspirin or during pregnancy.

Pharmacy only: Yes

RALGEX CREAM
SSL Healthcare Ireland Ltd

PA No: 618/22/1

■40g or 100g tube of cream.

☑Glycol monosalicylate 10% w/w, methyl nicotinate 1% w/w, capsicum oleoresin 0.12% w/w.

▣For the relief of muscular pain and stiffness, including backache, sciatica, lumbago, fibrositis and rheumatic pain.

◩Adults: After trial use, rub into skin until absorbed. Repeat as necessary up to 4 times daily.

▪Not recommended for

children under 12 yrs except on medical advice.

Do not use on sensitive areas or broken skin.

Pharmacy only: No

Always Consult Your Pharmacist

RALGEX HEAT SPRAY
SSL Healthcare Ireland Ltd

PA No: 618/24/1

▭125ml aerosol can.

▮Glycol monosalicylate 6% w/v, methyl nicotinate 1.6% w/v.

For the relief of muscular pain and stiffness, including backache, sciatica, lumbago, fibrositis and rheumatic pain.

Adults and children 5yrs and over: Hold the container about 6ins from the skin and spray in 2-3 short bursts. Further applications may be made at intervals of not less than 2 hrs. May be repeated up to 4 times daily.

Not to be used on children under 5 yrs.

Do not spray on sensitive areas or on broken skin.

Pharmacy only: No

TRANSVASIN HEAT RUB
SSL Healthcare Ireland Ltd

PA No 618/1/1

▭40g or 80g tube of cream.

▮Ethyl nicotinate 2% w/w, n-hexyl nicotinate 2% w/w, tetrahydrofurfuryl salicylate 14% w/w.

Relief of rheumatic and muscular pain and the symptoms of sprains and strains.

Adults and children: Massage gently into affected area until entirely absorbed. Apply at least twice daily until symptoms abate.

Pharmacy only: No

If Symptoms Persist Consult Your Doctor

PERIOD PAIN

Simple or 'primary' period pain is caused by contractions of the womb, which occur as its lining is shed during menstruation. It tends to occur in the first one or two days of the period, although it may also precede it. It usually involves a 'colicky' pain in the lower part of the abdomen, often accompanied by back pain and sometimes by leg pain. Young women who have not had a child are particularly affected.

All the painkillers used to treat general pain (see **General Pain Relief**) are used to treat period pain, although those with an anti-inflammatory action (**aspirin** and **ibuprofen**) are especially suitable since they reduce the production of some of the substances that may be involved in producing the womb contractions. **Hyoscine** may also be included as a muscle relaxant.

Precautions and warnings

- Avoid hyoscine if you suffer from glaucoma or if you have a bladder problem
- If you experience a dull aching pain in the lower abdomen and back several days before a period, seek medical advice. This sort of pain may be caused by one of a number of disorders of the womb such as fibroids, endometriosis or inflammation.

ADVIL TABLETS
Whitehall Laboratories Ltd

PA No: 172/29/1

Blister packs of 10 or 20 pinkish-brown, sugar-coated tablets, printed with 'Advil'.

Ibuprofen 200mg.

For the symptomatic treatment of pain and fever conditions such as acute pain from period pain, dental pain, muscular pain, headaches, cold and flu symptoms and backache.

Adults, the elderly and persons over 12 yrs: 1 or 2 tablets should be taken every 4-6 hrs. Maximum 6 tablets in 24 hrs.

Not recommended for children under 12 yrs.

Not to be taken by patients with stomach ulcers or those allergic to aspirin or other similar medicines.

Patients who are pregnant, elderly, have asthma or are receiving regular treatment should consult the doctor before taking Advil.

Pharmacy only: Yes

ANADIN EXTRA
Whitehall Laboratories Ltd

PA No: 172/18/1

Packs of 8, 12 or 24 white, film-coated, capsule-shaped cylindrical tablets with breakbar on one side and 'ΛE' on the other.

Aspirin 300mg, paracetamol 200mg, caffeine 45mg.

For the relief of pain such as headache, neuralgia, muscle pain, rheumatism, toothache, period pain and symptoms of the common cold and influenza.

Adults: 1-2 tablets every 4 hrs. Maximum 6 tablets in 24 hrs.

Children: Over 12 yrs: 1-2 tablets every 4 hrs. Maximum 6 tablets in 24 hrs.

Not to be given to children under 12 yrs except on medical advice.

Prolonged use can be harmful. If symptoms persist or if taking any other medication consult physician.

Do not exceed stated dose.

Do not take with any other paracetamol-containing products.

Not to be taken by patients with stomach ulcers or those allergic to aspirin or other similar medicines.

Patients who are pregnant, breastfeeding, elderly, have asthma or are receiving regular treatment should consult the doctor before taking Anadin Extra.

Pharmacy only: No

Always Read The Label

FEMINAX
Roche Consumer Health

PA No: 32/2/2

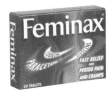

📦Packs of 20 capsule-shaped, white tablets with a breakline on one side and 'Feminax' on reverse.

💊Paracetamol 500mg, codeine phosphate 8mg, caffeine monohydrate equivalent to 50mg anhydrous caffeine, hyoscine hydrobromide 100µg.

❓Painkiller for the relief of period pain, stomach cramps, back pain and headache.

✅Adults and girls over 12 yrs: 1-2 tablets every 4 hrs. Maximum 6 tablets in 24 hrs.

❗Not to be taken by children under 12 yrs or by patients suffering from glaucoma.

May cause drowsiness.

Pharmacy only: Yes

IBUPROFEN 200MG
Clonmel Healthcare

PA No: 126/60/1

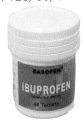

📦Tubs of 48 round, white, coated ibuprofen tablets printed with company logo and the code '244' on one side. For oral use.

💊Each tablet contains 200mg ibuprofen Ph Eur.

❓For the relief of headaches, dental pain, period pain, muscle strain and cold and flu symptoms.

✅Adults and children over 12 yrs: Initial dose of 2 tablets, then 1 or 2 tablets every 4 hrs if necessary.

❗Consult your doctor or pharmacist before taking any other medicine.

Ibuprofen used in combination with drugs to reduce blood clotting or thiazide diuretics increases the risk of unwanted effects.

Pharmacy only: Yes

NUROFEN PLUS
Boots Healthcare Ltd

PA No: 43/24/1

📦Packs of 12 or 24 white, capsule-shaped tablets with 'N+' printed on one side.

💊Ibuprofen 200mg, codeine phosphate 12.8mg.

❓For relief of migraine, cramping period pain, dental pain, sciatica, lumbago and rheumatic pain.

✅Adults and children 12 yrs and over: Swallow 2 tablets with water, then if necessary, take 1-2 tablets every 4-6 hrs. Do not exceed 6 tablets in 24 hrs.

❗Not suitable for children under 12 yrs (see Nurofen for Children).

Do not take Nurofen Plus if you have or ever had a stomach ulcer or other digestive system disorder, if you are allergic to any of the ingredients, to aspirin or to any other NSAIDs.

Consult your doctor before use if you are pregnant, breastfeeding, elderly, asthmatic or on any regular medication or treatment.

Pharmacy only: Yes

Always Consult Your Pharmacist

SKIN CARE

Antiseptics (Cuts, Burns, Scalds, Stings and Insect Bites)

Minor cuts and abrasions, burns or scalds, insect bites, cracked skin and blisters are traditionally treated with **antiseptics** which have an **antibacterial** action. There are many antiseptics in use but the common ones are **chlorhexidine**, **chloroxylenol**, **cetrimide**, **phenol**, **povidone iodine**, **benzalkonium chloride**, and **benzoyl peroxide**.

Caution

Antiseptic products are intended to prevent infection or to treat minor and superficial skin injuries. They are not suited to or intended for the treatment of anything other than superficial wounds.

The initial pain associated with a sting may be relieved by the application of a local anaesthetic (**benzocaine**). An **antihistamine** (**mepyramine**) will help to relieve itching. Insect repellants are useful to protect against bites from the gnat family of insects.

DETTOL ANTISEPTIC DISINFECTANT LIQUID
Reckitt Benckiser

PA No: 979/4/2

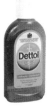

■125ml, 250ml, 500ml, 750ml or 4 litre bottles of light orange/brown liquid.

🗹Chloroxylenol BP 4.8% w/v.

🔲A medical antiseptic disinfectant for cuts, grazes, bites, stings and use in midwifery.

🗹Adults: Do not use undiluted. Dosage for 250ml, 500ml and 750ml bottles:
Medical: Cuts, grazes, bites and stings: 1 capful to ½ pint water. Cover with clean, dry dressing. Midwifery: 1 capful to 1 pint water for external antisepsis.
Personal hygiene: Bathing: 1-2 capfuls to bath water. Not to be used for babies under 9 months old except on medical advice. Dandruff: 1 capful to 1 pint warm water. Pour over scalp, leave for 10 mins before shampooing.
Spots and pimples: 1 capful to ½ pint warm water. Bathe affected area daily.
Dosage for 125ml bottle: Do not use undiluted.
Medical: Cuts, grazes, bites and stings: 2 capfuls to ½ pint water. Midwifery: 2 capfuls to 1 pint water for external antisepsis.
Personal hygiene: Bathing: 2-4 capfuls to bath water. Not to be used for babies under 9 months old except on medical advice. Dandruff: 2 capfuls to 1 pint warm water.
Spots and pimples: 2 capfuls to ½ pint warm water. Bathe affected area daily.
Dosage for 4 litre pack.
Medical: Cuts, grazes, bites and stings: 15ml to 300ml of water. Midwifery: 15ml to 600ml of warm water.
Personal hygiene: Bathing: 15ml to 30ml of bath water. Not to be used for babies under 9 months old except on medical advice.
Dandruff: 15ml to 600ml of warm water.
Spots and pimples: 15ml to 300ml of warm water.

▮For external use only. Not for eczematous conditions. Do not use undiluted.

Pharmacy only: No

If Symptoms Persist Consult Your Doctor

DETTOL ANTISEPTIC CREAM
Reckitt Benckiser

PA No: 979/4/1

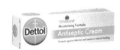

30g tube of antiseptic cream.

Chloroxylenol BP 0.3% w/w, triclosan 0.3% w/w, edetic acid (as potassium salt) 0.2% w/w.

For the treatment of cuts, grazes, bites and stings. Can also be used as an antiseptic hand cream.

Adults: Clean wound and surrounding area. Apply Dettol Antiseptic Cream directly or on lint or gauze. If necessary cover with plaster or dressing. Application may be repeated.

For external use only.

Pharmacy only: No

GERMOLENE CREAM
Bayer Ltd

PA No: 21/50/1

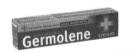

30g tube of antiseptic cream and local anaesthetic.

Phenol BP 1.2%, chlorhexidine gluconate BP 0.25% (w/w).

For the treatment of minor cuts, grazes, burns, scalds, blisters, insect bites, spots and rough skin.

Adults and children: Clean affected area, apply cream and rub in gently.

In the case of cuts or particularly tender areas rubbing may be avoided by applying liberally on a piece of white lint or gauze and covering with a light bandage or plaster.

Pharmacy only: No

GERMOLENE OINTMENT
Bayer Ltd

PA No: 21/49/1

27g tube of antiseptic ointment.

Anhydrous lanolin BP 35%, yellow soft paraffin BP 34.8%, white soft paraffin BP 1.13%, light liquid paraffin BP 7.9%, starch BP 10%, zinc oxide BP 6.55%, methyl salicylate BP 3%, octaphonium chloride BP 0.3%, phenol BP 1.19%.

For the treatment of minor cuts, burns and rough skin; also guards against infection.

Adults and children: Apply to affected area and rub gently.

In the case of cuts or particularly tender areas rubbing may be avoided by applying liberally on a piece of white lint or gauze and covering with a light bandage or plaster.

Pharmacy only: No

HIOXYL CREAM
Quinoderm Ltd

PA No: 308/8/1

Cream.

25g or 100g of hydrogen peroxide 1.5%.

For treatment of minor wounds, infections and leg ulcers.

Adults and children: Apply freely using lint or gauze.

Pharmacy only: Yes

SAVLON ANTISEPTIC CREAM
Novartis Consumer Health

PA No: 30/28/2

15g, 30g, 60g or 100g of smooth, white, homogenous cream with an antiseptic odour.

Cetrimide 0.5% w/w, chlorhexidine gluconate 0.1% w/w.

For the cleansing and prevention of superficial infections in skin tissue, minor skin disorders, blisters, minor burns and small wounds.

Adults and children: With clean hands, gently apply the cream over affected areas after cleansing.

Pharmacy only: No

Always Read The Label

SAVLON ANTISEPTIC WOUND WASH
Novartis Consumer Health

PA No: 30/25/1

▣100ml bottle of clear liquid.

☑Chlorhexidine gluconate solution 0.45% w/v.

☑Cleansing and disinfecting of minor wounds, cuts and grazes and minor abrasions including insect bites and stings, and minor burns and scalds.

☑Adults and children: Spray onto the affected area and flood the wound to wash away any dirt and debris. If necessary use a clean cloth or tissue to wipe away any excess dirt or liquid.

Pharmacy only: No

SAVLON CONCENTRATED
Novartis Consumer Health

PA No: 30/28/1

▣250ml, 500ml, 750ml or 5 litre bottles of clear liquid with a pine-like odour.

☑Cetrimide 2.25% w/v, chlorhexidine gluconate 0.225% w/v.

☑A general antiseptic for external first aid use.

☑Adults: Cuts, grazes, minor burns and bites: 2 capfuls to ½ a litre of warm water. Personal hygiene and midwifery: 2 capfuls to ½ a litre of warm water. Bathing: 5 capfuls to the bathwater.

Children: Cuts, grazes, minor burns and bites: 2 capfuls to ½ a litre of warm water. Personal hygiene: 2 capfuls to ½a litre of warm water. Bathing: 5 capfuls to the bathwater.

❗Keep out of eyes and ears.

Pharmacy only: No

SAVLON DRY
Novartis Consumer Health

PA No: 30/29/1

▣Orange/brown suspension in aerosol propellant.

☑Povidone iodine 1.14% w/v.

☑An antiseptic powder for the treatment of cuts, grazes, minor burns and scalds. Protects against infection.

☑Adults and children: Shake the can and spray affected area from a distance of 15-22cm (6-9 inches) until light dusting of powder is deposited. Do not use on babies under 1 month old.

❗Do not use near mouth, nose or eyes.

Pharmacy only: No

SUDOCREM
Tosara Products Ltd

PA No: 247/1/1

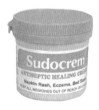

▣25g, 60g, 125g and 400g containers or 30g tube of cream emulsion.

☑Zinc oxide 15.25%, lanolin (hypoallergenic) 4%, benzyl benzoate 1.01%, benzyl cinnamate 0.15%, benzyl alcohol 0.39%.

☑For the treatment of nappy rash, bedsores, minor burns, eczema, acne, chilblains, surface wounds and sunburn.

☑Adults and children: Apply in a thin layer as required.

❗For external use only.

Pharmacy only: No

Always Read The Label

136

TCP FIRST AID CREAM
Pfizer/Warner Lambert Consumer Healthcare

PA No: 823/37/1

▭30mg tube of antiseptic cream.

▶Triclosan 0.3% w/w, chloroxylenol 0.5% w/w, TCP liquid antiseptic 25% w/w.

▢For the treatment of minor cuts, grazes, scratches, insect bites and stings, spots, pimples and blisters.

▨Adults and children: Clean wound and surrounding skin and apply directly or on to a dressing. Spots: Rub in gently.

Pharmacy only: No

TCP LIQUID ANTISEPTIC
Pfizer/Warner Lambert Consumer Healthcare

PA No: 823/37/2

▭50ml, 100ml or 200ml bottles of aqueous liquid antiseptic.

▶Phenol 0.175% w/v, halogenated phenols 0.68% w/v.

▢For the symptomatic relief of common mouth ulcers, cuts, grazes, bites and stings, boils, spots and pimples, and sore throat including those associated with colds and flu.

▨Adults: Gargle: Twice daily diluted 1:5 with water. Mouth ulcer: Apply undiluted 3 times daily. Spots: Apply undiluted every 4 hrs. Cuts: Apply diluted 1:1.

Pharmacy only: No

If Symptoms Persist Consult Your Doctor

FUNGAL INFECTION

Ringworm

Ringworm is caused by infection with a fungus, not a worm. It starts as a pink to red scaly rash that gradually expands outwards as the infection spreads. It then often clears in the centre to give the ring-like appearance that gives it its name. Infection may involve the body, hands (especially the palms), groin area or scalp, where it tends to produce a spreading bald patch containing broken hair stumps but with little inflammation. Athlete's foot (see **Foot Care**) is a form of ringworm.

Ringworm in the groin area can be produced following contact with an athlete's foot infection, so athlete's foot should not be regarded as trivial but should be actively treated. As well as being passed on by human contact, ringworm can be transmitted by animals. In particular, cattle ringworm produces a severe reaction with substantial inflammation, swelling and pus formation.

Until recently, ringworm spread through human contact was rare but it now appears to be on the increase in urban areas, being spread through schools. The reason for this is unknown.

Treatment

The same antifungal agents that are used for athlete's foot are effective against ringworm with **miconazole** or **econazole** being preferred. Treatment should be continued for at least a week after the infection has cleared. In order to prevent re-infection from fungal spores on the skin surrounding the infected area, the medication should be applied well beyond it.

Scalp ringworm usually affects children prior to puberty. It is resistant to treatment. Although it may initially appear to clear, the infection may get into the hair roots where it cannot be reached by a product applied to the skin. When the hair re-grows, the infection will reappear. Use of a shampoo containing **selenium sulphide** (see **Dandruff**) is a useful additional measure to prevent the spread of infection. However, early treatment is advisable to prevent subsequent baldness associated with scarring and medical attention is advised for all cases of scalp ringworm since it may be necessary to give a medicine which is active by mouth.

DAKTARIN CREAM
Janssen Pharmacy Healthcare

PA No: 748/16/1

▭30g tube of white, water-miscible cream.

▪Miconazole nitrate 20mg/g.

▯For the treatment of fungal and associated bacterial infections of the skin, such as athlete's foot, sweat rash, ringworm and infected nappy rash.

▪Adults and children: Apply once or twice daily to affected areas. Continue treatment for 10 days after lesions have disappeared.

Pharmacy only: Yes

DAKTARIN POWDER
Janssen Pharmacy Healthcare

PA No: 748/16/3

▭20g pack of white powder.

▪Miconazole nitrate 20mg/g, colloidal silicon dioxide, zinc oxide and talc.

▯For the treatment of fungal and associated bacterial infections of the skin, such as athlete's foot, sweat rash, ringworm and infected nappy rash.

▪Adults and children: Apply once or twice daily to affected area. Continue treatment until lesions have disappeared.

Pharmacy only: Yes

Always Read The Label

DESENEX
Roche Consumer Health

PA No: 72/8/2

◻55g tin of powder or 30g tube of ointment.

◼Zinc undecenoate 20%, undecenoic acid 2%.

◻For the treatment of athlete's foot.

Pharmacy only: Yes

MYCIL OINTMENT
Boots Healthcare Ltd

PA No: 43/17/1

◻25g of ointment.

◼Benzalkonium chloride 0.01% v/w, tolnaftate 1% w/w, polyethylene glycol, cetostearyl alcohol, dimethicone 20, glycerol, liquid paraffin.

◻For the treatment and prevention of athlete's foot.

◼Adults and children: Apply to the affected area morning and night. Continue treatment for at least a week after the infection has cleared up.

❗Do not use if sensitive to any of the ingredients.

Pharmacy only: Yes

MYCIL POWDER
Boots Healthcare Ltd

PA No: 43/16/1

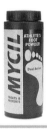

◻55g of powder.

◼Chlorhexidine hydrochloride 0.25% w/w, tolnaftate 1% w/w, silica, maize starch, purified talc.

◻For the treatment and prevention of athlete's foot.

◼Adults and children: Apply to the affected area morning and night. Continue treatment for at least a week after the infection has cleared up.

❗Do not use if sensitive to any of the ingredients.

Pharmacy only: Yes

MYCIL PUFFER PACK
Boots Healthcare Ltd

PA No: 43/16/1

◻55g powder puffer pack.

◼Chlorhexidine hydrochloride 0.25% w/w, tolnaftate 1% w/w, silica, maize, starch, purified talc.

◻For the treatment and prevention of athlete's foot.

◼Adults and children: Apply to the affected area morning and night. Continue treatment for at least a week after the infection has cleared up.

❗Do not use if sensitive to any of the ingredients.

Pharmacy only: Yes

MYCIL SPRAY
Boots Healthcare Ltd

PA No: 43/21/1

◻150ml spray.

◼Tolnaftate 1% w/w, butylated hydroxytoluene, dichlorodifluoromethane, polyethylene glycol, talc, trichlorofluoromethane.

◻For the treatment and prevention of athlete's foot.

◼Adults and children: Spray the affected area morning and night. Continue treatment for at least a week after the infection has cleared up.

❗Do not use if sensitive to any of the ingredients.

Pharmacy only: Yes

Always Consult Your Pharmacist

TINADERM CREAM
Schering-Plough Ltd

PA No: 277/2/2

■ 15g tube of white cream.

■ Tolnaftate 1% w/w.

▨ For the treatment of athlete's foot and other skin infections due to fungi.

▨ Adults and children: Apply topically twice daily to the affected area after thorough

washing and drying.

Pharmacy only: Yes

TINADERM PLUS POWDER
Schering-Plough Ltd

PA No: 277/62/1

■ 50g plastic bottle of white powder.

■ Tolnaftate 1.0% w/w.

▨ For the treatment of athlete's foot and other skin infections due to fungi.

▨ Adults and children: Apply topically twice daily to affected area after thoroughly washing and drying the areas concerned. Sprinkle into shoes,

socks and stockings to combat reservoirs of infection.

Pharmacy only: Yes

INSECT REPELLENTS

AUTAN ACTIVE AEROSOL
Bayer Ltd

PA No: N/A

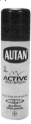

■ 100ml aerosol spray.

▨ Aqua, 1-piperidineecarboxylic acid 2-(2-hydroxyethyl)-1-methylpropylester, alcohol denat., glycerin, tridecyl stearate, tridecyl trimellitate, aloe barbadensis, dipentaerythrityl hexcaprylate/hexacaprate, sodium carbomer, acrylates/C10-30 akryl acrylates crosspolymer, parfum.

▨ Apply evenly to all exposed areas of the skin and under thin clothing. Reapply as necessary. Protects from biting insects for up to 8 hrs.

▮ Do not use on children under 2 yrs.

Do not use on severely sunburnt/blistered/broken skin.

For external use only.

Pharmacy only: No

AUTAN ACTIVE PUMP SPRAY
Bayer Ltd

PA No: N/A

■ Pump spray 100ml.

▨ Aqua, 1-piperidineecarboxylic

acid 2-(2-hydroxyethyl)-1-methylpropylester, alcohol denat., citric acid, parfum.

▨ Apply evenly to all exposed areas of the skin and under thin clothing. Reapply as necessary. Protects from biting insects for up to 8 hrs.

▮ Do not use on children under 2 yrs.

Do not use on severely sunburnt/blistered/broken skin.

For external use only.

Pharmacy only: No

If Symptoms Persist Consult Your Doctor

AUTAN ACTIVE STICK
Bayer Ltd

PA No: N/A

50ml stick.

Aqua, 1-piperidineecarboxylic acid, 2-(2-hydroxyethyl)-ester 1-methylpropyl-ester, alcohol

denat., citric acid, parfum.

Apply evenly to all exposed areas of the skin and under thin clothing. Reapply as necessary. Protects from biting insects for up to 8 hrs.

Do not use on children under 2 yrs.

Do not use on severely sunburnt/blistered/broken skin.

For external use only.

Pharmacy only: No

AUTAN BITE-EASE
Bayer Ltd

PA No: N/A

8ml micropump.

Aqua, alcohol denat., laureth 9, glycerine, tannic acid, menthyl lactate, panthenol,

menthol, camphor, bisabolol, dipotassium glycyrrhizate.

Dab onto infected area. Do not rub in as this may irritate your skin.

Do not use on children under 2 yrs.

Do not use on severely sunburnt/blistered/broken skin.

For external use only.

Pharmacy only: No

AUTAN FAMILY LOTION
Bayer Ltd

PA No: N/A

100ml of lotion.

Aqua, 1-piperidineecarboxylic acid 2-(2-hydroxyethyl)-1-methylpropylester, alcohol denat., glycerin, tridecyl stearate, tridecyl trimellitate, aloe

barbadensis, dipentaerythrityl hexcaprylate/hexacaprate, sodium carbomer, acrylates/C10-30 akryl acrylates crosspolymer, parfum.

Apply evenly to all exposed areas of the skin and under thin clothing. Reapply as necessary. Protects from biting insects for up to 4 hrs.

Do not use on children under

2 yrs.

Do not use on severely sunburnt/blistered/broken skin.

For external use only.

Pharmacy only: No

MIJEX EXTRA ROLL-ON FORMULA 3535
Intrapharma/Dugdale/J Pickles Healthcare

PA No: N/A

Roll-on. Contains no DEET.

15% Merck 3535.

Insect repellant.

Pharmacy only: Yes

MIJEX EXTRA SPRAY FORMULA 35454
Intrapharma/Dugdale/J Pickles Healthcare

PA No: N/A

Spray. Contains no DEET.

15% Merck 3535.

Insect repellent.

Pharmacy only: Yes

Always Read The Label

MIJEX GEL
Intrapharma/Dugdale/J Pickles Healthcare

PA No: N/A

Gel.

35g 20% DEET.

Effective insect repellent. Safe

for children.

Pharmacy only: Yes

MIJEX ROLL-ON
Intrapharma/Dugdale/J Pickles Healthcare

PA No: N/A

Roll-on.

50ml 60% DEET.

Effective, super strength insect

repellent.

Pharmacy only: Yes

MIJEX SPRAY
Intrapharma/Dugdale/J Pickles Healthcare

PA No: N/A

Plastic bottle with modern pump action spray.

60ml OFCF see 50% DEET.

A liquid repellent against mosquitos and midges.

Pharmacy only: Yes

MIJEX STICK
Intrapharma/Dugdale/J Pickles Healthcare

PA No: N/A

Mijex Stick.

17g 10% DEET.

Mosquito, midge and insect

repellent in a handy stick form.

Pharmacy only: Yes

PSORIASIS, ECZEMA, DERMATITIS AND DRY SKIN

Psoriasis
Psoriasis occurs in between 1% and 3% of the population and there is some evidence that it runs in families. It takes the form of patches of affected skin (plaques) of varying size (from a few millimetres to several centimetres across) consisting of a red rash with a clear outline. Dry silvery white scales cover the affected area. The scales become more obvious if the surface of the rash is scraped. The rash is associated with an increase in skin production.

There is often no obvious cause of psoriasis but in some people the rash can appear where the skin is damaged. It may be made worse by some prescribed medicines or by anxiety. In children and adolescents a smaller sized rash which looks like droplets (**guttate psoriasis**) but which usually clears in a few months, is an indication that the more common plaque form is likely to appear in later life.

Treatment
Coal tar preparations have been used to treat psoriasis for many years. **Salicylic acid** is sometimes included to remove scales and is particularly useful in scalp psoriasis (see **Hair and Scalp**).

Creams containing **hydrocortisone** are less messy than coal tar and are, perhaps, more suitable to apply to areas where the rash is visible. However, they are only suited to short term use (see **Eczema**).

Always Consult Your Pharmacist

Psoriasis is often improved by exposure to sunlight and many people find that their psoriasis improves while sunbathing on holiday. Supervised UVB treatment may be useful at other times, especially in winter.

Precautions and Warnings
- If you are unsure that your rash is psoriasis or if psoriasis affects anything other than a small area, seek medical advice. More potent medicines are available on prescription
- If you experience joint pain seek medical advice
- Ordinary sun beds are not suitable for treatment of psoriasis as they do not produce light at the correct wavelength.

ECZEMA, DERMATITIS AND DRY SKIN

The terms eczema and dermatitis are used to describe the same skin reaction. It starts as a red rash with an unclear outer margin and can progress to blistering, weeping, cracking and peeling. Irritant eczema may follow exposure of the skin to an irritant substance such as a detergent, an irritant industrial solvent or ammonia (see **Nappy Rash**).

Eczema can also occur as an allergic response to such contact. The elderly and anyone with a family history of asthma or hayfever are more likely to have such a reaction. Detergents and industrial chemicals – chromium in cement and resin based adhesives – are common causes of contact eczema but there are many others including nickel on jewellery or items of clothing such as jean buttons or bra fastenings. Preservatives and wool alcohols used in perfumes and cosmetics are also often involved. The initial reaction is at the point of contact but the rash may spread and become persistent so that early identification of the cause is important.

Another form of allergic eczema (**atopic eczema**) is possible in those with a family history of asthma, hayfever or urticaria. This often starts in babies as a rash on the cheeks and upper body and it settles in childhood on the backs of the knees and the fronts of the elbows, wrists and ankles. In adulthood, the face and body can become affected.

Treatment
Irritant eczema is treated by the use of **barrier creams** that protect against the irritant substance. Contact allergic eczema is best dealt with by avoiding the substance which causes the allergy. Protective clothing should be worn if appropriate.

Dry skin and atopic eczema are treated by washing and bathing using moisturising agents (**emollients**) which incorporate oily materials, especially **liquid paraffin** and **soft paraffin**, or other natural oils which hydrate and soften the skin. There are numerous OTC preparations of this type. It is important to note that not all of these products are medicines, and so they do not require a product authorisation (**PA**) number from the Irish Medicines Board (see **Introduction**). If you are not sure which product to choose, ask your pharmacist's advice.

Although steroid creams containing **hydrocortisone** can also improve eczema, they are only suited to short term use. In atopic eczema, which requires long term treatment, steroids should only be used under medical supervision.

Precautions and Warnings
- Do not use hydrocortisone cream for longer than three weeks
- Hydrocortisone cream should only be applied to the affected area
- Do not apply a steroid cream to the eyes, face, anal or genital area or to broken or infected skin.

If Symptoms Persist Consult Your Doctor

ALCODERM CREAM 60G
Intra Pharma Ltd

PA No: 590/1/1

60g tube of emollient.

Moisturises dry skin.

Pharmacy only: Yes

CALMURID CREAM 100G/500G
Intra Pharma Ltd

PA No: 590/8/1

Skin emollient. A white, shiny cream in a stabilising emulsified base.

Carbamide (urea) BP 10%, lactic acid EP 5%.

Eczema.

A thick layer is applied twice daily after washing affected area. Leave on for 3-5 mins then wipe off with tissue.

Pharmacy only: Yes

E45 CREAM
Boots Healthcare Ltd

PA No: 43/7/1

50g, 125g or 500g containers of dermatological cream.

Hypoallergenic anhydrous lanolin 1.0% w/w, light liquid paraffin 12.6% w/w, white soft paraffin 14.5% w/w, cetyl alcohol, citric acid, monohydrate, sodium lauryl sulphate, sodium hydroxide, methyl hydroxybenzoate, propyl hydroxybenzoate.

For the symptomatic relief of dry skin conditions, including flaking, itching, chapped skin, eczema and contact dermatitis.

Adults and children: Apply to affected area 2-3 times daily.

Pharmacy only: Yes

EPI-SHIELD
Shield Health Ltd

PA No: N/A

100ml cream.

Aqua, propylene glycol, stearic acid, glyceryl stearate, triethanolamine, acetylated naturally occurring alcohols including cetyl acetate and oleyl acetate, dimethicone, triclosan, dichlorobenzyl alcohol.

Skin protection and emollient cream for the protection of the skin, especially the hands, from the irritants that may cause contact dermatitis. Also for the relief of dry skin conditions.

Adults and children: Apply every 4 hrs.

Pharmacy only: Yes

OILATUM JUNIOR FLARE-UP
Stiefel Laboratories (Ireland) Ltd

PA No: 144/18/2

150ml bottle of colour free, fragrance free, antiseptic bath emollient for children.

Light liquid paraffin 52.5%, benzalkonium chloride 6.0%, triclosan 2.0%.

Oilatum Junior Flare-Up relieves itching, helps reduce redness, soothes and softens the skin. It is an effective cleanser and should not be used with soap.

Adults and children: 1 capful to a 10cm bath. 2 capfuls to a 20cm bath. Soak for 10-15 mins, gently pat the skin dry with a soft clean towel. Use once daily.

Infants: 1ml mixed well with water. Soak for 10-15 mins, gently pat the skin dry with a soft, clean towel. Use once daily.

Not recommended for children under 6 months.

Take care to avoid slipping in the bath.

Pharmacy only: Yes

Always Read The Label

OILATUM PLUS
Stiefel Laboratories (Ireland) Ltd

PA No: 144/18/1

▣ 500ml bottle of antiseptic emollient bath additive.

▣ Light liquid paraffin 52.5%, benzalkonium chloride 6.0%, triclosan 2.0%.

▣ Oilatum Plus is an antiseptic bath emollient for eczema, including eczema at risk from infection. *Staphylococcus aureus* (*Staph. aureus*) is a major cause of atopic eczema flare-up. Oilatum Plus contains two antiseptics which reduce *Staph. aureus* count whilst bathing and also carry on working after the bath. Oilatum Plus also relieves irritation and rehydrates the skin.

▣ Adults and children: 1 capful to a 10cm bath. 2 capfuls to a 20cm bath. Soak for 10-15 mins, gently pat the skin dry with a soft clean towel. Use once daily.

Infants: 1ml mixed well with water. Soak for 10-15 mins, gently pat the skin dry with a soft, clean towel. Use once daily.

▣ Not recommended for babies under 6 months.

Take care to avoid slipping in the bath.

Pharmacy only: Yes

OILATUM SHOWER GEL FORMULA
Stiefel Laboratories (Ireland) Ltd

PA No: 144/22/2

▣ 125g tube of concentrated emollient gel for use in the shower.

▣ Light liquid paraffin 70%.

▣ Oilatum Shower Gel Formula is formulated for treating dry skin and eczema in the shower. It is also particularly suitable for treating localised dermatitis, for example on the hands or elbows.

▣ Adults and children: First shower or wash in the normal way (using a mild cleanser such as Oilatum Soap), then massage small amounts of the gel onto the affected areas while the skin is still wet. Rinse off any excess gel using warm water and pat the skin dry with a soft, clean towel.

Always apply to wet skin. If applying the gel onto someone else, your hand, as well as the area being treated, should be wet.

▣ Take care to avoid slipping in the shower.

Pharmacy only: Yes

PROCAM LOTION
Perrans Distributors Ltd

PA No: N/A

▣ 100ml bottle of cream-based lotion.

▣ For relief of dry skin conditions. Rehydrates the skin and then forms a barrier to prevent against further drying.

▣ Apply liberally to the affected area twice daily. Gently massage into the skin.

▣ For external use only. Always patch test before using for the first time. Avoid contact with eyes. Not recommended for children under 3 yrs. Keep out of reach of children. Do not use during pregnancy. Local irritation may occur in rare cases. If this continues, cease product use. Do not use if there is a known sensitivity to any ingredient.

Pharmacy only: No

Always Consult Your Pharmacist

SCABIES

Scabies is caused by a common mite which burrows under the skin. The initial symptoms are of intense itching, especially at night, between the fingers, on the wrists, at the back of the elbows or on the buttocks or genitals. If the infection is ignored the itching may become widespread. If untreated, the burrow of the mite becomes infected and fills with pus. People who are run down or who have a deficient immune system are at increased risk of a more severe and widespread form of scabies.

Treatment

Treatment of scabies consists of the use of **insecticidal lotions** including **malathion** or **lindane**. These lotions should be applied liberally to the skin of the whole body except the face and scalp. A bath is not necessary prior to the application. A paintbrush is a useful applicator. The lotion should be left on the skin for 8-12 hours (lindane) or 24 hours (malathion) and then washed off by bathing. A second application may be necessary after one to two weeks. Infants should only be treated under medical supervision and the head and neck may also require treatment. Because it may take several weeks before itching signals that scabies is present, all close contacts should be treated simultaneously. Infestation is not passed on through bedding or clothing.

Precautions and Warnings

- Because the rash produced by scabies looks like that produced in eczema, scabies is sometimes misdiagnosed. Treatments intended for eczema will not cure scabies so if a persistent rash is present, medical advice should always be sought
- Treat all close contacts
- Infants should only be treated under medical supervision.

ASCABIOL EMULSION
Aventis Pharma Ltd

PA No: 40/62/1

100ml bottle.

Benzyl benzoate BP 25% w/v. Also contains stearic acid, triethanolamine, terpineol and oil cinnamon, leaf carbon, silicone MS antifoam A and water.

For the treatment of scabies and pediculosis.

Adults: Scabies: After total bathing Ascabiol Emulsion should be applied to the whole body except the head and face. A second application may be repeated within five days or,

alternatively, treatment may be applied on 3 occasions at 12-hourly intervals.

Children: Scabies: After total bathing apply Ascabiol Emulsion to the whole body except the head and face. Pediculosis: The affected region should be coated with Ascabiol followed by a wash 24 hrs later.

Ascabiol Emulsion must not be allowed to come in contact with the eyes.

May cause skin irritation and transient burning sensations. In the event of this being severe, it should be washed off using soap and warm water.

Store below 25°C. Shake bottle before use.

Pharmacy only: Yes

DERBAC-M LIQUID
SSL Healthcare Ireland Ltd

PA No: 618/14/1

◻50ml or 200ml bottles of white, creamy, liquid emulsion.

◪Malathion 0.5% w/v.

◪For the eradication of head and pubic lice and their eggs. For treatment of scabies.

◪Adults and children over 6 months: Head lice: Apply liberally and leave to dry naturally. Shampoo hair after 12 hrs. Use nit comb while hair is still wet. Pubic lice: Apply to all areas including beard and moustache, leave for 1-12 hrs before washing off. Scabies: Apply liberally after thorough cleansing and leave for 24 hrs before washing off.

In adults it may not be necessary to apply above the neck, but children under 2 yrs should have a thin film applied to the scalp, face and ears, avoiding the eyes and mouth.

❚Not recommended for children under 6 months.

Avoid contact with eyes.

Pharmacy only: Yes

QUELLADA LOTION
Stafford-Miller/Intra Pharma

PA No: N/A

◻100ml or 500ml bottles of white lotion.

◪Lindane 1%.

◪For the treatment of scabies.

◪Adults: Apply a thin layer to the whole body, excluding the face and scalp. Leave for 24 hrs then wash thoroughly. Repeat after 7 days if necessary.

Children: Over 6 months: As adults but under supervision. 1-6 months: Under medical supervision, wash off after 8-12 hrs.

❚Avoid contact with eyes or mucous membranes. Do not use on broken or infected skin.

Pharmacy only: Yes

Always Read The Label

SKIN IRRITATION

Allergic Skin Conditions (Hives/Nettle Rash/Urticaria)

Creams containing **antihistamines** (**diphenhydramine**, **mepyramine**) reduce the intense itching associated with rashes that are allergic in origin. However, they should not be used on broken or weeping skin or on blisters. These rashes develop quickly and consist of light pink or flesh coloured weals that may merge. They should also clear quickly. Long term use of antihistamines is not recommended as they can sensitise the skin and cause eczema or a sunburn-like reaction.

Caution

A rash that is widespread can be the result of an adverse reaction to a food or drug and it is important to consider whether such a cause is likely.

Precautions and Warnings

- If there is any swelling of the lips, face or throat, or any wheezing or shortness of breath, see your doctor.

ANTHISAN CREAM

Aventis Pharma

PA No: 40/39/4

- 25g tube of smooth, homogeneous cream.

- Mepyramine maleate 2% w/w, methylhydroxybenzoate.

For the treatment of allergic skin disorders such as the symptomatic relief of insect bites and stings.

- Adults and children: Apply to the affected area 2-3 times daily for up to 3 days or as directed by physician.

- Consult your doctor if symptoms persist.

Pharmacy only: Yes

BENADRYL SKIN ALLERGY RELIEF CREAM

Pfizer/Warner Lambert Consumer Healthcare

PA No: 823/16/1

- 42g tube of smooth, pink cream.

- Diphenhydramine hydrochloride Ph Eur 1%, zinc oxide Ph Eur 8%, racemic camphor Ph Eur 0.1%.

- For the treatment of the skin manifestations of allergy, e.g. sunburn, prickly heat and hives. It can also be used to relieve the itching and discomfort caused by insect bites, nettle stings, shingles and minor skin irritations.

- Adults and children: Apply cream 3-4 times daily.

- Do not use on raw or broken skin (cuts or grazes).

Pharmacy only: Yes

BENADRYL SKIN ALLERGY RELIEF LOTION

Pfizer/Warner Lambert Consumer Healthcare

PA No: 823/16/2

- 125ml botttle of smooth, pink, viscous lotion.

- Diphenhydramine hydrochloride Ph Eur 1%, zinc oxide Ph Eur 8%, racemic camphor Ph Eur 0.1%.

- For the treatment of the skin manifestations of allergy, e.g. sunburn, prickly heat and hives. It can also be used to relieve the itching and discomfort caused by insect bites, nettle stings, shingles and minor skin irritations.

- Adults and children: Apply lotion 3-4 times daily.

- Do not use on raw or broken skin (cuts or grazes).

Pharmacy only: Yes

Always Consult Your Pharmacist

BLISTEZE 5G
DDD Ltd

PA No: 302/4/1

◼5g tube of cream.

◼Strong ammonia solution 0.20%, aromatic ammonia solution 6.04%, liquefied phenol 0.494%.

◼Soothing and protective cream for sore, cracked and chapped lips.

◼Adults: Topical application to the lips every hour.

Children: Topical application to the lips every hour.

◼Keep out of the reach of children.

Pharmacy only: Yes

BURNEZE SPRAY
SSL Healthcare Ireland Ltd

PA No: 618/2/1

◼60ml spray cans.

◼Benzocaine 1% w/w.

◼For the symptomatic relief of pain from minor superficial burns and scalds where the skin is unbroken.

◼Adults and children: Hold nozzle 5 inches from the skin and spray once for 2-3 secs. Stop spraying immediately if white frost deposit appears. If necessary, the application may be repeated once only after 15 mins.

Pharmacy only: Yes

CALMURID HC CREAM 30G/100G
Intra Pharma Ltd

PA No: 590/9/1

◼White, shiny cream.

◼(Urea) BP 10%, lactic acid EP 5%.

◼For treatment of atopic eczema, neurodermatitis.

◼A thick layer applied twice daily. Leave for 3-5 mins then wipe off with tissue.

Pharmacy only: Yes

CETAPHIL 200ML
Galderma/Intra Pharma Ltd

PA No: N/A

◼Cleanser for sensitive skin.

◼Sensitive skin.

Pharmacy only: Yes

CORTOPIN HYDROCORTISONE CREAM
Pinewood Healthcare

PA No: 281/71/2

◼15g tube of smooth, white, homogeneous oil-in-water cream.

◼Hydrocortisone Ph Eur 0.5% w/w or 1% w/w, liquid paraffin, chlorocresol, white soft paraffin, cetostearyl alcohol, purified water.

◼For the topical treatment of contact dermatitis, irritant dermatitis, insect bite reactions and mild to moderate eczema.

◼Adults: Apply twice daily, massage well in, or as directed by the physician.

◼Contraindicated for use on the eyes, face, anogenital region, broken or infected skin including cold sores, acne and athlete's foot. Should not be recommended for children under 10 yrs or during pregnancy or breastfeeding without medical advice.

Pharmacy only: Yes

DERMIDEX DERMATOLOGICAL CREAM
SSL Healthcare Ireland Ltd

PA No: 547/2/1

◼30g or 50g tubes of cream.

◼Chlorbutanol hemihydrate 1% w/w, lidocaine 1.2% w/w, cetrimide 0.5% w/w, aluminium chlorhydroxyallantoinate 0.25% w/w.

◼Treatment of mild pain caused by minor skin cuts, scratches and grazes (chapping) and soreness caused by detergents, soaps, deodorants and jewellery, and bites and stings.

◼Adults and children: Apply to the affected area every 3 hrs.

◼Not recommended for children under 4 yrs.

Pharmacy only: Yes

If Symptoms Persist Consult Your Doctor

DRICLOR
Stiefel Laboratories (Ireland) Ltd

PA No: N/A

20ml roll-on applicator of clear, colourless, topical treatment for excessive perspiration.

Aluminium chloride hexahydrate 20%.

Driclor is an antiperspirant for the topical treatment of excessive perspiration of the armpits, hands and feet.

Adults: Apply to affected areas where necessary at night, wash off in the morning.

Avoid contact with eyes. Ensure area is dry and not shaved 12 hours before or after use.

Pharmacy only: Yes

E45 BATH
Boots Healthcare Ltd

PA No: N/A

250ml bottle of colourless, semi-dispersing bath oil.

Medicinal white oil 90.95% w/w and cetyl dimethicone 5% w/w.

E45 Emollient Bath Oil helps to prevent dry skin by retaining the skin's natural moisture.

Also recommended for bathing more serious dry skin conditions.

Adults: 15ml poured into warm bath water or applied on a wet sponge if showering.

Children: Pour 5-10mls into a small bath of warm water.

Pharmacy only: Yes

E45 SHOWER
Boots Healthcare Ltd

PA No: N/A

200ml hook pack of fragrance free, white, creamy emulsion.

Aqua, petrolatum, glycerin.

For cleaning dry, itchy skin. Suitable for people with eczema and dermatitis.

Apply to wet skin, massage gently then rinse off.

Pharmacy only: Yes

E45 WASH
Boots Healthcare Ltd

PA No: N/A

250ml pump containing white, creamy, perfume free liquid emulsion.

Paraffinum liquidum, petrolatum, cetyl dimethicone, cera microcrystallina.

E45 emollient cream wash cleans and moisturises dry skin without changing normal skin pH. It helps prevent dry skin by retaining the skin's natural moisture.

Also recommended instead of soap for washing more serious dry skin conditions.

Pharmacy only: Yes

EMULSIDERM EMOLLIENT
Dermal Laboratories

PA No: 278/8/1

300ml or 1L bottle with a measuring cap containing pale blue/green liquid emulsion.

Benzalkonium chloride 0.5%, liquid paraffin 25%, isopropyl myristate 25%.

For the treatment of dry skin conditions, including those associated with dermatitis and psoriasis. It permits rehydration of the keratin by replacing lost lipids, and its antibacterial properties assist in overcoming *Staphylococcus aureus*, the pathogen which often complicates atopic eczema and associated pruritus.

Adults and children: Shake bottle before use. Add 7-30ml to a bath of warm water. Soak for 5-10 mins. Pat dry. For application to the skin: Rub a small amount of undiluted emollient into the dry areas of skin until absorbed.

Pharmacy only: Yes

Always Read The Label

EUCERIN 3% UREA LOTION
Beiersdorf Ireland Ltd

PA No: N/A

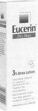

250ml bottle of light, non-greasy lotion.

Aqua, paraffinum liquidum, isohexadecane, PEG-7 hydrogenated castor oil, glycerin, urea, isopropyl palmitate, sodium lactate, benzyl alcohol, panthenol, ceresin, magnesium sulfate, lanolin alcohol (Eucerit®), bisabolol.

Binds moisture for effective relief of dry skin conditions. Fragrance and colourant free. For dry skin and eczema.

Adults: Apply sparingly twice daily.

Pharmacy only: Yes

EUCERIN 5% UREA CREAM
Beiersdorf Ireland Ltd

PA No: N/A

75ml tub of easily absorbed, non-greasy cream.

Aqua, paraffinum liquidum, urea, sodium lactate, polyglyceryl-3 diisostearate, magnesium stearate, ceresin, isopropyl palmitate, benzyl alcohol, panthenol, magnesium sulfate, lanolin alcohol (Eucerit®), bisabolol.

Binds moisture for effective relief of dry skin conditions and eczema. Fragrance and colourant free.

Adults: Apply sparingly twice daily.

Pharmacy only: Yes

EUCERIN BATH THERAPY
Beiersdorf Ireland Ltd

PA No: N/A

150ml bottle of lightly foaming bath oil.

Glycine soja, MIPA-laureth sulfate, ricinus communis, laureth-4, cocamide DEA, poloxamer 101, laureth-9, lanolin alcohol (Eucerit®), aqua, citric acid, diammonium citrate, BHT, propyl gallate.

Soothes, softens and protects dry skin and eczema.

Adults: Add 40ml into 8in bath and soak for 10-20 mins.

Children: Add 20ml to small bath of water.

Pharmacy only: Yes

EUCERIN SHOWER THERAPY
Beiersdorf Ireland Ltd

PA No: N/A

200ml bottle of lightly foaming shower oil.

Glycine soja, MIPA-laureth sulfate, ricinus communis, laureth-4, cocamide DEA, poloxamer 101, laureth-9, lanolin alcohol (Eucerit®), aqua, citric acid, diammonium citrate, BHT, propyl gallate.

Soothes, softens and protects dry skin. Gently cleanses without drying.

Adults and children: Apply to all affected areas and rinse under the shower.

Pharmacy only: Yes

Always Consult Your Pharmacist

EURAX CREAM
Novartis Consumer Health

PA No: 30/23/1

▭30g or 100g tubes.

▯Crotamiton 10% w/w.

▯For the symptomatic relief of pruritus of varying origins and for the treatment of scabies.

▯Adults and children: Pruritus: Apply to the affected area 2-3 times daily. Eurax will provide relief from irritation for 6-10 hrs after each application. Eurax can be used in children. There are no special dosage recommendations in the elderly. Scabies: After a thorough bath, Eurax should be applied to all areas below the chin with particular attention to interdigital areas. It is advisable to repeat the treatment 24 hrs later. A bath should be taken a day after with a change of clothes and bedding.

All contacts of patients with scabies should be treated simultaneously.

Pharmacy only: Yes

EURAX HC CREAM
Novartis Consumer Health

PA No: 30/18/1

▭15g tube of cream.

▯Crotamiton 10% w/w, hydrocortisone 0.25% w/w.

▯Relief of irritant contact dermatitis, allergic contact dermatitis, insect bite reactions, mild to moderate eczema.

▯Adults and children over 10 yrs: Apply sparingly over a small area twice a day for a maximum period of a week. Dressings should not be used.

▯Not recommended for children under 10 yrs.

Do not use on the eyes or face, the ano-genital region, or on broken, infected or weeping skin, including cold sores, acne and athlete's foot.

Pharmacy only: Yes

EURAX LOTION
Novartis Consumer Health

PA No: 30/23/2

▭100ml bottle.

▯Crotamiton 10% w/w.

▯For the symptomatic relief of pruritus of varying origins and for the treatment of scabies.

▯Adults and children: Pruritus: Apply to the affected area 2-3 times daily. Eurax will provide relief from irritation for 6-10 hrs after each application. Eurax can be used in children. There are no special dosage recommendations in the elderly. Scabies: After a thorough bath, Eurax should be applied to all areas below the chin with particular attention to interdigital areas. It is advisable to repeat the treatment 24 hrs later. A bath should be taken a day after with a change of clothes and bedding.

All contacts of patients with scabies should be treated simultaneously.

Pharmacy only: Yes

If Symptoms Persist Consult Your Doctor

HC45 HYDROCORTISONE CREAM 1%
Boots Healthcare Ltd

PA No: 43/23/1

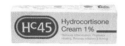

▣15g tube of cream.

▣Hydrocortisone acetate BP 1.0% w/w, water, white soft paraffin.

▣For the treatment of mild to moderate eczema, contact dermatitis from allergies or irritants, skin reactions to insect bites.

▣Adults: Use sparingly on small areas, once or twice daily, for a maximum of 7 days.

▣Do not use on eyes or face, anal or genital areas, or on broken or infected skin, including impetigo, cold sores, acne or athlete's foot. Do not use in pregnancy unless considered essential by the physician.

Not recommended for children under 10 yrs without medical advice.

Pharmacy only: Yes

HYDROCORTISYL
Aventis Pharma

PA No: 6/16/1

▣15g tube of skin cream (non-greasy base).

▣Hydrocortisone 1%.

▣For management of skin allergic disorders, contact dermatitis, eczemas, lichen simplex, pruritis and psoriasis.

▣Adults and children: Apply 1-4 times daily or as directed by the physician. Once improvement is evident, frequency of application should be gradually reduced.

▣Should not be used during pregnancy or breastfeeding unless considered essential by the physician. Continuous treatment for longer than 3 weeks should be avoided in patients under 3 yrs because of the possibility of adrenocortical suppression and growth retardation. Not for use on the eyes, face, in the anogenital region, on broken or infected skin including cold sores, acne and athlete's foot.

Pharmacy only: Yes

NIVEA CREME
Beiersdorf Ireland Ltd

PA No: N/A

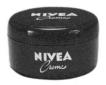

▣25ml pot, 50ml pot, 100ml tube, 200ml pot or 500ml pot.

▣Aqua (water), paraffinum liquidum, cera microcristallina, glycerin, ceresin, isohexadecane, lanolin alcohol (eucerit), paraffin, magnesium sulphate, decyl oleate, octyldodecanol, aluminium stearates, panthenol, citric acid, magnesium stearate, parfum (fragrance).

▣To prevent dry skin conditions resulting in such diseases as eczema and psoriasis, and to help maintain healthy skin.

Moisturises, nourishes and protects dry, rough and chapped skin.

▣Suitable for all ages.

Pharmacy only: No

OILATUM CREAM
Stiefel Laboratories (Ireland) Ltd

PA No: 144/23/2

▣40g tube of emollient cream.

▣Arachis oil 21%.

▣Oilatum Cream is an emollient cream used in the treatment of dry, sensitive skin conditions including ichthyosis. It coats the skin with a moisture-retaining film. Suitable for people allergic to lanolin.

▣Apply to the affected area, and rub in well. Use as often as required or as directed by doctor. Oilatum Cream is particularly effective when applied after washing.

Contains arachis oil.

Pharmacy only: Yes

Always Read The Label

OILATUM EMOLLIENT
Stiefel Laboratories (Ireland) Ltd

PA No: 144/22/1

■150ml, 250ml or 500ml bottles of water dispersible bath emollient.

☑Light liquid paraffin 63.4%.

▨Oilatum Emollient is a bath emollient for eczema and dry skin conditions. Its dual action provides soothing rehydration and helps prevent further drying. It disperses in bath water giving you a milky bath which also cleanses, so no soap is required.

▨Adults and children: Add 1-3 capfuls to a 20cm bath. Soak for 10-20 mins. Pat skin dry using a soft, clean towel. For maximum benefit use twice daily.

Infants: Add ½-2 capfuls to a small bath of water. Apply gently over body with a sponge. Pat skin dry using a soft, clean towel. For maximum benefit use twice daily.

Always use with water, either added to the bath or apply to wet skin.

▮Take care to avoid slipping in the bath.

Pharmacy only: Yes

OILATUM JUNIOR FLARE-UP
Stiefel Laboratories (Ireland) Ltd

PA No: 144/18/2

■150ml bottle of colour free, fragrance free, antiseptic bath emollient for children.

☑Light liquid paraffin 52.5%, benzalkonium chloride 6.0%, triclosan 2.0%.

▨Oilatum Junior Flare-Up relieves itching, helps reduce redness, soothes and softens the skin. An effective cleanser and should not be used with soap.

▨Adults and children: 1 capful to a 10cm bath. 2 capfuls to a 20cm bath. Soak for 10-15 mins, gently pat the skin dry with a soft clean towel. Use once daily.

Infants: 1ml mixed well with water. Soak for 10-15 mins, gently pat the skin dry with a soft, clean towel. Use once daily.

▮Not recommended for children under 6 months. Take care to avoid slipping in the bath.

Pharmacy only: Yes

OILATUM PLUS
Stiefel Laboratories (Ireland) Ltd

PA No: 144/18/1

■500ml bottle of antiseptic emollient bath additive.

☑Light liquid paraffin 52.5%, benzalkonium chloride 6.0%, triclosan 2.0%.

▨Oilatum Plus is an antiseptic bath emollient for eczema, including eczema at risk from infection. *Staphylococcus aureus* (*Staph. aureus*) is a major cause of atopic eczema flare-up. Oilatum Plus contains two antiseptics which reduce *Staph. aureus* count whilst bathing and also carry on working after the bath. Oilatum Plus also relieves irritation and rehydrates the skin.

▨Adults and children: 1 capful to a 10cm bath. 2 capfuls to a 20cm bath. Soak for 10-15 mins, gently pat the skin dry with a soft clean towel. Use once daily.

Infants: 1ml mixed well with water. Soak for 10-15 mins, gently pat the skin dry with a soft, clean towel. Use once daily.

▮Not recommended for babies under 6 months. Take care to avoid slipping in the bath.

Pharmacy only: Yes

Always Consult Your Pharmacist

OILATUM SHOWER GEL FORMULA
Stiefel Laboratories (Ireland) Ltd

PA No: 144/22/2

▢125g tube of concentrated emollient gel for use in the shower.

▣Light liquid paraffin 70%.

▢Oilatum Shower Gel Formula is specially formulated for treating dry skin and eczema in the shower. It is also particularly suitable for treating localised dermatitis, for example on the hands or elbows.

▣Adults and children: First shower or wash in the normal way (using a mild cleanser such as Oilatum Soap), then massage small amounts of the gel onto the affected areas while the skin is still wet. Rinse off any excess gel using warm water and pat the skin dry with a soft, clean towel.

▣Always apply to wet skin. If applying the gel onto someone else, your hand, as well as the area being treated, should be wet. Take care to avoid slipping in the shower.

Pharmacy only: Yes

OILATUM SOAP
Stiefel Laboratories (Ireland) Ltd

PA No: 144/22/3

▢100g bar of mild cleanser for dry, sensitive skin.

▣Light liquid paraffin 7.5%.

▢Oilatum Soap cleanses skin gently without causing dryness as ordinary soap can. It also leaves a protective layer on the skin after washing to protect against any further moisture loss.

▣Adults and children: Use as ordinary soap for washing, bathing and showering.

Pharmacy only: Yes

ROWAROLAN POWDER
Rowa® Pharmaceuticals Ltd

PA No: 74/46/1

▢20g of exudate absorbent powder.

▣Calcium carbonate 90%, silica colloidal anhydrous 5%, purified talc 5%.

▢For the treatment of leg ulcers, bed sores and similar conditions.

▣Adults: Sprinkle powder at least 3 times daily on affected area.

Pharmacy only: Yes

TCP FIRST AID CREAM
Pfizer/Warner Lambert Consumer Healthcare

PA No: 823/37/1

▢30mg tube of antiseptic cream.

▣Triclosan 0.3% w/w, chloroxylenol 0.5% w/w, TCP liquid antiseptic 25% w/w.

▢For the treatment of minor cuts, grazes, scratches, insect bites and stings, spots, pimples and blisters.

▣Adults and children: Clean wound and surrounding skin and apply directly or on to a dressing. Spots: Rub in gently.

Pharmacy only: No

TCP LIQUID ANTISEPTIC
Pfizer/Warner Lambert Consumer Healthcare

PA No: 823/37/2

▢50ml, 100ml or 200ml bottles of aqueous liquid antiseptic.

▣Phenol 0.175% w/v, halogenated phenols 0.68% w/v.

▢For the symptomatic relief of common mouth ulcers, cuts, grazes, bites and stings, boils, spots and pimples, and sore throat including those associated with colds and flu.

▣Adults: Gargle: Twice daily diluted 1:5 with water. Mouth ulcer: Apply undiluted 3 times daily. Spots: Apply undiluted every 4 hrs. Cuts: Apply diluted 1:1.

Pharmacy only: No

If Symptoms Persist Consult Your Doctor

WASP-EZE SPRAY
SSL Healthcare Ireland Ltd

PA No: 618/8/1

📼 30ml or 60ml aerosol spray can.

📼 Benzocaine 1% w/w,

mepyramine maleate 0.5% w/w.

❓ For the treatment of all insect bites and stings, nettle stings and jellyfish stings.

📼 Adults and children: Hold

nozzle approx 5 inches from skin and spray once for 2-3 secs. Stop spraying immediately if a white frost deposit appears. Repeat once after 15 mins, if necessary.

Pharmacy only: Yes

ZIRTEK
U.C.B. (Pharma) Ireland Ltd

PA No: 230/3/1

📼 Packs of 7 small, white, oblong tablets.

📼 Cetirizine dihydrochloride 10mg.

❓ For the symptomatic relief of hayfever, allergic rhinitis, urticaria and senile pruritus.

📼 Adults: 1 tablet daily.

Children: Not recommended for children under 12 yrs.

Pharmacy only: Yes

SKIN PROTECTANTS AND MOISTURISING CREAMS

BALNEUM BATH TREATMENT
Boots Healthcare Ltd

PA No: 54/85/1

📼 150ml bottle of liquid.

📼 Soya oil 84.75% w/w.

❓ For the management of ichthyosis and dry skin associated with eczema and dermatitis.

📼 Adults: Add 3 capfuls to a

full bath while water is running

Children: Add 1 capful to a bath while water is running. Soak for at least 10 mins. Rinse and pat dry with a towel.

Pharmacy only: Yes

BALNEUM PLUS BATH TREATMENT
Boots Healthcare Ltd

PA No: 54/74/1

📼 150ml bottle of liquid bath treatment.

📼 Soya oil 82.95% w/w, lauromacrogols 15% w/w.

❓ Provides relief from pruritus. It

is recommended for the treatment of dry skin conditions including those associated with eczema and dermatitis where pruritus is also experienced.

📼 Adults: Shake bottle before use. Pour 3 capfuls into a full bath of water as water is running. May also be used in shower with a flannel or

sponge, then rinse and pat dry with a towel.

Children: Add 1 capful to bath while water is running and soak for at least 10 mins. Rinse and pat dry with a towel.

Babies and infants: Daily application is recommended.

Pharmacy only: Yes

BLISTEZE 5G
DDD Ltd

PA No: 302/4/1

📼 5g tube of cream.

📼 Strong ammonia solution

0.20%, aromatic ammonia solution 6.04%, liquefied phenol 0.494%.

❓ A soothing and protective cream for sore, cracked and chapped lips.

📼 Adults and children: Topical application to the lips every hour.

❗ Keep out of the reach of children.

Pharmacy only: Yes

Always Read The Label

E45 BATH
Boots Healthcare Ltd

PA No: N/A

▭250ml bottle of colourless, semi-dispersing bath oil.

▪Medicinal white oil 90.95% w/w and cetyl dimethicone 5% w/w.

▪E45 Emollient Bath Oil helps prevent dry skin by retaining the skin's natural moisture.

Also recommended for bathing more serious dry skin conditions.

▪Adults: 15ml poured into warm bath water or applied on a wet sponge if showering.

Children: Pour 5-10ml into a small bath of warm water.

Pharmacy only: Yes

E45 CREAM
Boots Healthcare Ltd

PA No: 43/7/1

▭50g, 125g or 500g containers of dermatological cream.

▪Hypoallergenic anhydrous lanolin 1.0% w/w, light liquid paraffin 12.6% w/w, white soft paraffin 14.5% w/w, cetyl alcohol, citric acid, monohydrate, sodium lauryl sulphate, sodium hydroxide, methyl hydroxybenzoate, propyl hydroxybenzoate.

▪For the symptomatic relief of dry skin conditions, including flaking, itching, chapped skin, eczema and contact dermatitis.

▪Adults and children: Apply to affected area 2-3 times daily.

Pharmacy only: Yes

E45 LOTION
Boots Healthcare Ltd

PA No: N/A

▭200ml of lotion.

▪White soft paraffin 10% w/w, light liquid paraffin 4.0% w/w, hypoallergenic anhydrous lanolin 1.0% w/w.

▪Soothes and softens dry skin.

▪Adults and children: Use frequently on face, hands and body.

Pharmacy only: Yes

E45 SHOWER
Boots Healthcare Ltd

PA No: N/A

▭200ml hook pack of fragrance free, white, creamy emulsion.

▪Aqua, petrolatum, glycerin.

▪Gently cleanses dry, itchy skin. Suitable for people with eczema and dermatitis. The mild formulation does not foam. It cleans without drying, leaving skin soft and supple.

▪Apply to wet skin, massage gently then rinse off.

Pharmacy only: Yes

E45 WASH
Boots Healthcare Ltd

PA No: N/A

▭250ml pump of white, creamy, perfume free liquid emulsion.

▪Paraffinum liquidum, petrolatum, cetyl dimethicone, cera microcrystallina.

▪E45 emollient cream wash cleans and moisturises dry skin without changing normal skin pH. It helps prevent dry skin by retaining the skin's natural moisture.

Also recommended instead of soap for washing more serious dry skin conditions.

Pharmacy only: Yes

Always Consult Your Pharmacist

EMULSIDERM EMOLLIENT
Dermal Laboratories

PA No: 278/8/1

▣300ml or 1L bottle with a measuring cap containing pale blue/green liquid emulsion.

☑Benzalkonium chloride 0.5%, liquid paraffin 25%, isopropyl myristate 25%.

❓For the treatment of dry skin conditions, including those associated with dermatitis and psoriasis. It permits rehydration of the keratin by replacing lost lipids and its antibacterial properties assist in overcoming *Staphylococcus aureus*, the pathogen which often complicates atopic eczema and associated pruritus.

◪Adults and Children: Shake bottle before use. Add 7-30mls to a bath of warm water. Soak for 5-10 mins. Pat dry. For application to the skin: Rub a small amount of undiluted emollient into the dry areas of skin until absorbed.

Pharmacy only: Yes

EPI-SHIELD
Shield Health Ltd

PA No: N/A

▣100ml of cream.

☑Aqua, propylene glycol, stearic acid, glyceryl stearate, triethanolamine, acetylated naturally occurring alcohols including cetyl acetate and oleyl acetate, dimethicone, triclosan, dichlorobenzyl alcohol.

❓For the protection of the skin, especially the hands, from the irritants that may cause contact dermatitis. Also for the relief of dry skin conditions.

◪Adults and children: Apply every 4 hrs.

Pharmacy only: Yes

EUCERIN 3% UREA LOTION
Beiersdorf Ireland Ltd

PA No: N/A

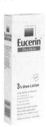

▣250ml bottle of light non-greasy lotion.

☑Aqua, paraffinum liquidum, isohexadecane, PEG-7 hydrogenated castor oil, glycerin, urea, isopropyl palmitate, sodium lactate, benzyl alcohol, panthenol, ceresin, magnesium sulfate, lanolin alcohol (Eucerit®), bisabolol.

❓Binds moisture for effective relief of dry skin conditions and eczema. Fragrance and colourant free.

◪Adults: Apply sparingly twice daily.

Pharmacy only: Yes

EUCERIN 5% UREA CREAM
Beiersdorf Ireland Ltd

PA No: N/A

▣75ml tub of easily absorbed, non-greasy cream.

☑Aqua, paraffinum liquidum, urea, sodium lactate, polyglyceryl-3 diisostearate, magnesium stearate, ceresin, isopropyl palmitate, benzyl alcohol, panthenol, magnesium sulfate, lanolin alcohol (Eucerit®), bisabolol.

❓Binds moisture for effective relief of dry skin conditions and eczema. Fragrance and colourant free.

◪Adults: Apply sparingly twice daily.

Pharmacy only: Yes

If Symptoms Persist Consult Your Doctor

EUCERIN BATH THERAPY
Beiersdorf Ireland Ltd
PA No: N/A

◻150ml bottle of lightly foaming bath oil.

🔲Glycine soja, MIPA-laureth sulfate, ricinus communis,

laureth-4, cocamide DEA, poloxamer 101, laureth-9, lanolin alcohol (Eucerit®), aqua, citric acid, diammonium citrate, BHT, propyl gallate.

▣Soothes, softens and protects dry skin with eczema.

▨Adults: Add 40ml into 8in bath and soak for 10-20 mins.

Children: Add 20ml to small bath of water.

Pharmacy only: Yes

EUCERIN SHOWER THERAPY
Beiersdorf Ireland Ltd
PA No: N/A

◻200ml bottle of lightly foaming shower oil.

🔲Glycine soja, MIPA-laureth sulfate, ricinus communis, laureth-4, cocamide DEA,

poloxamer 101, laureth-9, lanolin alcohol (Eucerit®), aqua, citric acid, diammonium citrate, BHT, propyl gallate.

▣Soothes, softens and protects dry skin. Gently cleanses without drying.

▨Adults and children: Apply to all affected areas and rinse under the shower.

Pharmacy only: Yes

HYDROMOL CREAM
Quinoderm Ltd
PA No: 308/14/1

◻50g, 100g tubes or 500g tub of cream.

🔲Arachis oil 10%, isopropyl myristate 5%, liquid paraffin 10%, sodium pyrrolidine carboxylate 2.5%, sodium lactate 1%.

▣Dry skin, including all forms of dermatitis, eczema, ichthyosis

and senile pruritis.

▨Adults and children: Apply liberally and massage in. Especially beneficial after bathing.

Pharmacy only: Yes

HYDROMOL EMOLLIENT
Quinoderm Ltd
PA No: 308/13/1

◻150ml, 350ml or 1 litre bottles of water-dispersable, oily solution.

🔲Light liquid paraffin 37.8%, isopropyl myristate 13%, isoctyl stearate 15.95%, dehydol LS3 11.25%, cetiol HE 22%.

▣For the treatment of dry skin conditions such as eczema, icthyosis and senile pruritus.

▨Adults: Added to bath (1-3 capfuls) or applied to wet skin.

❗Avoid contact with eyes.

Pharmacy only: Yes

LACTICARE
Stiefel Laboratories (Ireland) Ltd
PA No: 144/3/1

◻75g tube of moisturising cream.

🔲Sodium pyrrolidone carboxylate 2.5%, lactic acid 5%.

▣For the relief of dry, scaling skin conditions.

▨Adults and children: Apply to

the affected area as often as necessary and massage in carefully. The cream is particularly effective when applied directly after washing.

❗Do not apply to broken skin.

Pharmacy only: Yes

Always Read The Label

NIVEA CREME
Beiersdorf Ireland Ltd

PA No: N/A

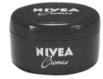

🔲25ml pot, 50ml pot, 100ml tube, 200ml pot or 500ml pot.

🔲Aqua (water), paraffinum liquidum, cera microcristallina, glycerin, ceresin, isohexadecane, lanolin alcohol (eucerit), paraffin, magnesium sulphate, decyl oleate, octyldodecanol, aluminium stearates, panthenol, citric acid, magnesium stearate, parfum (fragrance).

❓To prevent dry skin conditions resulting in such diseases as eczema and psoriasis, and to help maintain healthy skin.

Moisturises, nourishes and

protects dry, rough and chapped skin.

🔲Suitable for all ages.

Pharmacy only: No

OILATUM CREAM
Stiefel Laboratories (Ireland) Ltd

PA No: 144/23/2

🔲40g tube of emollient cream.

🔲Arachis oil 21%.

❓Oilatum Cream is an emollient cream used in the treatment of dry, sensitive skin

conditions including ichthyosis. It coats the skin with a moisture-retaining film. Suitable for people allergic to lanolin.

🔲Apply to the affected area, and rub in well. Use as often as required or as directed by doctor. Oilatum Cream is particularly effective when applied after washing.

⚠Contains arachis oil.

Pharmacy only: Yes

OILATUM EMOLLIENT
Stiefel Laboratories (Ireland) Ltd

PA No: 144/22/1

🔲150ml, 250ml or 500ml bottles of water dispersible bath emollient.

🔲Light liquid paraffin 63.4%.

❓Oilatum Emollient is a bath emollient for eczema and dry skin conditions. Its dual action provides soothing rehydration and helps prevent further drying. It disperses in bath water giving

you a milky bath which also cleanses, so no soap is required.

🔲Adults and children: Add 1-3 capfuls to a 20cm bath. Soak for 10-20 mins. Pat skin dry using a soft, clean towel. For maximum benefit use twice daily.

Infants: Add ½-2 capfuls to a small bath of water. Apply gently over body with a sponge. Pat skin dry using a soft, clean towel. For maximum benefit use twice daily.

⚠Always use with water, either added to the bath or apply to wet skin. Take care to avoid

slipping in the bath.

Pharmacy only: Yes

Always Consult Your Pharmacist

OILATUM JUNIOR
Stiefel Laboratories (Ireland) Ltd

PA No: 144/22/4

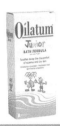

150ml or 300ml bottle of colour free, fragrance free emollient bath additive for children.

Light liquid paraffin 63.4%.

Oilatum Junior is for children with eczema and other dry skin conditions. It has a dual action which:i) soothes and rehydrates the skin to provide relief, and ii) helps protect against further drying.

Infants: $1/2$-2 capfuls to small bath of water. Apply gently over body with a sponge. Pat skin dry using a soft, clean towel. For maximum benefit use twice daily.

Children: 1-3 capfuls to 20cm bath. Soak for 10-20 mins. Pat skin dry using a soft, clean towel. For maximum benefit use twice daily.

Always use with water; either add to the bath or apply to wet skin. Take care to avoid slipping in the bath.

Pharmacy only: Yes

OILATUM JUNIOR CREAM
Stiefel Laboratories (Ireland) Ltd

PA No: N/A

150g of emollient cream.

Light liquid paraffin 6%, white soft paraffin 15%.

For the symptomatic relief of dry skin conditions. Suitable for use in eczema.

Use as required, especially after washing. Apply with clean hands to affected areas and rub in well.

Pharmacy only: Yes

OILATUM JUNIOR FLARE-UP
Stiefel Laboratories (Ireland) Ltd

PA No: 144/18/2

150ml bottle of colour free, fragrance free, antiseptic bath emollient for children.

Light liquid paraffin 52.5%, benzalkonium chloride 6.0%, triclosan 2.0%.

Oilatum Junior Flare-Up relieves itching, helps reduce redness, soothes and softens the skin. It is an effective cleanser and should not be used with soap.

Adults and children: 1 capful to a 10cm bath. 2 capfuls to a 20cm bath. Soak for 10-15 mins, gently pat the skin dry with a soft clean towel. Use once daily.

Infants: 1ml mixed well with water. Soak for 10-15 mins, gently pat the skin dry with a soft, clean towel. Use once daily.

Not recommended for children under 6 months. Take care to avoid slipping in the bath.

Pharmacy only: Yes

OILATUM PLUS
Stiefel Laboratories (Ireland) Ltd

PA No: 144/18/1

500ml bottle of antiseptic emollient bath additive.

Light liquid paraffin 52.5%, benzalkonium chloride 6.0%, triclosan 2.0%.

Oilatum Plus is an antiseptic bath emollient for eczema, including eczema at risk from infection. *Staphylococcus aureus (Staph. aureus)* is a major cause of atopic eczema flare-up. Oilatum Plus contains two antiseptics which reduce *Staph. aureus* count whilst bathing and also carry on working after the bath. Oilatum Plus also relieves irritation and rehydrates the skin.

Adults and children: 1 capful to a 10cm bath. 2 capfuls to a 20cm bath. Soak for 10-15 mins, gently pat the skin dry with a soft clean towel. Use once daily.

Infants: 1ml mixed well with water. Soak for 10-15 mins, gently pat the skin dry with a soft, clean towel. Use once daily.

Not recommended for babies under 6 months. Take care to avoid slipping in the bath.

Pharmacy only: Yes

If Symptoms Persist Consult Your Doctor

OILATUM SHOWER GEL FORMULA
Stiefel Laboratories (Ireland) Ltd

PA No: 144/22/2

▭125g tube of concentrated emollient gel for use in the shower.

☑Light liquid paraffin 70%.

▨Oilatum Shower Gel Formula is for treating dry skin and eczema in the shower. It is also particularly suitable for treating localised dermatitis, for example on the hands or elbows.

▨Adults and children: First shower or wash in the normal way (using a mild cleanser such as Oilatum Soap), then massage small amounts of the gel onto the affected areas while the skin is still wet. Rinse off any excess gel using warm water and pat the skin dry with a soft, clean towel.

❗Always apply to wet skin. If applying the gel onto someone else, your hand, as well as the area being treated, should be wet. Take care to avoid slipping in the shower.

Pharmacy only: Yes

OILATUM SOAP
Stiefel Laboratories (Ireland) Ltd

PA No: 144/22/3

▭100g bar of mild cleanser for dry, sensitive skin.

☑Light liquid paraffin 7.5%.

▨Oilatum Soap cleanses skin gently without causing dryness as ordinary soap can. It also leaves a protective layer on the skin after washing to protect against any further moisture loss.

▨Adults and children: Use as ordinary soap for washing, bathing and showering.

Pharmacy only: Yes

PROPY-LACTICARE
Stiefel Laboratories (Ireland) Ltd

PA No: N/A

▭150ml bottle of topical lotion.

☑Lactic acid 4.4%, propylene glycol 53.8%, glycerine 25.3%.

▨For the relief of very dry, scaling skin.

▨Adults: Intensive: Apply lotion to the affected areas twice daily. Use for 15 days.

Maintenance treatment: Use once daily.

❗Do not apply to broken skin.

Pharmacy only: Yes

TCP FIRST AID CREAM
Pfizer/Warner Lambert Consumer Healthcare

PA No: 823/37/1

▭30mg tube of antiseptic cream.

☑Triclosan 0.3% w/w, chloroxylenol 0.5% w/w, TCP liquid antiseptic 25% w/w.

▨For the treatment of minor cuts, grazes, scratches, insect bites and stings, spots, pimples and blisters.

▨Adults and children: Clean wound and surrounding skin and apply directly or on to a dressing. Spots: Rub in gently.

Pharmacy only: No

UNGUENTUM M
Boots Healthcare Ltd

PA No: 54/1/1

▭60g tube of cream.

☑Liquid paraffin, white soft paraffin.

▨For the symptomatic treatment of eczema, dermatitis, nappy rash, ichthyosis, protection of raw and abraded skin areas, pruritus and related conditions where dry, scaly skin is a problem.

▨Adults and children: A small amount of cream should be rubbed into the affected area of skin as often as necessary.

Pharmacy only: No

Spots

Acne

Common acne is caused by inflammation of the hair root and its associated gland. This causes increased secretion from the gland, which then plugs the hair shaft forming whiteheads or blackheads on the face, neck, shoulders, chest and upper back. The glands may then become infected by bacteria (especially by *Propionibacterium acnes*) leading to the formation of pus and further inflammation which produces the familiar spots of acne.

If you have acne it is important to avoid squeezing the spots but this advice is easier to give than to obey! In more severe acne (**cystic acne**) closed infected cavities (cysts) penetrate into the affected tissues and these may cause scarring.

Acne is associated with increased production of or sensitivity to a hormone produced at puberty and therefore usually first occurs at this time. It reaches a peak in girls at 16-17 years and in young men at 17-19 years, but clears in most people by the time they reach 23-25 years of age.

Treatment

Only mild acne is suitable for OTC treatment because of the danger of permanent scarring with the more severe forms. Because a bacterial infection is involved, **antiseptic** preparations (see **Antiseptics**) are usually the first option in treatment. Whatever treatment is used, progress is often slow, taking weeks or months, and the most important cause of treatment failure is failure to persist. Reassurance and support are important aspects of treatment.

Benzoyl peroxide has an antiseptic action and increases the rate of skin formation, which may be helpful. However, it can cause irritation, especially in the early stages of use, making the skin red and dry and causing it to peel. It is wise to start with a preparation containing a low concentration and work upwards. Peroxide will bleach fabric if it comes into contact with it. Abrasive agents containing **aluminium oxide** particles are also available as an aid to additional skin cleansing.

The treatment of severe acne should be medically supervised and may involve the use of **antibiotics** or other medicines that are only available on prescription.

ACNE AID SOAP
Stiefel Laboratories (Ireland) Ltd

PA No: 144/27/1

⬜ 100g soap bar.

🔲 Sulphonated vegetable oil 63.7%.

🔲 For use as a detergent soap for cleansing of the skin in greasy and hyperkeratotic conditions, including acne vulgaris.

🔲 Adults: Make a lather with warm water and massage into the affected skin using the finger tips or a face cloth. Rinse and repeat as necessary.

Pharmacy only: Yes

ACNECIDE GEL 5/10%
Intra Pharma Ltd

PA No: 5%: 590/7/1; 10%: 590/7/2

🔲 A smooth, white, aqueous gel intended for topical administration in human beings.

🔲 5 or 10% w/w benzoyl peroxide Ph Eur.

🔲 For treatment of acne vulgaris.

🔲 Keep from contact with eyes. If contact occurs, rinse with water; if undue redness or discomfort occurs, consult doctor.

Pharmacy only: Yes

Always Consult Your Pharmacist

BRASIVOL FINE/MEDIUM
Stiefel Laboratories (Ireland) Ltd

PA No: 144/25/2

■75g tube of scrub cleanser.

■Aluminium oxide particles 52%.

■For cleansing oily skin and for the management of acne vulgaris.

■Adults: Brasivol should always be applied to wet skin. Massage into the skin, using circular motion, for 15-20 secs, rinse with warm water and dry the skin carefully. Use once or twice daily replacing normal soap and water.

■Do not apply to broken or irritated skin.

Pharmacy only: Yes

BREVOXYL CREAM
Stiefel Laboratories (Ireland) Ltd

PA No: 144/33/1

■40g tube of topical anti-acne cream.

■Benzoyl peroxide 4% w/w in a hydrophase base.

■Brevoxyl Cream is used for the treatment of mild to moderate acne. Benzoyl peroxide is an oxidising agent with antibacterial activity against Propionibacterium acnes (P. acnes). The benzoyl peroxide is kept in solution as it is adsorbed. This minimises irritation and maximises the cream's potential to destroy P. acnes (the main bacteria involved in acne).

■Adults: Apply to the whole of the affected area once or twice daily. Wash with soap and water prior to application. Improvement can generally be seen after 4-6 weeks of treatment. However, longer use may be necessary.

■Patients with known hypersensitivity to any of the ingredients should not use the product. Avoid contact with eyes, mouth and other mucous membranes. Care should be taken when applying the product to the neck and other sensitive areas. The product may bleach hair and coloured or dyed fabrics.

Pharmacy only: Yes

HEALTHCRAFTS VITAMIN E OIL
Perrans Distributors Ltd

PA No: N/A

■8ml bottle with roll-on applicator.

■Vitamin E (d-alpha tocopheryl acetate), soya bean oil.

■ Natural form vitamin E oil. For the treatment of dry skin and lips.

■Adults: Rub into affected area as required.

Pharmacy only: No

PANOXYL ACNEGEL 5
Stiefel Laboratories (Ireland) Ltd

PA No: 144/11/5

■40g tube of topical anti-acne gel.

■Benzoyl peroxide 5%.

■PanOxyl Acnegel 5 is used for the treatment of acne. It has an antibacterial action and reduces the number of all surface bacteria. It also reduces the number of comedones (blackheads and whiteheads) and damps down inflammation.

■Adults: Apply a small amount of the gel once daily to the area of skin which has acne, not just individual spots.

Washing prior to application greatly enhances use.

■Avoid contact with eyes, mouth and other mucous membranes.

Pharmacy only: Yes

If Symptoms Persist Consult Your Doctor

PANOXYL ACNEGEL 10
Stiefel Laboratories (Ireland) Ltd

PA No: 144/11/6

▣40g tube of topical anti-acne gel.

☑Benzoyl peroxide 10%.

❓PanOxyl Acnegel 10 is used for the treatment of acne. It has an antibacterial action and reduces the number of all surface bacteria. It also reduces the number of comedones (blackheads and whiteheads) and damps down inflammation.

☑Adults: Apply a small amount of the gel once daily to the area of skin which has acne, not just individual spots. Washing prior to application greatly enhances use.

⚠Avoid contact with eyes, mouth and other mucous membranes.

Pharmacy only: Yes

QUINODERM CREAM
Quinoderm Ltd

PA No: 308/1/1

▣25g or 50g of cream.

☑Benzoyl peroxide 10%, potassium hydroxyquinoline sulphate 0.5%.

❓For the treatment of acne vulgaris, acneform eruptions, folliculitis.

☑Adults: Massage over affected areas 2-3 times daily.

Children: Massage over affected areas 2-3 times daily.

⚠Should not be used on acne rosacea.

Pharmacy only: Yes

QUINODERM CREAM 5%
Quinoderm Ltd

PA No: 308/1/2

▣50g of cream.

☑Benzoyl peroxide 5%, potassium hydroxyquinoline sulphate 0.5%.

❓For treatment of acne vulgaris, acneform eruptions, folliculitis.

☑Adults: Gently massage over affected area 1-3 times daily.

Children: Gently massage over affected area 1-3 times daily.

⚠Not recommended for use on acne rosacea.

Pharmacy only: Yes

QUINODERM LOTIO-GEL 5%
Quinoderm Ltd

PA No: 308/7/2

▣30ml thixotropic gel.

☑Benzoyl peroxide 5%, potassium hydroxyquinoline sulphate 0.5%.

❓For the treatment of acne vulgaris, acneform eruptions, folliculitis.

☑Adults and children: Massage over the affected area, apply sparingly 1-3 times daily.

Pharmacy only: Yes

TCP FIRST AID CREAM
Pfizer/Warner Lambert Consumer Healthcare

PA No: 823/37/1

▣30mg of antiseptic cream.

☑Triclosan 0.3% w/w, chloroxylenol 0.5% w/w, TCP liquid antiseptic 25% w/w.

❓For the treatment of minor cuts, grazes, scratches, insect bites and stings, spots, pimples and blisters.

☑Adults and children: Clean wound and surrounding skin and apply directly or on to a dressing. Spots: Rub in gently.

Pharmacy only: No

Always Read The Label

TCP LIQUID ANTISEPTIC
Pfizer/Warner Lambert Consumer Healthcare

PA No: 823/37/2

◻️50ml, 100ml or 200ml bottles of aqueous liquid antiseptic.

☑️Phenol 0.175% w/v, halogenated phenols 0.68% w/v.

🔲For the symptomatic relief of common mouth ulcers, cuts, grazes, bites and stings, boils, spots and pimples, and sore throat including those associated with colds and flu.

◼️Adults: Gargle: Twice daily diluted 1:5 with water. Mouth ulcer: Apply undiluted 3 times daily. Spots: Apply undiluted every 4 hrs. Cuts: Apply diluted 1:1.

Pharmacy only: No

STEROID CREAMS

HC45 HYDROCORTISONE CREAM 1%
Boots Healthcare Ltd

PA No: 43/23/1

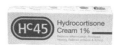

◻️15g tube of cream.

☑️Hydrocortisone acetate BP 1.0% w/w, water, white soft paraffin.

🔲For the treatment of mild to moderate eczema, contact dermatitis from allergies or irritants, skin reactions to insect bites.

◼️Adults: Use sparingly on small areas, once or twice daily, for a maximum of 7 days. Do not use on eyes or face, anal or genital areas, or on broken or infected skin, including impetigo, cold sores, acne or athlete's foot.

❗Do not use in pregnancy unless considered essential by the physician.

Not recommended for children under 10 yrs without medical advice.

Pharmacy only: Yes

HYDROCORTISYL
Aventis Pharma

PA No. 6/16/1

◻️15g tube of skin cream (non-greasy base).

☑️Hydrocortisone 1%.

🔲For management of allergic disorders, contact dermatitis, eczemas, lichen simplex, pruritis and psoriasis.

◼️Adults and children: Apply 1-4 times daily or as directed by the physician. Once improvement is evident, frequency of application should be gradually reduced.

❗Should not be used during pregnancy or breastfeeding unless considered essential by the physician. Continuous treatment for longer than 3 weeks should be avoided in patients under 3 yrs because of the possibility of adrenocortical suppression and growth retardation. Not for use on the eyes, face, in the anogenital region, on broken or infected skin including cold sores, acne and athlete's foot.

Pharmacy only: Yes

Always Consult Your Pharmacist

WARTS AND VERRUCAE

Warts are caused by a viral infection. They are most likely to occur where the skin is likely to suffer damage, such as the fingers, because the virus is able to penetrate the damaged skin. If warts are untreated, they are likely to spread by contact so that they can often be found on two fingers that have rubbed together. With time, immunity develops to the virus that causes warts and they may disappear. This gives rise to various folklore tales concerning cures.

Verrucae are warts on the sole of the foot. Once again, they are likely to occur on this area because the skin is subject to damage (see **Foot Care**).

Treatment

Treatment consists of the use of concentrated **salicylic acid**, which dissolves the wart. Measures to prevent the infection from spreading are also important. These include covering the wart with a plaster, which also aids penetration of the salicylic acid, or using a preparation that forms a protective film over the wart.

Washing with hot water to soften the skin before applying the treatment and carefully rubbing the affected area with a pumice stone or emery board after drying also speeds up treatment. It will usually take up to eight weeks of daily treatment before the warts disappear.

Medical treatment of warts consists of freezing (**cryotherapy**). A home-based form of cryotherapy, using a single application of a freezing aerosol, is available.

Precautions and Warnings

- Warts are infectious so prompt treatment is necessary
- All products used to dissolve or freeze skin should be applied only to the affected area since they may damage normal skin.

COMPOUND W
SSL Healthcare Ireland Ltd

PA No: 618/43/1

◨6.5ml bottle of faintly yellow, viscous liquid.

☑Salicylic acid 17% w/w.

❓Topical keratolytic for the treatment of warts and verrucae.

☑Adults and children over 6 yrs: Gently rub the hard skin from the surface of the wart/verruca with a pumice stone or emery board. Apply one drop at a time with dropper-rod until wart is covered. Allow to dry completely. Avoid contact with the surrounding skin. Repeat application daily, with regular washing, for up to 4 weeks.

▯Children under 6 yrs: do not use except on medical advice.

If there is doubt as to the diagnosis consult the doctor. Avoid contact with eyes, mouth, mucous membranes or healthy skin. Keep out of reach of children.

Pharmacy only: Yes

DUOFILM
Stiefel Laboratories (Ireland) Ltd

PA No: 144/1/1

◨15ml bottle of colourless or pale yellow/brown evaporative wart/verruca paint.

☑Salicylic acid 16.7%, lactic acid 16.7%.

❓Treatment for warts and verruca.

☑Adults: Apply to warts once daily, according to the following instructions: i) Soak the warts/verruca in hot water for 5 mins and dry well. ii) Rub the surface of the warts/verruca carefully with a pumice stone or manicure emery board. iii) Apply solution, taking care to avoid normal skin. iv) Allow to dry thoroughly and cover with a plaster if the wart is large or if it is a verruca on the foot. v) Continue treatment until the wart/verruca is completely cleared and the ridge lines of the skin have been restored.

▯Not suitable for children under 2 yrs. Children under 12 yrs should only use the product under supervision. Care must be taken to apply to wart/verruca only.

Pharmacy only: Yes

If Symptoms Persist Consult Your Doctor

SALACTOL WART PAINT
Dermal Laboratories

PA No: 278/6/1

10ml bottle of colourless or pale yellow/brown evaporative wart paint with spatula.

Salicylic acid 16.7%, lactic acid 16.7%.

For the topical treatment of warts, verrucae, corns and calluses.

Adults: Soak the affected site in warm water and pat dry. Gently rub the surface of the wart, verruca, corn or callus with a pumice stone or manicure emery board to remove any hard skin. Using the applicator provided, carefully apply a few drops to the lesion, taking care to localise the application to the affected area. Plantar warts should be covered with an adhesive plaster. Leave for 24 hrs. Repeat the procedure daily, removing old collodion on each occasion. Treatment may take 8 weeks.

Children: As per adult dose.

Not for use on or near the face, intertriginous or anogenital regions. Not suitable for diabetics or individuals with impaired peripheral blood circulation. Keep away from eyes and mucous membranes. Avoid spreading onto surrounding normal skin.

Pharmacy only: Yes

SALATAC WART GEL
Dermal Laboratories

PA No: 278/15/1

Collapsible tube containing 8g of clear colourless, collodion-like gel, complete with special applicator, emery board and instructions.

Salicylic acid BP 12% w/w, lactic acid BP 4% w/w.

For the topical treatment of warts, verrucae, corns and calluses.

Adults, children and the elderly: Once daily application, removing old elastic film formed from previous application on each occasion. No adhesive plaster is required.

Keep away from eyes, mucous membranes, cuts and grazes. Avoid spreading onto surrounding normal skin. Highly flammable - keep away from flames. Replace cap tightly after use. Not to be used on or near the face, intertriginous or anogenital regions, or by diabetics or individuals with impaired peripheral blood circulation.

Pharmacy only: Yes

WARTNER
Shield Health

PA No: N/A

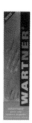

Home-based freezing kit for removal of warts and verrucas. Consists of a 35ml aerosol container, 10 foam applicators and a holder.

Dimethylether and propane.

For the treatment of warts and verrucas by freezing.

Should require only 1 application per wart or verruca. Adults and children over 4 yrs: Fit a foam applicator onto the holder. Place the holder (with applicator) into the opening on top of the aerosol. Press down firmly for 3 seconds. Place the tip of the foam applicator onto the wart or verruca for 20 seconds. In persistent cases, repeat treatment after 10 days.

Not suitable for children under 4 yrs.

Not suitable for areas of tender skin or for patients with diabetes.

If no improvement after 3 treatments, consult your doctor.

Pharmacy only: Yes

Always Read The Label

WOUND TREATMENT

SEAL ON STOPS BLEEDING SPRAY
Alltracel Pharma Limited

PA No: N/A

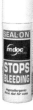

■80ml aerosol can. Approximately 20 applications per can.

☑Calcium/sodium salt of microdispersed oxidised cellulose (m.doc®) 2.5g.

▣Stops capillary bleeding from cuts, grazes and surface wounds quickly and efficiently (within 1-2 minutes).

☑Adults and children: Shake the can well and spray sufficient powder to uniformly cover the wound area from a distance of 15cm. On more profusely bleeding wounds, spray onto gauze and then place onto wound, applying temporary pressure if needed.

■Avoid contact with the eyes. In the event of prolonged bleeding seek medical advice.

Pharmacy only: No

Always Consult Your Pharmacist

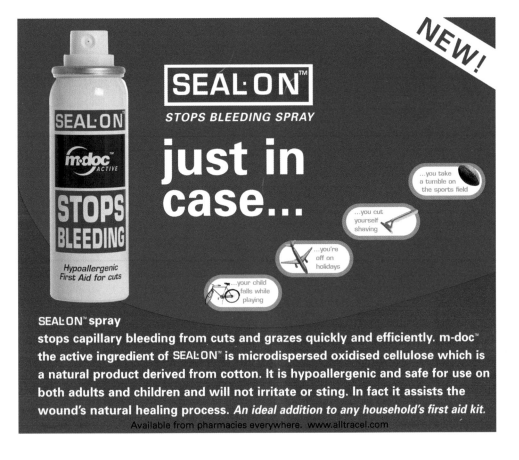

SLEEPING

General Information

A number of devices are available over the counter to aid those who have difficulty sleeping. However, it should be recognised that sleep quality is a highly subjective phenomenon.

MAX LITE EARPLUGS

Intrapharma/Howard Leight

PA No: N/A

■ Blister card containing 5 pairs of ear plugs.

🔲 Allow peaceful sleep, undisturbed by snoring partners or noisy neighbours. Soft and pliable. Anti-stress factor.

🔲 Suitable for adults and children.

Pharmacy only: Yes

SNOREEZE

Shield Health

PA No: N/A

■ 60ml liposome spray container.

🔲 Contained in a patented liposome base: Water, glycerine, olive oil, sunflower oil, peppermint oil, almond oil, sesame oil, vitamin E, vitamin B. Helps to keep the soft palate moistened during the night.

🔲 Coats and lubricates the soft tissues at the back of the throat, thus helping to reduce the vibrations that cause the snoring noise.

🔲 Adults: Use nightly. Shake the bottle, tilt head back, spray 3 times towards the inside upper part of the mouth, hold for 20 seconds and swallow.

🔲 Do not eat or drink after application (repeat spray if so). May not be effective if used within 1 hr of consuming alcohol.

Pharmacy only: Yes

SMOKING CESSATION

In recent times, much improved products and protocols have been devised to help people to give up smoking. These are based essentially on recognising the problem of nicotine dependence and reducing the craving and the withdrawal response that would occur if smoking is suddenly stopped. This is achieved by replacing the nicotine delivered by the cigarette with nicotine delivered through the soft tissues of the mouth by chewing gum, by using an inhaler or a microtab, or through the skin by means of a patch.

A vital feature of this treatment is the gradual reduction of the nicotine dosage over several weeks. This ensures that nicotine intake is gradually tapered off so that there is no withdrawal reaction. It is therefore very important to closely follow the dosage instructions on your chosen product.

Stopping smoking requires considerable self-determination and willpower. The evidence is that those who receive support in their efforts from friends or relatives do much better than those who go it alone.

Precautions and Warnings
- Use of nicotine replacement products is not recommended if you are pregnant or breastfeeding. Some authorities, however, consider that the use of such products is preferable to smoking.

CRAFE AWAY
Perrans Distributors Ltd

PA No: N/A

☐ Single wrapped mock plastic cigarette with tobacco flavour.

☐ Anti-smoking device to alleviate the physical rather than chemical addiction.

❗Not recommended for use during pregnancy.

Pharmacy only: No

NICORETTE DAYTIME PATCH
Pharmacia Consumer Healthcare

PA No: 936/2/3-5

☐ Packs of 7 or 14 x 15mg, 7 x 10mg or 7 x 5mg 16 hour nicotine patches (1 week's use).

☐ Nicotine replacement as an aid to smoking cessation.

☑ Adults: All users should begin with the 15mg patch and follow the Nicorette 12 week patch course. The 15mg patch should be used for 8 weeks, followed by 10mg patch for 2 weeks and then 5mg patch for 2 weeks. The patch should be applied first thing in the morning, and removed before retiring for the night. It should be applied to a completely clean, dry area of hairless skin on the front of the chest, upper arm or hip.

❗For waking hours only.

Not recommended for use while pregnant or breastfeeding.

Pharmacy only: Yes

NICORETTE GUM
Pharmacia Consumer Healthcare

PA No: 936/2/1, 2, 6, 7, 10, 11

☐ 30 pack, 105 pack or 210 pack of nicotine gum, available as 2mg or 4mg strengths, in classic, mint and citrus flavours.

☐ Nicotine replacement as an aid to smoking cessation.

☑ Adults: Those who smoke 20 or more cigarettes daily should use 4mg gum, otherwise 2mg gum is sufficient. Gum should be used at regular intervals during the day; usually 10 pieces daily are necessary.

Maximum of 15 daily. Gum should be used for a minimum of 3 months to ensure smoking habit is broken.

❗Not recommended for use while pregnant or breastfeeding.

Pharmacy only: Yes

Always Read The Label

NICORETTE INHALER
Pharmacia Consumer Healthcare

PA No: 936/2/9

Nicotine inhaler. Starter pack contains a holder, mouthpiece and 6 cartridges. Refill pack contains a spare mouthpiece and 18 or 42 cartridges.

10mg nicotine, with an available dose of 5mg nicotine per cartridge.

Nicotine replacement as an aid to smoking cessation. Designed to address the behavioural aspect of smoking cessation.

Suitable for adults who smoke 20 cigarettes per day or less.

A 3 month course, 6-12 cartridges daily for 8 weeks, followed by gradual reduction in the number of cartridges used to zero at 12 weeks. Each cartridge will last for 20 mins continuous puffing but this is not meant to be used up in one go, e.g. 4 x 5 mins or 2 x 10 mins.

Not recommended for use while pregnant or breastfeeding.

Pharmacy only: Yes

NICORETTE MICROTAB
Pharmacia Consumer Healthcare

PA No: 936/2/12

30 pack and 105 pack containing Nicorette sublingual tablet. Both packs contain dispensers.

2mg nicotine.

Nicotine replacement as an aid to smoking cessation.

Adults: Suitable for both low dependent smokers and high dependent smokers. Those who smoke less than 20 cigarettes per day use 1 Microtab every hr. If 1 Microtab per hr is not relieving cravings, dosage can be increased to 2 Microtabs per hr. Those who smoke 20 or more cigarettes per day should use 2 Microtabs per hr (maximum dose is 40 Nicorette Microtabs per day).

Not recommended for use while pregnant or breastfeeding.

Pharmacy only: Yes

Always Consult Your Pharmacist

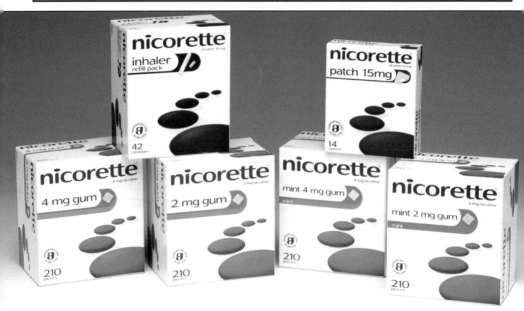

nicorette® beat cigarettes one at a time

NICOTINELL GUM
Novartis Consumer Health

PA No: Fruit 2mg: 30/21/4;
Fruit 4mg: 30/21/5; Mint
2mg: 30/21/6; Mint 4mg:
30/21/7

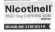

🔲Fruit and mint flavoured
chewing gum. 2mg packs
contain 12, 24 or 96 pieces.
4mg packs contain 12, 24 or
96 pieces.

🔲2mg and 4mg nicotine in
fruit and mint flavours.

🔲For the relief of nicotine
withdrawal symptoms in nicotine
dependency as an aid to
smoking cessation. The 4mg
gum is particularly suitable
when severe withdrawal
symptoms are experienced.

🔲One piece of gum to be
chewed when the user feels the
urge to smoke. Normally 8-12
pieces per day up to a
maximum of 25 pieces of 2mg
gum per day or 15 pieces of
4mg gum per day. After 3
months the user should gradually
cut down the number of pieces
chewed.

🔲For use in pregnancy or
whilst breastfeeding only on
medical advice.

Pharmacy only: Yes

NICOTINELL LOZENGE
Novartis Consumer Health

PA No: 30/21/8

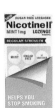

🔲Packs of 12, 36 or 96 mint-
flavoured lozenges.

🔲Nicotine 1mg.

🔲Relief of nicotine withdrawal
symptoms in nicotine
dependency as an aid to
smoking cessation.

🔲Adults: 1 lozenge to be
sucked when the user feels the
urge to smoke. Initially, 1
lozenge should be taken every
1-2 hrs. The usual dosage is 8-
12 lozenges per day. Maximum
25 lozenges in 24 hrs.

🔲For use in pregnancy or while
breastfeeding only on medical
advice.

Pharmacy only: Yes

If Symptoms Persist Consult Your Doctor

NICOTINELL PATCH
Novartis Consumer Health

PA No: TTS10: 30/21/1;
TTS20: 30/21/2; TTS30:
30/21/3

📱Round, flat, self-adhesive, transdermal patch. NICOTINELL TTS 10, 20, 30: Average absorption rate of 7, 14 and 21mg nicotine per 24 hrs respectively. Packs of 7 patches (TTS 10, 20, 30).

Packs of 21 patches (TTS 30 only).

Also available in 2-day starter packs (TTS 20 and TTS 30 only).

📱For the treatment of nicotine dependence as an aid to smoking cessation.

📝Adults: Individuals smoking 20 cigarettes or more a day: It is recommended that treatment be started with NICOTINELL TTS 30 once daily, applied to a dry, non-hairy area of the skin on the trunk or upper arm. Those smoking less than 20 daily: Start with NICOTINELL TTS 20. Sizes of 30cm², 20cm² and 10cm² are available to permit gradual withdrawal of

nicotine replacement, using treatment periods of 3-4 weeks for each size. Maximum continuous treatment period: 3 months. Patch size may be adjusted according to individual response, maintaining or increasing the dose if abstinence is not achieved or if withdrawal symptoms are experienced.

❗Not recommended for use during pregnancy or breastfeeding.

Pharmacy only: Yes

NIQUITIN CQ
GlaxoSmithKline

PA No: 678/71/3

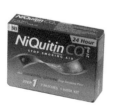

📱Niquitin CQ is a three step programme designed to support smoking cessation. Patches are designed to supply the body with the correct amount of nicotine, which decreases from step 1 to step 3.

📱Each 22cm² patch, for application to the skin, contains 114mg nicotine, and delivers 21mg of nicotine in 24 hrs. Each patch also contains ethylene/vinyl acetate copolymer, polyethylene/aluminium/ polyethylene terephthalate layer, polyethylene film, polyisobutyene and printing ink.

📱An aid to smoking cessation.

📝Those who smoke more than 10 cigarettes a day should start with step 1 for 6 weeks, then step 2 for 2 weeks, and step 3 for 2 weeks.

❗Not suitable for children under 18 yrs.

Not to be used by non-smokers or occasional smokers; by those with serious heart disease or who have had a recent stroke; with other nicotine-containing patches or gum.

Pharmacy only: Yes

Always Read The Label

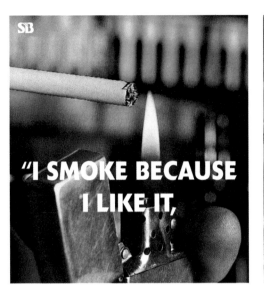

"I SMOKE BECAUSE I LIKE IT,

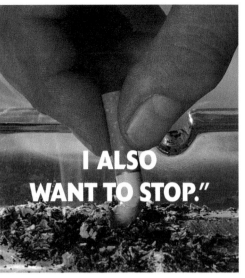

I ALSO WANT TO STOP."

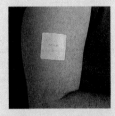
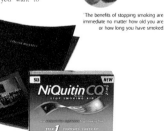

STOMACH UPSETS

CONSTIPATION

Constipation is defined as the infrequent passage of a hard motion. It may be accompanied by a sensation of incomplete evacuation of the bowel or discomfort felt in the lower part of the abdomen or the anus. It is important to recognise that regularity rather than frequency of bowel habit is what matters. 'Normal' frequency of defaecation may range from three times per day to once every three days.

The causes of constipation are too numerous to list here but among the most important are insufficient fibre and/or fluid intake, lack of exercise or immobility, medicines, pregnancy, diabetes, or an underactive thyroid gland. Travelling may also interfere with a regular bowel habit. If there is an identifiable cause for your constipation, it is best to treat this cause first.

Irritable bowel syndrome (IBS) is a disorder in which constipation, abdominal discomfort or pain, and a feeling of bloating or incomplete evacuation are prominent symptoms. Constipation may alternate with diarrhoea. It is estimated that up to 20% of the population suffer from IBS to some degree.

Treatment of constipation

If you are constipated, you need to firstly increase the **fibre** content of your diet, because fibre swells in contact with water and produces a softer, more easily passed stool. However, some people find high fibre cereals unpalatable, and a dietary approach may not be enough to cure constipation if it occurs as a side effect of some medicines. If you do not like high fibre cereal, an alternative is provided by medicines which contain material that is not digested (**ispaghula** or **methyl-cellulose**) and which work in the same way as fibre.

Laxative medicines

Herbal products which have been used as laxatives for a long time, and have a relatively gentle action, include **senna** and **frangula**. These substances, as well as **sodium picosulphate** and **lactulose**, are broken down by natural bacteria in the lower part of the bowel and therefore take 10-12 hours to work. **Bisacodyl** is a stronger laxative medicine with a slightly faster action when taken by mouth. In suppository form it acts faster still. **Magnesium hydroxide** (see **Indigestion and Heartburn**) also works as a laxative. **Liquid paraffin** and **glycerol** lubricate the passage of the motion and glycerol also increases its water content, making it softer.

Enemas containing some of the above ingredients are available but it is best to seek medical advice before using these.

Caution

Because the range of medicines sold as laxatives is confusing, you may wish to ask your pharmacist for advice as to which product best suits your particular need.

Unless there is a particular medical need, such as the regular consumption of prescription medicines which have constipation as a side effect, it should not be necessary to take laxatives on a regular basis.

Precautions and warnings

- Medicines containing ispaghula or methyl-cellulose should be taken with plenty of water, well before bedtime
- You may need to take fibre or lactulose for several days before they have a laxative effect

Always Consult Your Pharmacist

- Medicines taken by mouth containing senna, frangula, sodium picosulphate, lactulose and bisacodyl take time to work, so they are best taken last thing at night
- Do not use laxatives as a means of losing weight. The only weight lost is water and if you misuse laxatives continuously you may seriously damage your kidneys
- It is generally advised that children should not require regular laxatives. The routine administration of laxatives as a weekly ritual to clear the bowel should be discouraged
- Avoid laxatives containing sodium if you have high blood pressure and those containing magnesium if you have kidney disease (see **Indigestion and Heartburn**)
- Some laxative products contain sugar. Ask your pharmacist about this if you are diabetic.

BABYLAX
Pharma Global Ltd

PA No: *141/15/1*

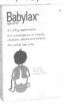

▭Applicators, containing faecal softener/lubricant.

▓Glycerol 1.8g, benzalkonium chloride 0.36g, 3.6g solution in rectal applicator.

▨Constipation in adults, the elderly and children of any age.

▨Adults and the elderly: 1-2 applicators.

Children: Under 3 months: ½-1 applicator. 3 months-6 yrs: 1 applicator. Over 6 yrs: 1-2 applicators.

▪For single use only.

Pharmacy only: Yes

CALIFIG
Merck Consumer Healthcare

PA No: *N/A*

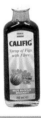

▭55ml or 110ml bottles, containing golden yellow liquid.

▓Sucrose, maltodextrin (soluble fibre 25% w/v), aqueous soft extract of figs (10% w/v), flavours (caramel, clove oil, peppermint oil, cassia oil), ginger tincture, preservative (sodium benzoate), citric acid monohydrate.

▨Helps maintain regularity and contains added fibre.

▨Adults: 15-30ml (1-2 tbsp).

Children: 1-3 yrs: 2.5-5ml (½-1 tsp). 3-6 yrs: 5-10ml (1-2 tsp). 6-15 yrs: 7.5-15ml (1 ½-3 tsp).

Pharmacy only: Yes

COLPERMIN
Pharmacia Consumer Healthcare

PA No: *936/6/1*

▭Packs of 20 or 100 peppermint oil capsules.

▓0.2ml peppermint oil.

▨For the relief of symptoms of irritable bowel syndrome,

including abdominal pain, bloating and diarrhoea and/or constipation.

▨Adults: 1 capsule 3 times daily, taken 30-60 mins before food, with a small quantity of water. The capsules should not be taken immediately after food. The dose may be increased to 2 capsules 3 times daily when discomfort is

more severe.

▪Children: There is no experience of the use of these capsules in children under the age of 15 yrs.

Not recommended for use by those allergic to menthol, or those with heartburn.

Pharmacy only: Yes

If Symptoms Persist Consult Your Doctor

DULCO-LAX
Boehringer Ingelheim Self Medication

PA No: 7/54/1

⬛Packs of 10, 20 or 60 tablets.

🔻Bisacodyl 5mg.

💬For the relief of constipation.

⬛If laxatives are needed every day, or there is persistent pain, consult your doctor. Avoid prolonged use.

Pharmacy only: Yes

DULCO-LAX PERLES
Boehringer Ingelheim Self-Medication

PA No: 7/55/2

⬛Packs of 50 microcapsules.

🔻Sodium picosulphate 2.5mg.

💬Laxative.

✏Adults: 2-4 capsules to be taken before bed.

⬛Do not take if you are pregnant, are planning to

become pregnant, or are under the age of 10 yrs unless instructed by doctor.

Pharmacy only: Yes

DULCO-LAX SUPPOSITORIES
Boehringer Ingelheim Self-Medication

PA No: 5s: 7/54/2; 10s: 7/54/3; 50s: 7/54/3

⬛Packs of 5 x 5mg, 10 x 10mg or 20 x 10mg suppositories.

🔻Bisacodyl.

💬Laxative.

✏Adults and children over 10 yrs: 1 x 10mg suppository.

Children under 10 yrs: 1 x 5mg suppository under medical supervision only.

⬛Do not take if you are pregnant or planning to become pregnant. If laxatives are required daily, consult your

doctor.

Pharmacy only: Yes

DUPHALAC SOLUTION
Solvay Healthcare Ltd

PA No: 108/15/1

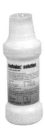

⬛300ml or 1 litre bottles, containing colourless/brownish-yellow, clear or not more than slightly opalescent solution.

🔻Lactulose 3.35g/5ml, lactose 0.35g/5ml and galactose 0.55g/5ml.

💬For treatment of constipation.

✏Adults and the elderly: Constipation: Initially 15ml twice daily.

Children: Constipation: 6-10 yrs: 10ml twice daily. 2-5 yrs: 5ml twice daily.

⬛May be used during pregnancy when considered

necessary by a physician.

Unlikely to adversely affect diabetics.

Pharmacy only: Yes

FYBOGEL ORANGE
Reckitt Benckiser

PA No: Orange: 979/9/2

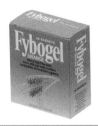

Packs of 10 or 30 sachets, containing buff coloured granules.

Ispaghula husk 3.5g.

For patients requiring a high fibre regimen.

Adults: 1 sachet morning and evening.

Children 6-12 yrs: ½-1 level 5ml spoonful of the granules (depending on age and size),

morning and evening. Children under 6 yrs: To be taken at doctor's advice: ½-1 level 5ml spoonful of the granules, (depending on age and size), morning and evening.

Pharmacy only: Yes

GLYCERINE SUPPOSITORIES
Martindale Pharmaceuticals

PA No: 396/7/3

12 x 4g suppositories. Also available as Glycerine Children's Suppositories and Glycerine Infant's Suppositories.

Glycerine 2.8g.

For treatment of constipation.

Adults: 1 as required.

Children under 12 yrs: Use children's formulation.

Pharmacy only: Yes

LAXOBERAL
Boehringer Ingelheim Self Medication

PA No: 100ml: 429/3/1; 30ml: 435/0/73

100ml or 300ml bottles, containing clear, yellowish-orange, fruit-flavoured liquid.

Sodium picosulphate 5mg per 5ml.

For the relief of constipation, either recent or chronic; whenever a stimulant laxative is required.

Adults: 5-15ml at night.

Children: 5-10 yrs: 2.5-5ml at night. 2-5 yrs: 2.5ml at night.

Should not be taken by those with undiagnosed abdominal pain or where intestinal obstruction is suspected.

Pharmacy only: Yes

LAXOSE
Pinewood Healthcare

PA No: 281/79/1

100ml, 300ml, 500ml or 1 litre bottles, containing colourless to brownish yellow, clear to slightly opalescent liquid.

Lactulose 3.3g per 5ml.

Constipation.

Adults: 15ml twice daily. Children: 5-10 yrs: 10ml twice daily. Children 2-5 yrs: 5ml twice daily.

Pharmacy only: Yes

MICROLAX
Pharmacia Consumer Healthcare

PA No: 936/4/1

Boxes of 4, 12 or 50 x 5ml microenemas.

A non-irritant faecal softener for the treatment of constipation.

Adults: One microenema when constipated.

Children: In children under the age of three, insert only half the nozzle length.

Not recommended for use in inflammatory bowel disease conditions.

Pharmacy only: Yes

Always Consult Your Pharmacist

MILK OF MAGNESIA
GlaxoSmithKline
PA No: 622/10/2

White liquid.

100ml or 300ml bottles containing 415mg of Magnesium hydroxide per 5ml spoonful.

For the relief of indigestion and constipation.

Adults: Indigestion: 5-10ml, maximum 60ml in 24 hrs. Constipation: 30-45ml at bedtime.

Children: Indigestion: 6-12 yrs: 5ml, maximum 30ml in 24 hrs. Constipation: Over 2 yrs: 5-10ml at bedtime.

Do not exceed the stated dose. Not suitable for use by those with kidney disease.

Pharmacy only: Yes

MILPAR
Merck Consumer Healthcare
PA No: 622/11/1

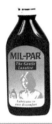

200ml or 500ml bottles of liquid.

Magnesium hydroxide 300mg, liquid paraffin 1.25ml per 5ml.

For the relief of constipation.

Adults: 15-30ml before breakfast or at bedtime.

Children: Over 7 yrs: 7.5-15ml at bedtime. 2-7 yrs: 5-10ml at bedtime.

Not recommended for children under 2 yrs.

Consult doctor before taking if suffering from kidney disease.

Pharmacy only: Yes

REGULAN, LEMON/ LIME FLAVOUR
Procter & Gamble (Health & Beauty Care) Limited
PA No: 441/34/1

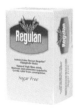

Premeasured, single-dose sachets of lemon and lime-flavoured, beige, fine ground powder, for oral solution to be reconstituted with water.

Isphagula husk 3.4g BP.

For the treatment of constipation and for patients who need to increase their daily fibre intake.

Adults: Usual dosage is the entire contents of 1 sachet taken 1-3 times daily.

Children 6-12 yrs: A reduced dosage based upon age and size of the child should be given: ½-1 level 5ml spoonful 1-3 times daily.

Regulan should always be taken as a liquid suspension and should be drunk immediately after mixing. The last dose should not be taken immediately before going to bed. May cause allergic reactions in people sensitive to inhaled or ingested isphagula powder.

It may be advisable to supervise treatment in the elderly or debilitated.

Contains 3mg of phenylalanine and this should be considered by phenylketonuric patients.

Pharmacy only: No

If Symptoms Persist Consult Your Doctor

REGULAN, ORANGE FLAVOUR
Procter & Gamble (Health & Beauty Care) Limited

PA No: 441/34/2

▣Premeasured, single-dose sachets of orange-flavoured, beige, fine ground powder, for oral solution to be reconstituted with water.

☑Isphagula husk 3.4g BP.

▣For the treatment of constipation and for patients who need to increase their daily fibre intake.

☑Adults: Usual dosage is the entire contents of 1 sachet taken 1-3 times daily.

Children 6-12 yrs: A reduced dosage based upon age and size of the child should be given: ½-1 level 5ml spoonful 1-3 times daily.

▮Regulan should always be taken as a liquid suspension and should be drunk immediately after mixing. The last dose should not be taken immediately before going to bed. May cause allergic reactions in people sensitive to inhaled or ingested isphagula powder.

It may be advisable to supervise treatment in the elderly or debilitated.

Contains 3mg of phenylalanine and this should be considered by phenylketonuric patients.

Pharmacy only: No

SENOKOT SYRUP
Reckitt Benckiser

PA No: 979/16/1

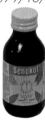

▣100ml bottle, containing brown, fruit-flavoured syrup.

☑Senna 7.5mg per 5ml.

▣Occasional use in the management of constipation.

☑Adults: 5-10ml taken at bedtime.

Pharmacy only: Yes

SENOKOT TABLETS
Reckitt Benckiser

PA No: 979/16/2

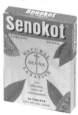

▣Blister packs of 20, 60 or 100 small, greenish-brown tablets.

☑Standardised senna 7.5mg per tablet.

▣Occasional use in the management of constipation.

☑Adults: 2 tablets at bedtime.

▮Children under 12 yrs: Consult your doctor (or only on medical advice).

Pharmacy only: Yes

DIARRHOEA

In a healthy adult, a brief bout of diarrhoea is usually more of a nuisance than a threat. In infants and the elderly however, it should be taken seriously because babies and the elderly are at greater risk of suffering from dehydration. Dehydration is the major problem associated with diarrhoea and it can cause serious illness. Therefore, you should always seek medical advice if infants or the elderly are affected. If you experience diarrhoea immediately after foreign travel, contact your doctor. If diarrhoea is prolonged (more than 24-48 hours), contact your doctor. If you pass blood in your diarrhoea, contact your doctor straight away.

Treatment of diarrhoea

Since the main danger of diarrhoea is dehydration, it is very important to maintain your **fluid** and **salt** intake. Diarrhoea causes a loss of salts, which are important for maintaining the natural salt balance in the body. Specially formulated **oral rehydration salts** provide a balanced mixture of salts. These are usually available in sachets, and should be diluted with water and sipped slowly. Flat Seven-Up, though a popular folklore remedy, does not provide this salt balance and is not recommended.

Today diarrhoea is seen as a natural protective mechanism which rids the bowel of infection or irritants. Your diarrhoea will usually stop in a few hours if the advice given above is followed. If absolutely necessary, salt replacement can be supplemented with an additional medicine which slows bowel movement. **Loperamide** is used for this purpose. **Kaolin** is a traditionally used remedy which provides bulk in the bowel and which is said to absorb toxins.

Caution

Many episodes of diarrhoea are caused by viruses rather than bacteria and will therefore not respond to antibiotics. Do not use antibiotics as an initial treatment for diarrhoea. In fact, some antibiotics may actually cause diarrhoea by upsetting the natural balance of bacteria in the intestine.

Precautions and warnings

- Seek medical advice if infants or the elderly are affected
- See your doctor if diarrhoea lasts more than 48 hours, if bleeding occurs or if you have recently returned from overseas
- If you are pregnant or breastfeeding avoid loperamide
- Avoid loperamide if you have an inflammatory bowel disease, such as ulcerative colitis, or liver disease.

ARRET CAPSULES

Janssen Pharmacy Healthcare

PA No: 748/22/1

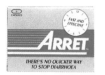

☐ Packs of 6 or 12 brown and turquoise, hard, gelatin capsules.

☑ Loperamide hydrochloride.

▨ For the treatment of acute diarrhoea, together with fluid and electrolyte replacement.

▨ Adults: 2 capsules initially then 1 after each episode of diarrhoea.

Children: Over 12 yrs: 2 capsules initially then 1 after each episode of diarrhoea.

Pharmacy only: Yes

Always Consult Your Pharmacist

DIORALYTE SACHETS
Aventis Pharma Ltd

PA No: Plain: 468/1/1;
Blackcurrant: 468/34/1;
Citrus: 468/34/2

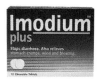

Carton containing 20 sachets of powder for reconstitution.

Sodium chloride Ph Eur 0.47g, potassium chloride Ph Eur 0.30g, disodium hydrogen citrate Ph Eur 0.53g, glucose Ph Eur 3.56g, silicon dioxide Ph Eur 0.009g and saccharine sodium Ph Eur 0.006g.

Fast and effective treatment of lost water and body salts in infants, children and adults.

Adults: The contents of each sachet should be dissolved in 200ml of fresh drinking water. The solution should be made up immediately before use and stored for no longer than 24 hrs.

Children: The contents of each sachet should be dissolved in 200ml of fresh drinking water. For infants and where drinking water is unavailable, water should be freshly boiled and cooled.

Sachets should be stored in a cool dry place below 20°C. There are no known contra-indications to Dioralyte. However, there may be a number of conditions where treatment is inappropriate, e.g. intestinal obstruction requiring surgery. Cow's milk and artificial milk feeds in infants should be stopped for 24 hrs and gradually re-introduced.

Pharmacy only: Yes

ELECTROLADE
Eastern Pharmaceuticals/ Intra Pharma Ltd

PA No: Banana: 739/1/1;
Blackcurrant: 739/1/3;
Melon: 739/001/002;
Orange: 739/1/4

Sachets of oral rehydration powder in a variety of flavours.

Sodium chloride 236mg, potassium chloride 300mg, sodium bicarbonate 500mg, anlysous dextrate 4g.

Fluid and mineral replacement following diarrhoea or vomiting.

Adults: 1-2 sachets, total 16 in 24 hrs.

Children: 1 sachet, total 12 in 24 hrs.

Children under 2 yrs should be under medical supervision. If symptoms persist, consult a doctor.

Pharmacy only: Yes

IMODIUM PLUS
Janssen Pharmacy Healthcare

PA No: 755/3/1

Packs of 12 chewable tablets.

Loperamide hydrochloride 2mg, simethicone 125mg.

Stops diarrhoea. Also relieves stomach cramps, wind and bloating.

Adults: 2 tablets initially.

Children: 12-18 yrs: 1 tablet initially, followed by 1 tablet after each bowel movement.

Pharmacy only: Yes

If Symptoms Persist Consult Your Doctor

RAPOLYTE
ERGHA Healthcare Ltd

PA No: 294/10/1

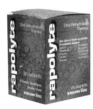

Packs of 25 foil laminated sachets containing a white powder with a raspberry odour.

Potassium chloride 0.30g, sodium citrate 0.60g, sodium chloride 0.35g, anhydrous glucose 4.0g.

Oral rehydration for the correction of fluid and electrolyte loss in the management of watery diarrhoea.

Adults and children over 12 yrs: The contents of a single sachet reconstituted in 200ml of freshly boiled and cooled water. The solution must not be boiled after reconstitution. The solution is given ad lib for 4 to 6 hrs then as required for fluid replacement.

Infants: The solution is substituted for milk feed.

Pharmacy only: Yes

REHIDRAT LEMON/LIME, REHIDRAT ORANGE
Pharmacia Consumer Healthcare

PA No: 778/9/1, 778/9/2

Packs of 24 foil laminate sachets containing either a greyish-white powder with green particles, or a white granular powder with yellow particles.

Sodium chloride 0.44g, potassium chloride 0.38g, sodium bicarbonate 0.42g, citric acid 0.44g, glucose 4.09g, sucrose 8.07g.

Oral rehydration therapy for the prevention and correction of fluid and electrolyte loss in the management of diarrhoea.

Adults and children over 12 yrs: The contents of 1 sachet should be dissolved in 250ml drinking water. The solution should be freshly made prior to use. The solution is given ad lib over 4-6 hours, then as required for fluid replacement.

Infants: Dissolve 1 sachet in 250ml freshly boiled water and substitute for milk feed.

Pharmacy only: Yes

INDIGESTION AND HEARTBURN

Unfortunately, indigestion is a very common experience. If you eat a very large meal or one with a high fat content, if you drink alcohol with your meal and if you also smoke, you are likely to pay for it later, since these are the risk factors for indigestion and heartburn.

Indigestion is often accompanied by upward movement (**reflux**) of the acidic stomach contents into the tube which connects the mouth to the stomach (the oesophagus). This produces the burning sensation in the centre of the chest known as heartburn. Up to 30% of people over 50 years old suffer occasionally from indigestion/heartburn and usually this is of no medical significance. If you are a sufferer, lifestyle changes such as weight loss, avoiding foods which are associated with your symptoms and stopping smoking may reduce the problem.

Heartburn often occurs in the later stages of pregnancy because of the hormonal changes that occur in pregnancy and because of the physical presence of the developing infant. Heartburn at night, which comes on after lying down in bed, may be associated with hiatus hernia, a tear in the muscle surrounding the lower part of the oesophagus. Heartburn is a common condition in middle age which can often be helped by the lifestyle changes mentioned above, and avoiding late night meals or, if necessary, raising the head of the bed.

If your symptoms are persistent or severe, or if you have any difficulty in swallowing, it is important to seek medical advice.

Treatment of indigestion and heartburn

Antacids are the most common form of over the counter (OTC) treatment. The stomach produces a strong acid (hydrochloric acid) after a meal, which can irritate the stomach lining. Antacids are alkaline substances which can neutralise this excess acid. Numerous antacids are available, including **calcium** or **magnesium carbonate, sodium bicarbonate, aluminium hydroxide, magnesium trisilicate** and **magnesium hydroxide**.

Caution re antacids

Some prescribed medicines are specially made to release their active ingredients into the bowel rather than into the stomach. This release is triggered by the relatively alkaline conditions in the bowel, so taking antacids at the same time as these medicines may trigger this release prematurely. Some antacids will also prevent certain prescribed medicines from being absorbed, and will therefore greatly reduce their effect. If you are taking prescribed medicines, you should therefore consult your pharmacist before taking antacids.

If you have high blood pressure you should avoid antacids which contain sodium (salt) because increased salt intake raises blood pressure. If you have kidney disease, you should avoid antacids containing magnesium because damaged kidneys may not be able to fully remove the additional magnesium from the bloodstream.

Stopping acid production

Recently, substances which are very powerful inhibitors of acid production have become available as OTC treatments for indigestion. These include **famotidine** and **ranitidine**. These substances stop acid production for a longer period. Medicines containing higher doses of these substances are available on prescription to treat ulcers.

Caution

If you have an ulcer, do not use these OTC preparations as substitutes for your prescribed ulcer treatment. The best way to avoid indigestion is with sensible eating habits. It is not a good idea to take one of these very strong substances as a preventive before binge eating.

Always Consult Your Pharmacist

HEARTBURN

If you have heartburn, look for a product which contains **alginate** or **alginic acid**. This forms a viscous barrier which floats on the surface of the stomach contents. This barrier helps to prevent reflux into the oesophagus.

WIND (FLATULENCE)

If wind or bloating is a particular problem, an **antiflatulent** agent may help. Examples of such agents are **dimethicone** and **simethicone**. Another way to treat bloating is to speed up the passage of food through the stomach. **Domperidone** is a substance which does this.

Precautions and Warnings

- Prescribed medicines which include iron, and some medicines used to treat asthma and arthritis, may cause indigestion or heartburn
- Antacids may interfere with the absorption of some prescribed medicines
- Antacids may cause the premature release of active ingredients from some prescribed medicines
- If you are taking prescribed medicines, consult your pharmacist before taking antacids or domperidone
- Do not take antacids and domperidone at the same time
- Avoid medicines containing sodium if you have high blood pressure
- Avoid medicines containing magnesium if you have kidney disease
- If you have severe liver or kidney disease do not take domperidone except under medical supervision
- If you are pregnant or breastfeeding, antacids, alginate and antiflatulent agents are safe to take. Other medicines should be avoided.

ACIDEX
Pinewood Healthcare

PA No: 281/75/1

200ml or 500ml bottles, containing pink, aniseed-flavoured suspension. Gluten and sugar free.

Each 5ml contains sodium bicarbonate BP 133.5mg, sodium alginate BP 250mg, calcium carbonate BP 80mg.

Each 10ml contains 141mg sodium.

For the management of reflux disease, hiatus hernia and heartburn of pregnancy.

Adults and children over 12 yrs: 2-4 5ml spoonfuls.

Children 6-12 yrs: 1-2 5ml spoonfuls.

Not recommended for children under 6 yrs.

Doses should be taken after meals and at bedtime.

Do not take in the case of incipient cardiac, liver or kidney failure and hypertension.

Pharmacy only: Yes

ACIDOPINE
Pinewood Healthcare

PA No: 976/3/1

Packs of 6 or 12 x 10mg mottled round uncoated tablets embossed with F1 10 on one side and plain on reverse.

Each tablet contains 10mg famotidine.

Short-term relief of heartburn and/or excess acid.

Adults and children 16 yrs and older: 10mg when necessary to relieve symptoms associated with eating and drinking 15 minutes before a meal.

When symptoms may be expected to disturb sleep: 1 hr before the evening meal.

Maximum dosage per 24 hrs: 20mg.

Do not take in cases of moderate or severe kidney failure, liver impairment, or history of gastroduodenal ulcer or reflux oesophagitis.

Pharmacy only: Yes

If Symptoms Persist Consult Your Doctor

ANDREWS ANTACID
GlaxoSmithKline

PA No: 678/48/1

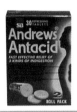

Packs of 30 or 60 tablets.

Calcium carbonate Ph Eur 600mg, heavy magnesium carbonate Ph Eur 125mg per tablet.

For the relief of acid indigestion, heartburn and trapped wind.

Adults: Suck or chew 1-2 tablets as required. Maximum 12 tablets in 24 hrs.

Not recommended for children.

Do not exceed the stated dose.

Not suitable for use by those with kidney disease.

Pharmacy only: No

ANDREWS ANTACID FRUIT FLAVOUR
GlaxoSmithKline

PA No: 678/48/2

Packs of 30 fruit-flavoured tablets.

Calcium carbonate Ph Eur 600mg, heavy magnesium carbonate Ph Eur 125mg per tablet.

For the relief of heartburn, acid indigestion and trapped wind.

Adults: Suck or chew 1-2 tablets as required. Maximum 12 tablets daily.

Children: Not recommended.

Do not exceed the stated dose.

Not suitable for use by those with kidney disease.

Pharmacy only: No

ANDREWS LIVER SALTS
GlaxoSmithKline

PA No: 678/43/1

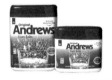

113g and 227g tins of powder.

Sodium bicarbonate Ph Eur 22.6%, citric acid Ph Eur 19.5%, magnesium sulphate Ph Eur 17.4% w/w.

For the relief of upset stomach, indigestion and constipation.

Adults: Indigestion: 5-10ml in water up to 4 times daily. Constipation: 10ml in water before breakfast or at bedtime.

Children: Over 6 yrs: Half adult dose. Not suitable for children under 6 yrs.

Do not exceed the stated dose.

Not suitable for use by those with kidney disease.

Pharmacy only: No

BISODOL ANTACID POWDER
Whitehall Laboratories Ltd

PA No: 172/10/1

50g or 100g packs of white, sugar-free powder with a slight odour and taste of peppermint.

Sodium bicarbonate 532mg, light magnesium carbonate 345mg, heavy magnesium carbonate 18mg per 5ml.

For the relief of symptoms of indigestion, heartburn, acidity and flatulence.

Adults: 1 level teaspoon stirred into $\frac{1}{3}$ of a tumbler of water after meals or as required.

Not suitable for use by those with kidney disease.

Consult doctor before use if pregnant or breastfeeding.

Pharmacy only: No

Always Read The Label

BISODOL EXTRA STRONG MINT TABLETS
Whitehall Laboratories Ltd

PA No: 172/10/4

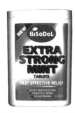

⬛Packs of 30 circular, smooth, white, bevel-edged tablets impressed 'BiSoDol ESM' on both sides.

⬛Sodium bicarbonate 64mg, calcium carbonate 522mg, light magnesium carbonate 68mg.

⬛Relief of symptoms of indigestion, heartburn, acidity and flatulence.

⬛Adults and children over 12 yrs: 1 or 2 tablets as required.

⬛Not suitable for use by those with kidney disease.

Antacids are known to reduce the absorption of certain medicines. This may be avoided if such drugs are not administered within 2 hours of taking Bisodol Extra Strong Mint tablets.

Pharmacy only: No

BISODOL TABLETS
Whitehall Laboratories Ltd

PA No: 172/10/2

⬛Packs of 30 or 100 circular, smooth, white, bevelled tablets, marked 'BiSoDol' on both surfaces.

⬛Sodium bicarbonate 64mg, calcium carbonate 522mg, light magnesium carbonate 68mg.

⬛For the relief of symptoms of indigestion, heartburn, acidity and flatulence.

⬛Adults: 2 tablets as required.

⬛Not suitable for use by those with kidney disease.

If symptoms persist consult your doctor.

Pharmacy only: No

DENTINOX INFANT COLIC DROPS
DDD Ltd

PA No: 302/3/1

⬛100ml bottle, containing translucent, white, emulsified liquid with aroma of dill.

⬛Activated dimethicone 21mg per 2.5ml dose.

⬛For the gentle relief of wind and griping pains caused by accumulation of ingested air.

⬛Infants from birth onwards: 2.5ml with or after each feed.

⬛If symptoms persist seek medical advice.

Pharmacy only: Yes

GAVISCON 250MG TABLETS
Reckitt Benckiser

PA No: Mint: 979/11/4;
Lemon: 979/11/5

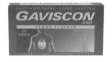

⬛Packs of 24 white, circular tablets, available in mint and lemon flavours.

⬛Alginic acid Ph Eur 250mg, sodium bicarbonate Ph Eur 85mg, aluminium hydroxide dried gel Ph Eur 50mg, magnesium trisilicate Ph Eur 12.5mg per tablet.

⬛Treatment of heartburn, indigestion and symptoms of reflux disease. Alginate is not absorbed and consequently can be taken during pregnancy and breastfeeding.

⬛Adults: 1-2 tablets after meals and at bedtime.

⬛Children under 12 yrs: Not recommended.

Pharmacy only: Yes

Always Consult Your Pharmacist

GAVISCON LIQUID
Reckitt Benckiser

PA No: Liquid: 979/15/3;
Suspension: 979/15/1

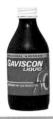

🔲 200ml or 500ml bottles, containing pink, fennel-flavoured suspension.

✅ Sodium alginate 500mg, sodium bicarbonate 267mg, calcium carbonate 160mg per 10ml dose.

❓ Treatment of heartburn, indigestion and symptoms of reflux disease. Alginate is not absorbed and consequently can be taken during pregnancy and breastfeeding.

✅ Adults and children over 12 yrs: 10-20ml after meals and at bedtime.

Children 6-12 yrs: 5-10ml after meals and at bedtime.

❗ Not recommended for children under 6 yrs.

Pharmacy only: Yes

GAVISCON LIQUID PEPPERMINT FLAVOUR
Reckitt Benckiser

PA No: 979/15/2

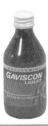

🔲 200ml bottles, containing white peppermint-flavoured suspension.

✅ Sodium alginate 500mg, sodium bicarbonate 267mg, calcium bicarbonate 160mg per 10ml dose.

❓ Treatment of heartburn, indigestion and symptoms of reflux disease. Alginate is not absorbed and consequently can be taken during pregnancy and breastfeeding.

✅ Adults and children over 12 yrs: 10-20mls after meals and at bedtime.

Children 6-12 yrs: 10mls after meals and at bedtime.

❗ Not recommended for children under 6 yrs.

Pharmacy only: Yes

GAVISCON TABLETS
Reckitt Benckiser

PA No: Mint: 979/11/2

🔲 Packs of 60 white, circular, mint-flavoured tablets (three tubes of 20 tablets per pack).

✅ Alginic acid Ph Eur 500mg, magnesium trisilicate Ph Eur 25mg, aluminium hydroxide dried gel Ph Eur 100mg, sodium bicarbonate Ph Eur 170mg per tablet.

❓ Treatment of heartburn, indigestion and symptoms of reflux disease. Alginate is not absorbed and consequently can be taken during pregnancy and breastfeeding.

✅ Adults and children over 12 yrs: 1-2 tablets after meals and at bedtime.

❗ Not recommended for children under 12 yrs.

Pharmacy only: Yes

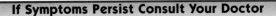

If Symptoms Persist Consult Your Doctor

MAALOX
Aventis Pharma

PA No: 468/16/4

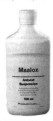

□500ml bottles of Maalox Suspension and packs of 50 Maalox No. 2 Tablets.

☑Suspension: Per 5ml: Dried aluminium hydroxide gel 225mg, magnesium hydroxide 200mg. Tablets: Dried aluminium hydroxide gel 400mg, magnesium hydroxide 400mg.

▣For relief of heartburn, indigestion and hyperacidity.

☑Adults and the elderly: 10-20ml or 1-2 tablets chewed 20-60 mins after meals and at bedtime.

Pharmacy only: Yes

MAALOX PLUS
Aventis Pharma

PA No: Suspension: 468/8/1; Tablets: 468/8/2

□355ml bottles of Maalox Plus Suspension (white, lemon/cream-flavoured oral suspension), and packs of 20 or 50 Maalox Plus Tablets (pale yellow/white tablet).

☑Suspension: Per 5ml: Dried aluminium hydroxide gel BP 220mg, magnesium hydroxide BP 195mg, simethicone 25mg. Tablets: Dried aluminium hydroxide gel BP 20mg, magnesium hydroxide BP 200mg, simethicone 25mg.

▣For relief of heartburn and indigestion. Contains simethicone as an antiflatulent for relief of wind.

☑Adults and the elderly:

Suspension: 5-10ml 4 times daily (after meals and at bedtime) or as required. Tablets: 1-2 tablets 4 times daily (after meals and at bedtime) or as required.

▣Should not be used in patients who are severely debilitated or suffering from kidney failure.

Pharmacy only: Yes

MILK OF MAGNESIA
GlaxoSmithKline

PA No: 622/10/2

□White liquid.

▣100ml or 300ml bottles containing 415mg of magnesium hydroxide per 5ml spoonful.

▣For the relief of indigestion and constipation.

☑Adults: Indigestion: 5-10ml, maximum 60ml in 24 hrs. Constipation: 30-45ml at bedtime.

Children: Indigestion: 6-12 yrs: 5ml, maximum 30ml in 24 hrs. Constipation: Over 2 yrs: 5-10ml at bedtime.

▣Do not exceed the stated dose.

Not suitable for use by those with kidney disease.

Pharmacy only: No

MOTILIUM TABLETS
Janssen Pharmacy Healthcare

PA No: 748/32/5

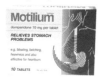

□Packs of 10 white, circular, biconvex, film-coated tablets marked with 'M/10' on one side and 'Janssen' on the other.

▣Domperidone 10mg.

▣For relief of stomach problems such as bloating, heaviness and belching; also for heartburn.

☑Adults: 1 tablet 3 times daily 15-30 mins before meals.

Children: Over 12 yrs: 1 tablet 3 times daily 15-30 mins before meals.

Pharmacy only: Yes

Always Read The Label

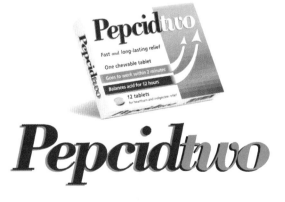

PEPCID AC
Janssen Pharmacy Healthcare

PA No: 755/1/1

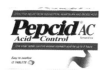

Packs of 6, 12 or 18 easy-to-swallow tablets.

10mg famotidine USP, hydroxypropylcellulose EP, magnesium stearate EP, hydroxypropyl methylcellulose EP, microcrystalline cellulose EP, pregelatinised maize starch BP, red iron oxide, talc EP, titanium dioxide EP.

For effective long-term relief from the symptoms of heartburn, indigestion and excess acid.

Adults (including the elderly) and children 16 yrs or older: 1 tablet to relieve symptoms, or 1 tablet 15 mins before eating to prevent symptoms for up to 12 hrs. Maximum 2 tablets in 24 hrs.

Not recommended for children under 16 yrs.

Do not take for more than 2 weeks continuously.

Consult a physician before taking these tablets if: you have unintended weight loss associated with indigestion; kidney or liver problems; any other illness; persistent stomach pains; you are middle-aged or older and have indigestion symptoms for the first time or symptoms that have recently changed; you are pregnant or breastfeeding; you are allergic to famotidine or any other ingredient in this product.

Pharmacy only: Yes

PEPCIDTWO
Janssen Pharmacy Healthcare

PA No: 755/4/1

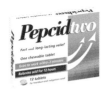

Packs of 6 or 12 mint-flavoured, chewable tablets.

Famotidine 10mg, calcium carbonate 800mg, magnesium hydroxide 165mg.

One chewable tablet provides relief from indigestion, heartburn and acid regurgitation or reflux symptoms. Pepcidtwo starts to neutralise acid within two minutes and balances acid for 12 hrs throughout the day or night.

Adults 16 yrs and over: Chew 1 tablet thoroughly and swallow, preferably with water. Repeat the dose if symptoms return.

Do not take more than 2 tablets in 24 hrs.

Not suitable for children under 16 yrs.

Pepcidtwo, like all indigestion remedies, is designed for short-term treatment of symptoms. Therefore, if after two weeks of continuously using Pepcidtwo you still suffer continuous symptoms, consult pharmacist or doctor before further treatment.

Pharmacy only: Yes

REMEGEL
SSL Healthcare Ireland Ltd

PA No: 618/38/1

Packs of 8 or 24 light green, soft, chewable tablets with a peppermint menthol taste.

Calcium carbonate 800mg.

For the relief of indigestion and heartburn.

Adults: Chew 1-2 pieces as symptoms occur. Repeat hourly as necessary up to a maximum of 12 pieces in 24 hrs.

Not recommended for children.

Pharmacy only: No

Always Consult Your Pharmacist

REMEGEL ALPINE MINT WITH LEMON
SSL Healthcare Ireland Ltd

PA No: 618/38/2

▣Packs of 8 or 12 light green, soft, chewable tablets with a mint and lemon-taste

▣Calcium carbonate 800mg.

▣For the relief of acid indigestion and heartburn.

▣Adults: Chew 1-2 pieces as symptoms occur. Repeat hourly if symptoms return up to a maximum of 12 pieces in 24 hrs.

▮Not recommended for children.

Pharmacy only: No

RENNIE DEFLATINE
Roche Consumer Health

PA No: 50/145/1

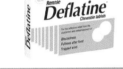

▣Packs of 18 white, round, chewable tablets with a mint and lemon flavour (3 foil strips per pack, 6 tablets per foil strip).

▣Simethicone USP 25mg, calcium carbonate Ph Eur 680mg, heavy magnesium carbonate Ph Eur 80mg.

▣For fast, effective relief from indigestion, the discomfort and embarrassment of bloatedness, fullness after food and trapped wind.

▣Adults: As soon as any discomfort is felt, suck or chew one or two tablets.

▮Not recommended for children.

Maximum dosage 16 tablets in one day. If taking antibiotics or other prescribed medicines consult your doctor or pharmacist before taking Rennie Deflatine.

Pharmacy only: No

RENNIE DIGESTIF
Roche Consumer Health

PA No: 32/20/3

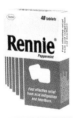

▣Roll wrap of 12 white, square, dimpled tablets with 'Digestif Rennie' stamped on both faces. Mint flavoured. Also available as blister packs of 24, 48 or 96 tablets.

▣Calcium carbonate 680mg, light magnesium carbonate 80mg, sucrose, saccharin (spearmint only).

▣For relief of acid indigestion, heartburn, acidity and flatulence.

▣Adults: 1-2 tablets to be sucked or chewed. Maximum of 16 tablets in 24 hrs.

▮Not recommended for children.

Pharmacy only: No

RENNIE DUO
Roche Consumer Health

PA No: 50/140/1

▣50ml, 180ml or 500ml bottles, containing peppermint-flavoured, cream-coloured liquid.

▣Calcium carbonate 600mg, magnesium carbonate 70mg, sodium alginate 150mg, sodium content 60mg/5ml.

▣For relief of heartburn and acid indigestion.

▣Adults and children over 12 yrs: 10ml after meals and at bedtime. Maximum 8 x 10ml doses per day.

▮Not recommended for children under 12 yrs.

Do not exceed the stated dose.

Not suitable for use by those with kidney disease.

Pharmacy only: Yes

If Symptoms Persist Consult Your Doctor

RENNIE RAP-EZE
Roche Consumer Health

PA No: 50/124/1

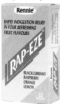

⬜Packs of 8 or 32 fruit-flavoured, coloured, square, dimpled tablets with 'Rap-Eze' stamped on one face and 'Rennie' on the other.

☑Calcium carbonate 500mg.

🔲Relief from indigestion, flatulence and indigestion during pregnancy.

🔲Adults: 1-2 tablets to be sucked or chewed. Maximum 16 tablets in 24 hrs.

🔲Not recommended for children.

Pharmacy only: No

ZANTAC 75™ DISSOLVE
GlaxoSmithKline

PA No: 44/76/10

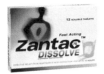

⬜Packs of 12 effervescent tablets.

☑Each tablet contains 75mg ranitidine hydrochloride.

🔲For the treatment of heartburn, excess acid and dyspepsia.

🔲Adults, the elderly and children 16 yrs and over: Dissolve 1 tablet completely in at least 75ml of water. Swallow all of the solution. If symptoms persist for more than 1 hr or return, another tablet can be taken.

🔲Do not take more than 2 tablets in 24 hrs. If symptoms persist for more than 2 weeks, consult your doctor.

Seek doctor's or pharmacist's advice before taking Zantac 75 Dissolve if you are allergic to any of the ingredients, have a peptic or duodenal ulcer, are pregnant or breastfeeding, have kidney or liver problems or are taking any other medication.

Pharmacy only: Yes

ZANTAC 75™ TABLETS
GlaxoSmithKline

PA No: 44/76/9

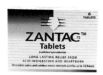

⬜Packs of 6, 12 or 24 tablets.

☑Ranitidine hydrochloride. Each tablet contains 75mg ranitidine as ranitidine hydrochloride.

🔲Effective relief from the symptoms of heartburn and acid indigestion for up to 12 hrs.

🔲Adults and children over 16 years: 1 tablet with water when symptoms occur. Dose may be repeated after 12 hrs if symptoms return.

🔲Do not take more than 2 tablets in 24 hrs.

If symptoms persist for more than 2 weeks, please consult your doctor.

Pharmacy only: Yes

Always Read The Label

WORM TREATMENT

Infection with **threadworms (enterobiasis)** is the most common worm infection in children. It is easily discovered because the usual sign of infection is a child scratching his or her bottom at night. This happens because the worms lay their eggs around the anus at night causing intense itching.

The infection can be picked up by eating food contaminated with threadworm eggs. Infection is easily transmitted if hygiene is poor because the scratching transfers the eggs to the fingers. If you look carefully, worms 3-8 millimetres in length can sometimes be seen moving in the child's bowel movements.

Treatment is necessary to stop the infection since some of the newly hatched worms will migrate from the anal area back into the intestine. If worm infection is not treated it may lead to loss of sleep, irritability, loss of appetite and weight loss. Infection in adults can occur but it is much less common.

Treatment of Threadworms

Threadworms can be treated with **piperazine**, which paralyses the worms and allows them to be expelled. To assist in their removal process, a **laxative (sennoside** from **Senna** - see **Constipation)** is incorporated into the product. The treatment must be repeated after 14 days to ensure complete elimination of the infection.

An alternative threadworm treatment is with **mebendazole**, which kills the worms. Because of the danger of re-infection, repeat treatment is again strongly recommended two and four weeks after the initial treatment.

Hygiene/Advice

Good hygiene is important in order to avoid re-infection. Children should be supervised to ensure that they wash their hands thoroughly. Pyjamas etc. should be thoroughly washed in a very hot wash. Do not be embarrassed about seeking advice from your pharmacist about worm infection. It is a common problem and it will be dealt with sympathetically and professionally.

TOXOCARIASIS

Toxocariasis is a common roundworm infection in puppies and it is occasionally seen in cats. Children may be infected through contact with eggs in soil or sandpits contaminated with dog or cat faeces. Infection through stroking the animals is unlikely because there is an incubation period of two weeks before the eggs of the worm become mature.

Although infection in humans often produces no symptoms and clears spontaneously without treatment, there is a danger that the worms may enter vital organs such as the eye where they may cause blindness, or the liver where they may cause significant damage.

Toxocariasis remains a serious public health issue in Europe. Blood tests which detect previous infection show that between 5% and 30% of the population have been infected. Therefore, prevention of toxocariasis is preferable to treatment. Do not allow young children to play in areas which are contaminated by dog or cat faeces. It is vital that any susceptible animals in your household are wormed regularly. This particularly includes young puppies or pregnant bitches, but worming of other dogs and domestic cats/kittens is also advisable. See your pharmacist or vet for advice.

OTHER WORM INFECTIONS

There are a variety of much less common worm infections which are often found in countries with warm or humid climates. Infection may be transmitted through contact with soil or from eating undercooked food - especially pork. These infections may not be associated with any obvious symptoms. Piperazine is effective against one such infection, namely hookworm, and mebendazole is effective against many different worm infections. However, because careful diagnosis is essential, you should not attempt to treat these more exotic infections on an over-the-counter basis.

Precautions and Warnings

- If you are breastfeeding or are pregnant, seek medical advice before taking any worm preparation
- Anyone with epilepsy should avoid piperazine
- If you are taking **cimetidine** on prescription, avoid mebendazole
- Seek medical advice if you think that you might have picked up a worm infestation after overseas travel.

PRIPSEN POWDER
SSL Healthcare Ireland Ltd

PA No: 618/31/1

☐Dual dose pack of powder.

☑Piperazine phosphate 4g, sennoside B (as total sennosides) 15.3mg.

☐For the eradication of threadworms and roundworms.

☑Adults and children over 6 yrs: 1 sachet repeated after 14 days.

Children: 1-6 yrs: $\frac{2}{3}$ of sachet. Infants: 3 months-1 yr: $\frac{1}{3}$ of sachet. All to be repeated after 14 days to eliminate reinfestation.

❗Special precautions: Breastfeeding, epilepsy.

Pharmacy only: Yes

VERMOX SUSPENSION
Janssen Pharmacy Healthcare

PA No: 545/15/1

☐30ml bottle, containing banana-flavoured, white suspension.

☑Mebendazole 20mg per ml.

❓Used to treat threadworms and roundworms. Kills worms. Also used under medical supervision to treat many other worm infections including those from areas with humid or tropical climcates.

☑Adults: 5ml (repeat treatment strongly recommended after 2 and 4 weeks).

❗Not for use during pregnancy or breastfeeding.

Pharmacy only: Yes

VERMOX TABLETS
Janssen Pharmacy Healthcare

PA No: 748/42/2

☐Packs of 6 orange-flavoured, sugar-free, chewable tablets.

☑Mebendazole 100mg.

❓Used to treat threadworms and roundworms. Kills worms. Also used under medical supervision to treat many other worm infections including those from areas with humid or tropical climcates.

☑Adults: 1 tablet (repeat treatment strongly recommended after 2 and 4 weeks).

❗Not for use during pregnancy and breastfeeding.

Pharmacy only: Yes

If Symptoms Persist Consult Your Doctor

Tonics have a long history of traditional use for the promotion of well-being in people who are debilitated, for example by illness or old age. There are two main groups of products, one containing a mixture of vitamins, minerals and bitter tasting substances, and the other containing the herbal product **ginseng**.

Evidence for the effectiveness of this category of medicines is not as clear cut as it is in many other cases. It is a fact, however, that many people feel better, even if they are given a medicine which contains no active ingredients. This 'placebo effect' is more powerful than is commonly recognised.

While there is some evidence for a specific beneficial effect of ginseng, herbal does not necessarily mean harmless. There is some evidence of an effect on hormone balance, blood pressure and blood sugar control.

Precautions and Warnings
- Do not take ginseng if you have high blood pressure, diabetes, or if you are pregnant.

EFFICO TONIC
Pharmax Ltd

PA No: 609/2/1

300ml or 500ml bottles of liquid, available in orange and mixed fruit flavours.

In 5ml: Vitamin B1 (thiamine) 0.18mg, nicotinamide 2.1mg, caffeine 20.2mg, gentian infusion 0.669% w/v.

A tonic when tired, listless or run down.

Adults: 10ml 3 times daily before meals.

Children over 6 yrs: 2.5-5ml 3 times daily before meals.

May be diluted with water.

Do not take Effico if pregnant or breastfeeding unless recommended by a doctor.

Pharmacy only: Yes

FERYBAR ELIXIR
Pinewood Healthcare

PA No: N/A

Iron tonic with liver extract.

Liver extract, thiamine, riboflavine, pyridoxine, nicotinamide, calcium pantothenate, sodium gylcerophosphate, potassium glycerophosphate, manganese sulphate, ferric ammonium, citric acid, ethanol.

May be helpful to those prone to anaemia, suffering blood loss or exhaustion.

Adults: 10-20ml 3 times daily.

Children: 5-10ml 3 times daily.

Pharmacy only: Yes

FOSFOR SYRUP
TP Whelehan Ltd

PA No: N/A

200ml bottle of raspberry-flavoured liquid. Amino acid compound.

Phosphorylcolamine.

For use during recovery from illness or surgery and when appetite is poor.

Adults: 20ml 3 times daily.

Children: 10ml 3 times daily.

Pharmacy only: Yes

Always Read The Label

METATONE TONIC
Pfizer/Warner Lambert Consumer Healthcare

PA No: 823/12/1

300ml bottle of clear, red syrup.

Thiamine hydrochloride 0.5mg, calcium glycerophosphate 45.6mg, potassium glycerophosphate 45.6mg, sodium glycerophosphate 22.8mg, manganese glycerophosphate NFX 697mg per 5ml.

For the management of convalescence and debility.

Adults: 5-10ml diluted 2-3 times daily before meals.

Children: Over 6 yrs: 5ml diluted 2-3 times daily before meals.

Pharmacy only: Yes

SEVEN SEAS VITAMIN & MINERAL TONIC
Seven Seas Ireland Ltd

PA No: N/A

150ml or 300ml bottles of orange-flavoured liquid.

Manganese sulphate monohydrate 0.76mg, vitamin D 130IU, copper sulphate 1mg, calcium glycerophosphate 22.5mg, potassium glycerophosphate solution 4.5mg, iron 24mg, vitamin A, alcohol 1,300IU.

Vitamin and mineral supplement.

Adults: 10ml 3 times daily after meals.

Pharmacy only: Yes

Always Consult Your Pharmacist

TRAVEL SICKNESS

Travel or motion sickness is thought to occur when the brain receives conflicting signals from the eyes and the organs of balance in the inner ear. The sort of motion that can occur during a sea journey is particularly likely to produce motion sickness. There is also a strong psychological component to feeling sick so that someone who has previously experienced motion sickness may be inclined to suffer on a subsequent occasion. Young infants do not get motion sickness so they do not require treatment.

Treatment

Effective medicines for motion sickness comprise either **hyoscine** or **antihistamines (dimenhydrinate, meclizine, cinnarizine)**. These are preventive rather than curative and should be taken before the journey as they are much less effective once vomiting starts. However, if vomiting has started, a useful tip is to dissolve a tablet under the tongue.

Hyoscine is particularly effective for short sea journeys but its effect only lasts for about three hours before a second dose is required. A second dose is likely to make your mouth dry and occasionally it may disturb vision. Antihistamines are longer acting, with cinnarizine and dimenhydrinate lasting four to six hours and meclizine lasting 12 hours or more. Your choice of treatment may therefore depend on the duration of your intended journey.

It is very important to bear in mind that antihistamines may cause drowsiness and are therefore not suitable if you intend to drive. Alcohol strongly increases this effect and should be absolutely avoided.

Precautions and Warnings

- Avoid hyoscine if you suffer from glaucoma or if you have a bladder or prostate problem
- Avoid antihistamines if you intend to drive or if you are taking any prescribed medicine that may cause sedation. If in doubt, ask your pharmacist
- Avoid alcohol if you are taking an antihistamine.

DRAMAMINE
Pharmacia Consumer Health
PA No: 936/5/1

⬜Pack of 10 white, round, biconvex tablets.

☑Dimenhydrinate BP 50mg.

▢For the treatment of motion sickness. To be taken half an hour before start of journey.

☑Adults: 1-2 tablets 2-3 times daily.

Children 7-12 yrs: ½-1 tablet 2-3 times daily.

❗May cause drowsiness.

Pharmacy only: Yes

JOY-RIDES
Stafford Miller/Intra Pharma
PA No: 125/1/1

⬜Carton containing 12 tablets, individually sealed in an aluminium foil strip.

☑0.15mg hyoscine hydrobromide EP.

▢For the treatment and prevention of travel sickness.

☑Adults: 2 tablets, repeated in 6 hrs if necessary, up to a maximum of 4 tablets in 24 hrs.

Children: 3-4 yrs: ½ a tablet, repeated in 6 hrs if necessary, up to a maximum of 1 tablet in 24 hrs. 4-7 yrs: 1 tablet, repeated in 6 hrs if necessary, up to a maximum of 2 tablets in 24 hrs. 7-12 yrs: 1-2 tablets, repeated in 6 hrs if necessary, up to a maximum of 2 tablets in 24 hrs. 13+: 2 tablets, repeated in 6 hrs if necessary, up to a maximum of 4 tablets in 24 hrs.

❗Children under 3 yrs: Do not take without consent of doctor.

Pharmacy only: Yes

If Symptoms Persist Consult Your Doctor

KWELLS
Roche Consumer Health

PA No: 32/12/2

◻Packs of 12 round, pinkish tablets, plain on one side with a breakline on the other.

◼Hyoscine hydrobromide

300µg.

◻For the treatment and prevention of travel sickness.

◪Adults: 1 tablet every 6 hrs, if required. Maximum 3 tablets in 24 hrs.

Tablets to be taken up to 30

mins before travelling or at onset of nausea.

◼Not to be taken by persons suffering from glaucoma or with hypersensitivity to hyoscine.

Pharmacy only: Yes

SEA-LEGS
SSL Healthcare Ireland Ltd

PA No: 618/36/1

◻Packs of 12 tablets.

◼Meclizine hydrochloride 12.5mg.

◻Travel sickness.

◪Adults: 2 tablets 1 hr before travel or the night before. Maximum 2 tablets in 24 hrs.

Children: 6-12 yrs: 1 tablet 1 hr before travel or the night

before. 2-6 yrs: ½ tablet 1 hr before travel or the night before.

◼Children under 2 yrs: Not recommended.

Pharmacy only: Yes

STUGERON TABLETS 15S
Janssen Pharmacy Healthcare

PA No: 545/19/3

◻Packs of 15 white, circular, biconvex tablets engraved with

S/15 on one side and Janssen on the other.

◼Cinnarizine 15mg.

◻For the prevention and control of motion sickness.

◪Adults: 2 tablets 2 hrs before travelling, then 1 tablet every 8

hrs during the journey.

Children: 5-12 yrs: Half adult dose.

◼Do not exceed the stated dose.

Pharmacy only: Yes

TRAVEL SICKNESS DEVICES

ROUND TRIP
Intrapharma/Sea Band

PA No: N/A

◻2 pairs of adhesive patches

per box.

◻Disposable patches use the principle of acupressure for effective relief of nausea

associated with travel.

◪Suitable for children.

Pharmacy only: Yes:

SEA BAND (TRAVEL AND MORNING SICKNESS)
Intrapharma/Sea Band

PA No: N/A

◻Box containing 1 pair of wristbands.

◻Effective use of acupressure in eliminating nausea associated with travel and morning sickness.

Pharmacy only: Yes

Always Read The Label

VAGINAL THRUSH

Vaginal thrush is an infection that most women will suffer from at some time in their life. Typically the symptoms consist of itching and a vaginal discharge, which is usually a thick white discharge (like cottage cheese or curdled milk) but is occasionally watery. It is usually odourless. Occasionally, the infection may cause burning or external pain in the vaginal area during urination and intercourse may be painful.

In about one-third of women, the yeast *Candida albicans* is found in the vagina. As with other Candidal infections, it does no harm unless circumstances arise which permit it to overgrow (see **Mouth Care – Thrush**). The organism is normally present in faeces. It may therefore be transferred to the vagina because of poor hygiene.

Minor injury during sexual intercourse may produce a flare-up but other trigger factors are often more important. These include diabetes, pregnancy, use of some higher dose oral contraceptives or oral steroid treatment, antibiotic treatment or a deficient immune system. Irritation, caused by the use of vaginal deodorants or wearing tight clothing, may also trigger infection.

Candidal infections are most common in women of childbearing age and are unusual in children or in women after the menopause. In women of childbearing age the vagina tends to be acidic. A natural bacterium (lactobacillus) converts carbohydrate generated in vaginal cells by an action of female hormone into lactic acid. While these acid conditions favour the overgrowth of Candida, the lactobacillus normally competes with it and keeps it in check.

Treatment

Treatment of vaginal thrush is by means of either a cream with a vaginal applicator or a pessary (tablet intended for insertion into the vagina) containing the anti-yeast agent **clotrimazole**. The treatment should be inserted as deeply as is comfortable. The pessaries are available for either three day dosage or in a single use dose.

Precautions and Warnings

- If you have not had thrush before, if you are unsure about whether you have thrush, or if you are pregnant seek medical advice
- If have thrush and you are under 16 or over 60, seek medical advice
- Seek medical advice if you have any pain other than external pain or if there is any bleeding
- If you have vaginal thrush more than twice in any six month period, consult your doctor, as repeated infection may indicate some causative factor which should be identified
- If symptoms do not disappear within seven days, seek medical advice
- Creams used to treat thrush may weaken some contraceptive devices.

CANESTEN 100MG PESSARY
Bayer Ltd

PA No: 21/4/1

■6 white pessaries sealed in a bubble pack and an applicator for insertion into the vagina. Patient information leaflet is included.

■Clotrimazole BP 100mg.

■Treatment of vaginal thrush.

■Adults: Insert 1 pessary into vagina daily, at night, for 6 consecutive days or 2 pessaries for 3 days.

■Not recommended for children.

Medical advice should be sought if the patient is suffering symptoms for the first time or is pregnant.

Pharmacy only: Yes

Always Consult Your Pharmacist

CANESTEN 200MG PESSARY

Bayer Ltd

PA No: 21/4/8

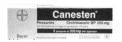

3 pessaries sealed in a bubble pack and an applicator for insertion into the vagina. Patient information leaflet included.

Clotrimazole BP 200mg.

Treatment of vaginal thrush.

Adults: Insert 1 pessary into the vagina daily, at night, for 3 consecutive days.

Not recommended for children.

Medical advice should be sought if the patient is suffering symptoms for the first time or is pregnant.

Pharmacy only: Yes

CANESTEN 500MG PESSARY

Bayer Ltd

PA No: 21/4/10

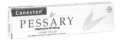

1 pessary sealed in foil and an applicator for insertion into the vagina. Patient information leaflet is included.

Clotrimazole BP 500mg.

Treatment of vaginal thrush.

Adults: Insert pessary into vagina at night using applicator.

Not recommended for children due to vaginal applicator.

Medical advice should be sought if the patient is suffering symptoms for the first time or is pregnant.

Pharmacy only: Yes

If Symptoms Persist Consult Your Doctor

VITAMINS, MINERALS AND NUTRITIONALS

VITAMINS

Carbohydrate, fat and protein are the main dietary constituents. However, if we are to thrive and maintain normal health we require a supply of other essential nutrients. Vitamins and minerals are examples of this. International authorities set recommended dietary allowances (RDAs) for vitamins and minerals which are reviewed from time to time. Within the European Union, the European Scientific Committee on Food is currently reviewing RDAs for a new Food Supplement Directive.

In most cases, a balanced diet will provide all the necessary vitamins and minerals. There are circumstances, however, when a supplement may be required. Such circumstances include pregnancy, where the additional demands of the developing infant must be catered for. In pregnancy, there is a particular additional requirement for **folic acid** because this substance is essential for the formation of nucleic acids. Nucleic acids are essential for cell division and for the growth of the developing infant. Most importantly, it has been shown that a deficiency of folic acid is associated with spina bifida.

It is therefore now regarded as essential that women who are planning to conceive take additional folic acid on a daily basis. Ideally, they should begin before they become pregnant, and should continue through the first three months of pregnancy when the development of the baby is at a critical stage. Despite the fact that this has been widely advertised, it is still clear that many would-be mothers are not doing as they should.

Folic acid is also used to treat a rare metabolic disease, homocysteinuria. It reduces abnormally high levels of the amino acid, homocysteine, which is associated with this disease. Blood levels of this amino acid vary within the normal population and a high blood level has been identified as a possible risk factor in heart disease. It is not yet clear whether additional folic acid intake will reduce the risk of heart disease.

Other circumstances in which additional vitamins may be useful include periods of rapid growth, such as in adolescence. Vitamin supplements may be needed if someone is not eating properly, for example an elderly person or an alcoholic. Vegetarians and vegans may also need to supplement their diet. Additional intake should, of course, be balanced and reasonable.

Precautions

Excessive intake of vitamins can be damaging since large doses can cause toxic effects. Excessive amounts of vitamins A and D in particular can cause such problems. It is not recommended that extra vitamin A should be taken in pregnancy because some substances which resemble vitamin A can cause birth defects. Some authorities go so far as recommending that pregnant women do not eat liver since it contains a large amount of vitamin A.

There is evidence that additional vitamin B6 (pyridoxine) may reduce premenstrual symptoms, at least on a temporary basis. However, there is also some controversy about it causing temporary nerve damage (tingling) if it is taken in large doses.

New Research about Vitamins

In recent times, evidence has arisen to suggest that certain reactive molecules, known as free

---

Always Read The Label

radicals – produced during normal body metabolism or by smoking – can damage tissues and are implicated in heart artery disease and in certain cancers. Some vitamins (A, C and E) have anti-oxidant activity and can mop up these free radicals.

Great excitement was generated when it was discovered that low blood levels of vitamin E in particular, but also vitamin C and beta-carotene (a substance in the body from which vitamin A is made) were associated with an increased risk of heart disease. Evidence was also found of links between lower blood levels of vitamin E and some cancers. However, the evidence that extra intake of these vitamins protects against cancer or heart disease is still not clear cut, even after very large trials have been conducted.

By comparison, there is much better evidence that an increased intake of oily fish such as salmon and mackerel, or fish oils, is beneficial in protecting against heart disease and an increased fruit, vegetable and fibre intake appears to give some protection against bowel cancer.

B COMPLEX VITAMINS

BECOSYM FORTE
Roche Consumer Health

PA No: 50/54/3

Packs of 100 tablets.

Vitamin B1 (thiamine hydrochloride) 15mg, vitamin B2 (riboflavine) 15mg, vitamin B6 (pyridoxine hydrochloride) 10mg, nicotinamide 10mg.

Vitamin B supplement.

Adults: 2-3 tablets daily.

Pharmacy only: Yes

BENERVA
Roche Consumer Health

PA No: 50/56/5

Tablets.

Vitamin B1 (thiamine hydrochloride) 50mg. Benerva compound: Vitamins B2, B3.

Vitamin B dietary supplement.

Adults and elderly: Mild chronic deficiency: 25mg daily.

Severe deficiency: 200-300mg daily.

Not recommended for children.

Pharmacy only: Yes

CARDIO-GUARD
Clonmel Healthcare

PA No: N/A

Packs of 28 tablets.

Folic acid 0.4mg.

To normalise homocysteine

levels in the blood.

One daily.

Pharmacy only: Yes

CLONFOLIC
Clonmel Healthcare

PA No: 126/95/1

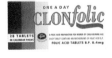

Calendar packs of 28 or 98 pale yellow, circular, biconvex tablets.

Folic acid 0.4mg.

For the prevention of first occurrence neural tube defects in the foetus. For use in patients who are planning a pregnancy.

Adults: 1 tablet daily.

Supplementation should begin 3 months before the woman conceives and be continued for at least the first 12 weeks of pregnancy.

Do not use if hypersensitive to folic acid or have vitamin B12 deficiency.

Pharmacy only: Yes

Always Consult Your Pharmacist

HEALTHCRAFTS VITAMIN B6 50MG 60S
Perrans Distributors Ltd

PA No: N/A

▣Packs of 60 tablets.

▣Dicalcium phosphate, microcrystalline cellulose, vitamin B6 (as pyridoxine hydrochloride) 50mg, hydrogenated vegetable oil, magnesium stearate.

▣Vitamin B6 supplement.

▣Adults: 1 tablet daily with food.

Pharmacy only: Yes

HEALTHCRAFTS VITAMIN B12 90S
Perrans Distributors Ltd

PA No: N/A

▣Packs of 90 tablets.

▣Dicalcium phosphate, microcrystalline cellulose, vitamin B12 (as cyanocobalamin prep.), hydrogenated vegetable oil, magnesium stearate.

▣Vitamin B12 supplement.

▣Adults: 1 tablet daily with food.

Children: Over 12 yrs: As per adult dose.

Pharmacy only: No

HEALTHCRAFTS VITAMIN B COMPLEX 30S
Perrans Distributors Ltd

PA No: N/A

▣Packs of 30 tablets.

▣Dicalcium phosphate, microcrystalline cellulose, soya fibre, tablet coating

(hydroxypropylmethylcellulose, glycerin), colours (iron oxides, titanium dioxide, talc), niacin 18mg (as niacinamide), hydrogenated vegetable oil, magnesium stearate, pantothenic acid 6mg (as calcium pantothenate), vitamin B6 2mg (as pyridoxine hydrochloride), thiamin hydrochloride 1.4mg, riboflavin 1.6mg, vitamin B12 1µg (as cyanocobalamin prep.), folacin 200µg (as folic acid), biotin 0.15mg.

▣Vitamin B complex supplement to help maintain healthy nervous, digestive and blood systems.

▣Adults: 1 tablet daily with food.

Pharmacy only: No

SANATOGEN B COMPLEX TABLETS
Roche Consumer Health

PA No: N/A

▣Bottles of 60 orange/peach-speckled, biconvex, film-coated tablets.

▣Vitamin B1 (thiamine) 12mg, vitamin B2 (riboflavin) 1.6mg, niacin 18mg, vitamin B6 2mg, folic acid 300µg, vitamin B12 2µg.

▣Vitamin B complex supplement.

▣Adults: 1 tablet daily.

Pharmacy only: Yes

SEVEN SEAS SUPER VITAMIN B6 CAPSULES
Seven Seas Ireland Ltd

PA No: 416/4/1

▣Packs of 60 pink, oval capsules.

▣Vitamin B6 (pyridoxine hydrochloride) 10mg + 40mg.

▣Vitamin B6 supplement.

▣Adults: 1 capsule daily with liquid.

Pharmacy only: 10mg: No, 40mg: Yes

SEVEN SEAS VITAMIN B COMPLEX WITH BREWER'S YEAST
Seven Seas Ireland Ltd

PA No: 416/2/1

▣Packs of 30 oval capsules.

▣Vitamin B12 (cyanocobalamin) 1µg, vitamin B1 (thiamine hydrochloride) 1.4mg, vitamin B2 (riboflavin) 1.6mg, vitamin B6 (pyridoxine hydrochloride) 2mg, nicotinic acid (niacin) 20mg, pantothenic acid 6mg, folic acid 40µg, biotin 0.15mg, inositol 5mg, brewer's yeast 100mg.

▣Vitamin B complex and folic acid supplement to help maintain healthy nervous, digestive and blood systems.

▣Adults: 1 capsule daily.

Pharmacy only: No

If Symptoms Persist Consult Your Doctor

VICKS VITAL
Procter & Gamble (Health & Beauty Care) Limited

PA No: N/A

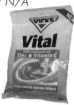

☐Orange- and lemon-flavoured liquid filled lozenges.

☑Per 4g lozenge: Vitamin C 20mg, zinc acetate 5mg, glucose syrup, sugar, water, glycerin, citric acid, flavourings, lactic acid, sodium lactate, menthol, colour: betacarotene, emulsifier: lecithin and vegetable oil.

☐Daily supplement to help maintain immune defence.

☑Adults and children over 6 yrs: 1-3 lozenges daily.

Pharmacy only: No

FISH OILS

EFAMOL EFAMARINE
Nutricia

PA No: N/A

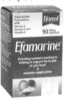

☐90 capsules in a jar contained within a cardboard carton.

☑2 capsules provides: Efamol pure evening primrose oil 860mg, Marine fish oil 214mg and vitamin E 20mg.

☐Dietary supplement providing nutrients involved in helping to support the health of the heart and joints. Triple action

formulation with omega 3, omega 6 and vitamin E.

☑2 capsules per day with food.

☐If you are using phenothiazine medication or have a history of epilepsy, consult your doctor before taking this medication.

Pharmacy only: No

HEALTHCRAFTS HIGH STRENGTH COD LIVER OIL
Perrans Distributors Ltd

PA No: N/A

☐Packs of 30 capsules.

☑Cod liver oil 1,000mg, eicosapentaenoic acid (EPA) 115mg, docosahexaenoic acid (DHA) 105mg, vitamin E 10mg (as d-alpha-tocopherol), vitamin A 800µg, vitamin D 5µg, capsule shell (gelatin, glycerin).

☐High strength vitamin

supplement to help maintain the health.

☑Adults: 1 capsule daily with food.

Children: As per adult dose.

Pharmacy only: No

OMEGA PLUS (EPO + FISH OIL) 60S
Intrapharma/Dugdale/Health Perception

PA No: N/A

☐Pack of 60 tablets.

☑Evening Primrose oil 500mg (45mg GLA), fish oil 500mg (90mg EPA, 60mg DHA).

☐Dietary supplement.

Pharmacy only: Yes

Always Read The Label

POWER HEALTH COD LIVER OIL ENRICHED WITH HALIBUT LIVER OIL
Power Health Products Ltd

PA No: N/A

🔲Pale, deep golden yellow, clear discap tin (spherical).

☑Cold-pressed cod and halibut liver oils providing 800µgs vitamin A and 5µgs vitamin D (on average).

☑Adults: 1 per day.

Children over 1 yr: 1 per day.

Pharmacy only: No

SEVEN SEAS ACTIVE 55 PURE COD LIVER OIL
Seven Seas Limited

PA No: N/A

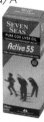

🔲300ml bottle containing a golden yellow liquid.

☑Cod liver oil enriched with fish oil omega 3 9.2g, omega 3 nutrients 2,800mg (providing EPA (eicosapentaenoic acid) and DHA (docosahexaenoic acid) 2,300mg), vitamin A (as palmitate prep) 800µg, vitamin D (as D3 prep) 5µg, vitamin E (dl a tocopheryl acetate) 10mg.

❓Helps to maintain healthy joints, fitness, health and vitality.

☑Adults: 10ml (2 tsps) daily.

Women who are pregnant, breastfeeding or likely to become pregnant: 5ml (1 tsp) daily.

Children over 12 yrs: 5ml (1 tsp) daily.

Pharmacy only: No

SEVEN SEAS ACTIVE 55 PURE COD LIVER OIL & GLUCOSAMINE
Seven Seas Limited

PA No: N/A

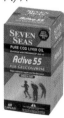

🔲Packs of 30 and 60 tablets.

☑Cod liver oil (triomega) blend 615mg, Omega 3 nutrients 200mg (providing EPA (eicosapentaenoic acid) and DHA (docosahexaenoic acid) 165mg), vitamin A (prep) 267µg, vitamin D (cholecalciferol) 1.67µg, vitamin E (dl a tocopheryl acetate) 1.37mg, glucosamine sulphate 100mg.

❓A special blend of health-promoting properties combining cod liver oil to help maintain all round general good health and healthy joints, plus the added benefit of glucosamine sulphate, which is involved in the formation and rebuilding of connective tissues such as cartilage.

☑Adults: 1 capsule daily.

Pharmacy only: No

SEVEN SEAS EXTRA HIGH STRENGTH COD LIVER OIL ONE-A-DAY
Seven Seas Ireland Ltd

PA No: N/A

🔲Packs of 30 or 60 capsules.

☑Cod liver oil enriched with fish oil Omega 3 (incl. EPA and DHA), vitamin A, vitamin D, vitamin E.

❓Helps maintain healthy joints, fitness, health and vitality.

☑Adults and children over 12 yrs: 1 capsule with liquid each day.

❗Do not exceed recommended daily intake.

Pharmacy only: No

Always Consult Your Pharmacist

SEVEN SEAS HIGH STRENGTH COD LIVER OIL ONE-A-DAY

Seven Seas Ireland Ltd

PA No: 417/6/1

Packs of 60 or 120 capsules.

Vitamin A acetate 800µg, vitamin D 5µg, vitamin E (natural source) 10mg, cod liver oil with fish oil EPA 1ml, eicosapentaenoic acid 120mg, docosahexaenoic acid 60mg.

For the treatment of vitamin A, D and E deficiencies.

Adults: 1 capsule daily with liquid.

Not recommended for children.

Pharmacy only: No

SEVEN SEAS HIGH STRENGTH PURE COD LIVER OIL

Seven Seas Ireland Ltd

PA No: N/A

150ml or 300ml bottles containing a golden-yellow liquid.

Vitamin A palmitate 800µg, vitamin E (dl-alpha-tocopherol acetate) 10mg, vitamin D3 (cholecalciferol) 5µg, cod liver oil with fish oil EPA 9.2mg, eicosapentaenoic acid 1,200mg, docosahexaenoic acid 600mg.

For the treatment of vitamin A, D and E deficiencies.

Adults: 10ml daily.

Children: Over 1 yr: 10ml daily.

Not recommended for children under 1 yr.

Pharmacy only: No

SEVEN SEAS ORANGE SYRUP AND COD LIVER OIL

Seven Seas Ireland Ltd

PA No: 716/2/1

150ml or 300ml bottles of orange syrup.

Vitamin C (ascorbic acid) 35mg, orange juice 700mg, vitamin B6 (pyridoxine hydrochloride) 0.7mg, vitamin A acetate 4,000IU, vitamin D 400IU, vitamin E (natural source) 3IU, cod liver oil 3ml, eicosapentaenoic acid 252mg, docosahexaenoic acid 224mg.

For the treatment of vitamin A, D and E deficiencies.

Adults: 10ml daily. During pregnancy or lactation: 5ml daily.

Children: Over 1 yr: 10ml daily. 1-6 months: 2.5ml. 6-12 months: 5ml diluted with previously boiled and cooled water or milk if desired.

Pharmacy only: No

SEVEN SEAS PULSE PURE FISH OIL CAPSULES

Seven Seas Ireland Ltd

PA No: 417/8/1

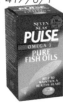

Packs of 60 or 120 capsules.

Vitamin E (natural source) 0.46mg, eicosapentaenoic acid 70mg, docosahexaenoic acid 45mg, fish oil 500mg.

Fish oil supplement.

Adults: 1 capsule daily.

Pharmacy only: No

If Symptoms Persist Consult Your Doctor

SEVEN SEAS PURE COD LIVER OIL & VITAMIN C

Seven Seas Ireland Ltd

PA No: N/A

Packs of 30 capsules.

Vitamin A Palmitate 800µg, vitamin D3 5µg, vitamin E (dl-alpha-tocopheryl acetate) 1.34mg, vitamin C (ascorbic acid) 250mg, cod liver oil 500mg, eicosapentaenoic acid 42.1mg, docosahexaenoic acid 37.4mg.

Cod liver oil and vitamin C supplement to help maintain healthy joints, skin, nails and a healthy heart.

Adults: 1 capsule daily.

Pharmacy only: No

SEVEN SEAS PURE COD LIVER OIL AND CALCIUM

Seven Seas Ireland Ltd

PA No: N/A

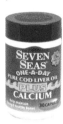

Packs of 30 capsules.

Vitamin A palmitate 800µg, vitamin E (dl-alpha-tocopherol acetate) 10mg, vitamin D3 (cholecalciferol) 5µg, calcium 267mg, cod liver oil 500mg, eicosapentaenoic acid 42.1mg, docosahexaenoic acid 37.4mg.

Vitamin and calcium supplement.

Adults: 1 capsule daily.

Pharmacy only: No

SEVEN SEAS PURE COD LIVER OIL AND EVENING PRIMROSE OIL

Seven Seas Ireland Ltd

PA No: N/A

Packs of 30 or 90 clear capsules.

Vitamin A palmitate 800µg, vitamin E (dl-alpha-tocopherol acetate) 0.33mg, evening primrose oil 200mg, vitamin D3 (cholecalciferol) 2.5µg, gamma-linolenic acid 15.2mg, cod liver oil 615mg, eicosapentaenoic acid 52.5mg, docosahexaenoic acid 46.7mg.

Cod liver oil and evening primrose oil supplement.

Adults: 1 capsule daily.

Pharmacy only: No

SEVEN SEAS PURE COD LIVER OIL AND MULTIVITAMINS

Seven Seas Ireland Ltd

PA No: N/A

Packs of 30 or 90 capsules.

Vitamin C (ascorbic acid) 30mg, vitamin A palmitate 800µg, vitamin E (dl-alpha-tocopherol acetate) 10mg, vitamin B12 (cyanocobalamin) 2µg, vitamin B2 (riboflavine) 1.6mg, vitamin B6 (pyridoxine hydrochloride) 2mg, nicotinamide 18mg, pantothenic acid 5mg, vitamin D3 (cholecalciferol) 2.5µg, vitamin B1 (thiamine mononitrate) 1.2mg, folic acid 400µg, biotin 10µg, cod liver oil 500mg, eicosapentaenoic acid 42.1mg, docosahexaenoic acid 37.4mg.

Multivitamin and cod liver oil supplement.

Adults: 1 capsule daily with liquid.

Pharmacy only: No

Always Read The Label

SEVEN SEAS PURE COD LIVER OIL AND ODOURLESS GARLIC
Seven Seas Ireland Ltd

PA No: N/A

Packs of 30 capsules.

Vitamin A palmitate 800µg, vitamin D3 (cholecalciferol) 5µg, cod liver oil 800mg, eicosapentaenoic acid 67mg, docosahexaenoic acid 60mg, vitamin E (dl-alpha-tocopherol) 1.34mg, garlic powder 6mg.

Cod liver oil and garlic

supplement.

Adults: 1 capsule daily.

Not recommended for children.

Pharmacy only: No

SEVEN SEAS PURE COD LIVER OIL AND VITAMIN E
Seven Seas Ireland Ltd

PA No: N/A

30 capsules in a plastic

container.

Pure cod liver oil 695mg, vitamin A 800µg, vitamin D 5µg, vitamin E 67.1mg; capsule shell (gelatin, glycerin).

Helps maintain skin and

nails, strong bones and teeth, healthy heart, joints and circulatory systems.

Adults: 1 capsule with liquid daily.

Pharmacy only: No

SEVEN SEAS PURE COD LIVER OIL CAPSULES
Seven Seas Ireland Ltd

PA No: 716/1/1

Packs of 60 or 120 capsules.

Vitamin A acetate 670IU, vitamin D 67IU, vitamin E (natural source) 0.3IU, cod liver oil 0.32ml, eicosapentaenoic acid 26mg, docosahexaenoic acid 24mg.

For the treatment of vitamin A, D and E deficiencies.

Adults: 2 capsules 3 times

daily. Pregnant or breastfeeding women: 1 capsule 3 times daily.

Children: Over 6 yrs: 2 capsules 3 times daily.

Not recommended for children under 6 yrs.

Pharmacy only: No

SEVEN SEAS PURE COD LIVER OIL CAPSULES ONE-A-DAY
Seven Seas Ireland Ltd

PA No: N/A

Packs of 30, 60 or 120

clear, oval, gelatin capsules.

Vitamin A acetate 800µg, vitamin D 2.5µg, vitamin E (natural source) 0.33mg, cod liver oil 0.54ml, docosaphexaenoic acid 39.3mg, eicosapentaenoic acid 43.9mg.

For the treatment of vitamin A, D and E deficiencies.

Adults: 1 capsule daily.

Pharmacy only: No

SEVEN SEAS PURE COD LIVER OIL LIQUID
Seven Seas Ireland Ltd

PA No: 716/1/2

170ml, 300ml or 450ml of clear, yellow liquid.

Vitamin A acetate 4,000IU, vitamin D 400IU, vitamin E (natural source) 10IU, cod liver oil 9.2g, eicosapentaenoic acid 828mg, docosahexaenoic acid 736mg.

For the treatment of vitamin A, D and E deficiencies.

Adults: 10ml daily. Pregnant or breastfeeding women: 5ml daily.

Children: Over 1 yr: 10ml daily. 7-12 months: 5ml daily. 0-6 months: 2.5ml daily.

Pharmacy only: No

Always Consult Your Pharmacist

MINERAL SUPPLEMENTS
(may also contain vitamins)

RDAs have been set for **calcium**, **iron** and **zinc**. There is good evidence that regular extra calcium intake (1 gram per day) offers some protection against osteoporosis (easily fractured bones) which is a problem for many women after the menopause. Additional vitamin D may also be helpful since this vitamin conserves calcium.

Additional iron intake may be required during pregnancy. However, it is better to allow your doctor to decide if this is the case by monitoring the haemoglobin in your blood. Young girls may need extra iron at adolescence because of the spurt in growth at that time and the additional iron lost in blood during menstruation. Iron intake needs to be prolonged to be effective but iron can produce stomach upset and constipation or diarrhoea if it is taken in effective doses. Anaemia should be medically managed by monitoring as above.

Zinc deficiency is rare. Some studies have shown that zinc can reduce the growth of the virus that causes colds but there is no firm evidence that it protects against colds.

CALCIA
Perrans Distributors Ltd

PA No: N/A

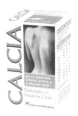

Packs of 90 tablets.

Calcium 800mg, iron 14mg, vitamin D 7.5µg, vitamin C and vitamin B6 2mg, vitamin B12 1µg.

A balanced calcium formulation especially for women.

Adults: 3 tablets daily.

Pharmacy only: No

CALCIA WITH GLUCOSAMINE & VITAMIN D
Perrans Distributors Ltd

PA No: N/A

Packs of 60 tablets.

Glucosamine 1,000mg, calcium 800mg, vitamin D 5µg.

Helps maintain healthy joints, muscles and bones.

Adults: 3 tablets daily with meals.

Pharmacy only: No

CALCICHEW
Shire Pharmaceuticals

PA No: 535/1/2

Pot of 100 white, chewable tablets.

Calcium carbonate 1.25g (equivalent to calcium 500mg).

Calcium deficiency, osteoporosis, osteomalacia, malabsorption and pregnancy. May be used as a phosphate binding agent in the management of kidney failure in patients on kidney dialysis.

Adults: 1-5 daily. Phosphate binder: dose as required by the individual patient depending on serum phosphate level.

Children: Half adult dose.

Pharmacy only: Yes

If Symptoms Persist Consult Your Doctor

CALCICHEW-D3
Shire Pharmaceuticals

PA No: 535/1/1

▭Pot of 100 white, chewable tablets.

▮Calcium carbonate 1.25g (equivalent to calcium 500mg), vitamin D3 200IU.

▨Calcium and vitamin D deficiency; as an adjunct to osteoporosis therapy; osteomalacia. May be used as a phosphate binding agent in the management of kidney failure in patients on kidney dialysis.

▨Adults: 2 tablets daily. Phosphate binder: dose as required by the individual patient depending on serum phosphate level.

Pharmacy only: Yes

CALCICHEW-D3 FORTE
Shire Pharmaceuticals

PA No: 535/1/3

▭Pot of 100 white, chewable tablets.

▮Calcium carbonate 1.25g (equivalent to calcium 500mg), vitamin D3 400IU.

▨Calcium and vitamin D deficiency; as an adjunct to osteoporosis therapy; osteomalacia.

▨Adults: 2 tablets daily.

Pharmacy only: Yes

CALTRATE
Whitehall Laboratories Limited

PA No: N/A

▭Packs of 60 tablets.

▮Calcium 600mg, vitamin D 5µg.

▨Helps replace vital calcium essential to bone health.

▨Adults and children over 11 yrs: Take 1 or 2 tablets daily or as directed by GP or dietitian.

Pharmacy only: Yes

CALTRATE PLUS
Whitehall Laboratories Limited

PA No: N/A

▭Packs of 60 tablets.

▮Calcium 600mg, vitamin D 5µg, magnesium 45mg, zinc 5mg, copper 1mg, manganese 1mg, boron 250µg.

▨A complete calcium supplement plus important nutrients essential for bone health.

▨Adults and children over 11 yrs: Take 1 or 2 tablets daily or as directed by GP or dietitian.

Pharmacy only: Yes

Always Read The Label

CALTRATE PLUS CHEWABLE
Whitehall Laboratories Limited
PA No: N/A

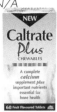

⬛Packs of 60 fruit-flavoured, chewable tablets.

🟦Calcium 600mg, vitamin D 5µg, magnesium 45mg, zinc 5mg, copper 1mg, manganese 1mg, boron 250µg.

❓A complete calcium supplement plus important nutrients essential for bone health.

◪Adults and children over 11 yrs: Take 1 or 2 tablets daily or as directed by GP or dietitian.

Pharmacy only: Yes

DECAL
Ricesteele Manufacturing
PA No: N/A

⬛Bottles of 50 chewable tablets.

🟦Calcium 120mg (as calcium lactate, calcium gluconate and calcium phosphate), vitamin D2 50IU.

❓Calcium and vitamin D supplement.

◪Adults: 1-6 tablets daily.

Children: 1-3 tablets daily.

❗Not recommended for patients with impaired kidney function, a history of kidney stone formation or patients receiving cardiac glycosides.

Pharmacy only: Yes

FEFOL
Celltech
PA No: 365/70/1

⬛Iron and folic acid preparation.

❓For prevention of iron and folic acid deficiency during pregnancy, after the first 13 weeks.

◪Adults: 1 capsule during pregnancy. Capsules should be swallowed whole, not chewed.

❗Nausea may be experienced.

Pharmacy only: Yes

FEOSPAN
Celltech
PA No: 365/73/1

⬛Iron preparation.

❓For treatment and prevention of iron deficiency.

◪Adults: 1-2 capsules daily.

Children: 1 capsule daily.

Capsules may be opened and pellets mixed with cool food.

❗Nausea may be experienced.

Pharmacy only: Yes

FERROGRAD
Abbott Laboratories
PA No: 38/21/1

⬛Blister packs of 3 x 10 sustained-release tablets.

🟦Ferrous sulphate.

❓For the prevention and treatment of iron deficiency and anaemia.

◪Adults: 1 tablet daily to be taken with food.

Pharmacy only: Yes

Always Consult Your Pharmacist

FERROGRAD C
Abbott Laboratories

PA No: 38/20/1

▣ Blister packs of 3x10 tablets.

▣ Ferrous sulphate, sodium ascorbate.

▣ Iron and vitamin C supplement for the prevention and treatment of iron deficiency and anaemia.

▣ Adults: 1 tablet daily to be taken with food.

Pharmacy only: Yes

FERROGRAD FOLIC
Abbott Laboratories

PA No: 38/22/1

▣ Blister packs of 3 x 10 sustained-release tablets.

▣ Ferrous sulphate, folic acid.

▣ For the prevention and treatment of iron and folic acid deficiency and anaemia.

▣ Adults: 1 tablet daily to be taken with food.

Pharmacy only: Yes

HEALTHCRAFTS CALCIUM WITH VITAMIN D 400MG 30S
Perrans Distributors Ltd

PA No: N/A

▣ Packs of 30 butterscotch-flavoured, chewable, calcium tablets.

▣ Calcium carbonate 400mg, sucrose, acacia powder, hydrogenated vegetable oil, calcium stearate, vitamin D 2.5µg (as D3 prep.), silica, flavouring (butterscotch, from natural source ingredients).

▣ Calcium and vitamin D supplement to help maintain healthy, strong bones and teeth, normal muscle, blood clotting and nerve functions.

▣ Adults: 1-2 tablets with food each day.

Children: As per adult dose.

Pharmacy only: No

HEALTHCRAFTS IRON PLUS WITH VITAMIN C 30S
Perrans Distributors Ltd

PA No: N/A

▣ Packs of 30 tablets.

▣ Dicalcium phosphate, microcrystalline cellulose, vitamin C 60mg, iron 14mg (as ferrous sulphate), hydrogenated vegetable oil, tablet coating (hydroxypropylmethylcellulose, glycerin), colour (iron oxide), magnesium stearate, soya bean oil.

▣ Iron and vitamin C supplement to help maintain healthy blood.

▣ Adults: 1 tablet daily with food.

Children: As per adult dose.

Pharmacy only: No

HEALTHCRAFTS KELP PLUS 30S
Perrans Distributors Ltd

PA No: N/A

▣ Packs of 30 tablets.

▣ Dicalcium phosphate, kelp (dried ascophyllum nodosum, brown seaweed), microcrystalline cellulose, iron (as ferrous sulphate) 12mg, hydrogentated vegetable oil, tablet coating (hydroxypropylmethylcellulose, glycerin), colours (titanium dioxide, curcumin, copper chlorophyllin, iron oxide), zinc 5mg, calcium 85mg, iodine 140µg.

▣ Kelp supplement enriched with calcium, iron and zinc to help maintain the body's metabolism.

▣ Adults: 1 tablet daily with food. Maximum 1 tablet in 24 hrs.

Children: As per adult dose.

Pharmacy only: No

If Symptoms Persist Consult Your Doctor

HEALTHCRAFTS SELENIUM (200µG) PLUS VITAMINS A, C & E 60S
Perrans Distributors Ltd

PA No: N/A

Packs of 60 tablets.

Vitamin A prep 450µg,

vitamin E (as d-alpha-tocopheryl acid succinate) 30mg, vitamin C prep 90mg, selenium 200µg, microcrystalline cellulose, dicalcium phosphate, selenomethionine prep, stearic acid, magnesium stearate, sodium carboxymethylcellulose, silicon dioxide.

Formulated for the immune system, with antioxidants to help protect the body from damaging free radicals.

Adults: Take 1 tablet daily with food.

Pregnant women should consult their doctor before taking this product.

Pharmacy only: No

HEALTHCRAFTS ZINC PLUS 15MG 30S
Perrans Distributors Ltd

PA No: N/A

Packs of 30 tablets.

Dicalcium phosphate, microcrystalline cellulose, zinc sulphate 15mg, tablet coating (hydroxypropylmethylcellulose, glycerin), colour (titanium dioxide), soya fibre, hydrogenated vegetable oil, copper gluconate 1mg, magnesium stearate.

Mineral supplement to help maintain healthy skin.

Adults: 1 tablet daily with food. Maximum 1 tablet in 24 hrs.

Children: As per adult dose.

Pharmacy only: No

NUTRICIA IRON FORMULA
Nutricia Ireland Ltd

PA No: N/A

Jar of 60 tablets in a cardboard carton. Tamper

evident seal on jar. Contains lactoferrin – an iron-binding, natural milk protein acting as an iron- and vitamin C-transporting carrier. Lactoferrin and vitamin C can together enhance iron absorption and thereby improve the iron status.

2 tablets provide: Vitamin C 60mg, lactoferrin 200mg, iron 15mg.

Dietary supplement.

2 tablets per day.

Pharmacy only: Yes

POWER HEALTH CALCIUM 400 TABLETS
Power Health Products Ltd

PA No: N/A

White, round, 13mm, uncoated tablets.

Calcium carbonate, providing 400mg calcium.

Adults: 2 tablets per day.

Pharmacy only: No

POWER HEALTH MAGNESIUM 300
Power Health Products Ltd

PA No: N/A

White, round, 13mm, uncoated tablets.

Magnesium oxide, providing 300mg magnesium.

Adults: 1 tablet per day.

Pharmacy only: No

POWER HEALTH ORAL ZINC
Power Health Products Ltd

PA No: N/A

Cream-coloured, multi-speckled, 13mm, round tablets.

Zinc gluconate 27mg providing 3.5mg zinc, rose hip powder 30mg, acerola powder 10mg.

Adults: 1 tablet every 2 hrs as required.

Maximum 4 tablets per 24 hrs.

Pharmacy only: No

Always Read The Label

SEVEN SEAS ANTIOXIDANT VITAMIN E CAPSULES
Seven Seas Ireland Ltd

PA No: 416/1/1

Orange-tinted, clear, oval capsules. 200IU (90 capsules), 400IU (60 capsules).

Vitamin E (dl-alpha-tocopherol acetate) 200IU + 400IU.

Vitamin E supplement.

Adults: 1 capsule daily with liquid.

Pharmacy only: No

SEVEN SEAS CHEWABLE CALCIUM PLUS VITAMIN D
Seven Seas Ireland Ltd

PA No: N/A

30 lemon-flavoured, chewable tablets in a plastic container.

Calcium carbonate, sorbitol corn starch, magnesium stearate, natural flavours (lemon flavour, lemon oil), glyceryl monostearate, artificial sweetener (aspartame), vitamin D preparation.

For maintenance of strong and healthy bones.

Adults: 1-2 tablets daily with liquid.

Pharmacy only: No

SEVEN SEAS CHEWABLE IRON PLUS VITAMIN C
Seven Seas Ireland Ltd

PA No: N/A

30 soft, citrus-flavoured, chewable capsules in a plastic container.

Vitamin C 30mg, iron 7mg, fractionated coconut oil, mannitol, glycerin, gelatin, hard vegetable fat, modified starch, hydrogenated vegetable oil, ferrous fumarate, flavouring (orange oil, grapefruit), citric acid, emulsifier (lecithin), artificial sweetener (aspartame) natural source colours (chlorophyll, titanium dioxide, black iron oxide).

Iron and vitamin C supplement essential for the transportation of oxygen in the blood, for the release of energy from food.

Adults: 1-2 capsules daily, to be chewed or swallowed whole with a cold drink.

Pharmacy only: No

SEVEN SEAS CHEWABLE ZINC PLUS VITAMIN C
Seven Seas Ireland Ltd

PA No: N/A

30 soft, fruit-flavoured, chewable capsules in a container.

Vitamin C 60mg, zinc 3.75mg, fractionated coconut oil, mannitol, glycerin, hard vegetable fat, gelatin, modified starch, ascorbic acid, hydrogenated vegetable oil, flavouring (forest fruits), emulsifier (lecithin), zinc sulphate, artificial sweeteners (aspartame and saccharin), natural source colours (black iron oxide, carmine red, titanium dioxide).

Zinc and vitamin C supplement to help maintain healthy skin.

Adults: 1-4 capsules daily to be chewed or swallowed whole with a cold drink.

Pharmacy only: No

Always Consult Your Pharmacist

SPATONE IRON+
IntraPharma

PA No: N/A

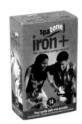

🔲Natural spa water containing iron already in solution. 20ml – 100% natural mineral-containing spa water in a sachet.

☑16.3mg Fe2+ (clinically proven up to 40% bioavailability in iron deficient subjects). No additives.

🔲One sachet of Spatone contains approximately 45% of the adult recommended dietary allowance (RDA) of iron. It can

provide the additional 2.4mg of iron necessary in young or pregnant women.

☑Adults and children: 1 sachet per day.

❗People who know they have genetic haemochromatosis or carry the haemochromatosis gene should not take iron supplements, including Spatone Iron+.

Pharmacy only: Yes

STREPSILS ZINC DEFENCE
Boots Healthcare Limited

PA No: N/A

🔲Packs of 24 blackcurrant-

flavoured lozenges.

☑Per lozenge: Zinc 3.0mg, vitamin C 12mg, menthol.

🔲To help maintain the body's immune system and provide support in its resistance to

infections.

☑Adults and children over 12 yrs: Dissolve 1 lozenge slowly in the mouth 5 times daily (this provides 100% of RDA).

Pharmacy only: No

MULTIVITAMINS WITH MINERALS

ANTIOXIDANTS/ MINERALS PLUS 60S
Intrapharma/Dugdale/Health Perception

PA No: N/A

🔲Packs of 60 tablets.

☑Betacarotene 10mg, vitamin E 50mg, vitamin C 500mg, vitamin D 10µg, vitamin B1 39mg, vitamin B2 20mg, vitamin B3 20mg, vitamin B5 10mg, vitamin B6 5mg, vitamin B12 25µg, zinc 1mg, manganese 1mg, selenium

32.5µg, iron 15mg, chromium 25µg, glutathione 20mg, folic acid 200µg, lycopene (grape seed and tomato extract) 20mg.

🔲Vitamin and mineral supplement.

Pharmacy only: Yes

BEROCCA
Roche Consumer Health

PA No: 50/143/1

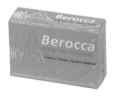

🔲Tube containing 20 effervescent, vitamin B complex tablets. Tropical flavoured.

☑Ascorbic acid (vitamin C) 1,000mg, vitamin B 15mg, vitamin B2 15mg, vitamin B3 50mg, vitamin B5 25mg, vitamin B6 10mg, vitamin B12 10µg, biotin 150µg, calcium 100g, magnesium 100mg.

🔲For a deficiency and/or increased requirement of vitamin

C, B vitamins, calcium and magnesium.

☑Adults and children over 12 yrs: Dissolve one tablet daily in a glass of water to make a tropical-flavoured drink.

❗Not recommended for children under 12 yrs.

Harmful for people with phenylketonuria.

Pharmacy only: Yes

If Symptoms Persist Consult Your Doctor

CENTRUM
Whitehall Laboratories Ltd

PA No: N/A

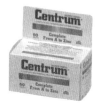

Packs of 30 or 60 orange-scored tablets, marked 'EC/1' on one side and 'W' on reverse.

Vitamin A 800µg, betacarotene 1,200µg, vitamin D 5µg, vitamin E 10mg, vitamin C 60mg, thiamin (B1) 1.4mg, riboflavin (B2) 1.6mg, niacin (B3) 18mg, vitamin B6 2mg, folic acid 200µg, vitamin B12 1µg, biotin 0.15mg, pantothenic acid 6mg, vitamin K 30µg, calcium 162mg, phosphorus 125mg, iron 14mg, magnesium 100mg, zinc 15mg, iodine 150µg, copper 2mg, manganese 2.5mg, potassium 40mg, chloride 36mg, chromium 25µg, molybdenum 25µg, selenium 25µg, nickel 5µg, tin 10µg, vanadium 10µg, boron 70µg, silicon 2µg.

Multivitamin and mineral supplement with the complete antioxidant group and folic acid.

Adults: 1 tablet daily with water.

Children: Over 12 yrs: As per adult dose.

Pharmacy only: Yes

CENTRUM SELECT 50+
Whitehall Laboratories Ltd

PA No: N/A

Packs of 30 or 60 grey-scored tablets, marked 'Select' on one side and 'W1' on reverse.

Vitamin A (retinol) 1,200µg, betacarotene 1,800µg, vitamin D 10µg, vitamin E 30mg, vitamin C 90mg, vitamin B1 (thiamin) 1.8mg, vitamin B2 (riboflavin) 3.2mg, vitamin B3 (niacin) 40mg, vitamin B6 (pyridoxine) 3mg, folic acid 400µg, vitamin B12 25µg, biotin 45µg, pantothenic acid 10mg, vitamin K 30µg, calcium 200mg, phosphorus 125mg, iron 4mg, magnesium 100mg, zinc 15mg, iodine 150µg, copper 2mg, manganese 5mg, potassium 80mg, chloride 72mg, boron 100µg, silicon 10µg, chromium 100µg, molybdenum 25µg, selenium 75µg, nickel 5µg, tin 10µg, vanadium 10µg.

Multivitamin and mineral supplement for adults over 50 yrs of age.

Adults: Over 50 yrs of age: 1 tablet daily with water. Under 50 yrs of age: Use Centrum.

Not recommended for children.

Pharmacy only: Yes

FORCEVAL
Unigreg

PA No: N/A

Packs of 30 or 90 red/brown gelatin capsules marked 'Forceval'.

Vitamin A 5,000IU, vitamin D2 600IU, vitamin B1 10mg, vitamin B2 5mg, vitamin B6 0.5mg, vitamin B12 2mg, vitamin C 50mg, vitamin E 10mg, nicotinamide 20mg, choline bitartrate 40mg, calcium pantothenate 2mg, L-lysine hydrochloride 60mg, inositol 60mg, calcium 70mg, iron 10mg, copper 0.5mg, phosphorus 55mg, magnesium 2mg, potassium 3mg, zinc 0.5mg, iodine 0.1mg, manganese 0.5mg.

Vitamin and mineral supplement.

Adults: 1 capsule daily.

Children: Use Forceval Junior capsules.

Pharmacy only: Yes

FORCEVAL JUNIOR
Unigreg

PA No: N/A

Packs of 30 small brown, oval-shaped soft gelatin capsules, numbered 571 in white on one side.

Vitamin A (as betacarotene) 1,250IU, vitamin D2 200IU (5µg), vitamin B1 1.5mg, vitamin B2 1mg, vitamin B6 1mg, vitamin B12 2mg, vitamin C 25mg, vitamin E 5mg, vitamin K 25µg, biotin 50µg, nicotinamide 7.5mg, pantothenic acid 2mg, folic acid 100µg, iron 5mg, copper 1mg, magnesium 1mg, zinc 5mg, iodine 75µg, manganese 1.25mg, selenium 25µg, chromium 50µg, molybdenum 50µg.

Vitamin and mineral supplement.

Children 5 yrs and over: 2 capsules per day or as prescribed by doctor.

Consult you doctor if you are taking other medication, including other vitamins or mineral products.

If you are a pregnant teenager, consult the doctor before using this product.

Pharmacy only: Yes

GINSANA CAPSULES
Boehringer Ingelheim Self Medication

PA No: 337/18/1

Packs of 30 or 60 soft, gelatin capsules; calorie- and sugar-free.

Standardised ginseng extract G115 100mg per 650mg.

Used as an adjunct in the management of patients with impaired general health or convalescing.

Adults: 2 capsules per day at breakfast or one each with breakfast and lunch.

Not recommended for children.

Consult doctor before use if receiving any other medications.

Pharmacy only: Yes

GINSANA TONIC
Boehringer Ingelheim Self Medication

PA No: 337/18/2

250ml bottle of tonic with natural aromatics.

Standardised ginseng extract G115 140mg, tonic wine, sorbitol, aromatics per 15ml.

Used as an adjunct in the management of patients with impaired general health or convalescing.

Adults: 15ml daily before or after meals, preferably at breakfast.

Not recommended for children.

Shake bottle well before use.

Consult a doctor before use if receiving medication.

Pharmacy only: Yes

HEALTHCRAFTS MULTIVITAMINS WITH IRON AND CALCIUM 30S
Perrans Distributors Ltd

PA No: N/A

Packs of 30 tablets.

Calcium carbonate 200mg, dicalcium phosphate, iron 14mg (as ferrous sulphate prep.), vitamin C 60mg, tablet coating (hydroxypropylmethylcellulose, glycerin), colour (titanium dioxide, iron oxide), soya fibre, niacin (as niacinamide), hydrogenated vegetable oil, vitamin E 10mg (as d-alpha-tocopherol acid succinate), hydroxypropylmethylcellulose, vitamin A 800µg (as acetate prep. with antioxidant d-alpha-tocopherol), magnesium stearate, pantothenic acid 6mg (as calcium pantothenate), vitamin B6 2mg (as pyridoxine hydrochloride), vitamin D 5µg (as D3 prep.), thiamin mononitrate 1.4mg, riboflavin 1.6mg, vitamin B12 1µg (as cyanocobalamin prep.), folacin 200µg (as folic acid).

Multivitamins with iron and calcium supplement to help maintain healthy growth of organs and tissues, maintaining the function of the body's digestive, nervous and immune systems.

Adults: Take 1 tablet with food daily. Do not exceed this amount if you are pregnant.

Children: As per adult dose.

Pharmacy only: No

Always Consult Your Pharmacist

IDÉOS
Helsinn Birex Pharmaceuticals

PA No: 737/1/1

▢Cartons of 4 tubes of 15 chewable tablets.

☑Calcium carbonate 1,250mg, cholecalciferol 10µg (corresponding to calcium 500mg and vitamin D3 400IU).

▨Vitamin D3 and calcium deficiency correction in the elderly. Also as an adjunct to specific therapy for osteoporosis.

▨Adults: 2 tablets to be chewed daily.

▍Not recommended for children.

Not recommended with treatment with the digitalis glycosides or thiazide diuretics. In cases of kidney impairment/long-term use; check calcium excretion and plasma calcium.

Pharmacy only: Yes

KIDDI PHARMATON
Boehringer Ingelheim Self Medication

PA No: 337/6/1

▢100ml or 200ml bottles of syrup.

☑Lysine hydrochloride 200mg, vitamin B1 10mg, vitamin B2 6mg, vitamin B6 3mg, vitamin B12 10µg, nicotinamide (PP) 6mg, panthenol 5mg, vitamin A 3,000IU, vitamin D2 400IU, calcium 39mg, phosphorus 61mg per 10ml.

▨Vitamin supplement. Also for convalescence of all age groups.

▨Adults: 15ml daily 1 hr before meals.

Children: Up to 5 yrs: 7.5ml daily. Over 5 yrs: 15ml daily 1 hr before meals.

▍Not recommended for patients receiving levodopa as vitamin B6 reduces the effect of levodopa.

Pharmacy only: Yes

NUTRICIA ANTIOXIDANT FORMULA
Nutricia Ireland Ltd

PA No: N/A

▢Jar of 60 capsules in a cardboard carton. Tamper evident seal on jar.

☑2 capsules provide: Vitamin E 268mg (400IU), mixed carotenoids 1.5mg (typically supplying alphacarotene 337µg, betacarotene 637µg, lycopene 281µg, lutein 187µg), vitamin C 200mg, copper 2mg, manganese 2mg, selenium 50µg, alpha lipoic acid 50mg, N-acetyl-l-cysteine 50mg, coenzyme Q-10 30mg, lactoferrin 50mg, citrus bioflavonoids 10mg (providing hesperidin 2.5mg), green tea (Camellia sinensis) 20mg, leaf extract (providing polyphenols) 16mg.

▨Dietary supplement to help maintain the immune system.

▨2 capsules per day.

Pharmacy only: Yes

If Symptoms Persist Consult Your Doctor

A new range of
multi-action supplements from Nutricia®

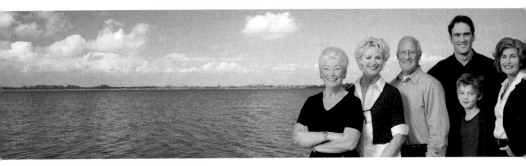

Introducing a new unique range of scientifically formulated,
multi-action supplements designed to safeguard key nutrients at different life stages.

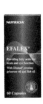

Nutricia Efalex –
◆ Provides high levels of fatty acids important for brain and eye function.
◆ Blend of high quality tuna oil and Efamol Pure Evening Primrose Oil (EPO).

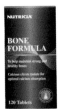

Nutricia Bone Formula –
◆ Unique formula to help maintain bone strength, density and integrity.
◆ Contains calcium citrate malate, shown in studies to be absorbed and retained better than other sources of calcium.
◆ Provides gamma linolenic acid (GLA) which assists calcium absorption.

Nutricia Multi-Fibre Formula –
◆ Formulated to help maintain healthy digestive function and regularity.
◆ Unique blend of 6 plant fibres – insoluble, soluble and fermentable.
◆ Provides 50% of daily dietary fibre requirements.
◆ Fructo-oligosaccharides of Inulin help maintain healthy intestinal flora.

Nutricia Efanatal –
◆ Provides long-chain polyunsaturated fatty acids for mother and baby before, during and after pregnancy.
◆ High quality tuna oil and Efamol Pure EPO for optimal levels of fatty acids.
◆ LCPs are important in last trimester of pregnancy for foetal eye/brain development.

Nutricia Efamol PMP –
◆ Providing nutrients for everyday of the monthly cycle.
◆ Blend of Efamol EPO and other key nutrients may help maintain hormonal balance.
◆ Contains vitamin B6 and magnesium that are important for menstruating women.

Nutricia Iron Formula –
◆ Highly absorbable form of iron due to lactoferrin and Vitamin C content.
◆ Very gentle on the stomach and digestive system.
◆ Lactoferrin also regulates iron uptake.
◆ Lactoferrin also has antioxidant properties.

Nutricia Antioxidant Formula –
◆ A very potent mix of 12 researched antioxidants.
◆ Synergistic combination helps provide protection to the whole body.
◆ Formula provides support to the immune function.

Nutricia Multiman Formula –
◆ Scientifically formulated to help safeguard the nutritional requirements of men.
◆ Contains over 30 key nutrients for optimal mens health.
◆ Includes saw palmetto, lycopene and Vitamin E.

Nutricia Multiwoman Formula –
◆ Scientifically formulated to help safeguard the nutritional requirements of women.
◆ Contains 31 nutrients for optimal women's health.
◆ Includes key nutrients for hormonal and bone health.
◆ Includes iron and folic acid.

NUTRICIA SUPPLEMENTS
The science of well-being

For further information, Freephone 1-800-923535

NUTRICIA MULTIMAN FORMULA

Nutricia Ireland Ltd

PA No: N/A

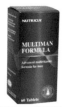

▣60 tablets in a jar in a cardboard carton. Tamper evident seal on jar.

▣2 tablets contain: Natural source mixed carotenoids (Betatene) providing typically betacarotene 3mg, alphacarotene 103.6µg, cryptoxanthin 31.4µg, zeaxanthin 15.7µg, lutein 15.7µg, vitamin C 120mg, vitamin D 5µg, vitamin E 67mg, vitamin K 25µg, thiamin 4.5mg, riboflavin 5.1mg, niacin (niacinamide) 19mg, vitamin B6 6mg, vitamin B12 6µg, folic acid 400µg, biotin 30µg, pantothenic acid 5mg, calcium 200mg, iodine 150µg, magnesium 100mg, zinc 15mg, selenium 100µg, copper 2mg, manganese 2mg, chromium 50µg, molybdenum

20µg, Saw palmetto 25mg, choline 10mg, boron 2mg, inositol 5mg, lycopene 500µg, lutein 500µg, vanadium 20µg, alpha-lipoic acid 10mg.

▣Multivitamin and mineral supplement for men.

▣2 tablets per day with a meal.

Pharmacy only: Yes

NUTRICIA MULTIWOMAN FORMULA

Nutricia Ireland Ltd

PA No: N/A

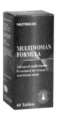

▣60 tablets in a jar in a cardboard carton. Tamper evident seal on jar.

▣2 tablets contain: natural source mixed carotenoids (providing typically: betacarotene 3mg, alphacarotene 103.6µg, cryptoxanthin 31.4µg, zeaxanthin 15.7µg, lutein 15.7µg), vitamin D 5µg (200IU), vitamin E 53.6mg (80IU), vitamin C 120mg, thiamin 3.3mg, riboflavin 3.9mg, niacin (niacinamide) 15mg, vitamin B6 4.8mg, folic acid 360µg, vitamin B12 6µg, biotin 30µg, pantothenic acid 5mg, vitamin K 20µg, calcium 200mg, iron 15mg, magnesium 100mg, zinc 12mg, iodine 150µg, boron 2mg, chromium 70µg, copper 2mg, manganese 2mg, molybdenum

20µg, selenium 100µg, choline 10mg, inositol 5mg, vanadium 20µg, lycopene 500µg, lutein 500µg, alpha-lipoic acid 10mg.

▣Multivitamin and mineral supplement for women.

▣2 tablets per day with a meal.

Pharmacy only: Yes

Always Read The Label

NUTRICIA PRENATAL FORMULA
Nutricia Ireland Ltd

PA No: N/A

🔲60 tablets in a jar in a cardboard carton. Tamper evident seal on jar.

🔳2 tablets provide: Natural source mixed carotenoids (equivalent to vitamin A 502µg typically providing betacarotene 3.7mg, alphacarotene 137.2µg, cryptoxanthin 39.2µg, zeaxanthin 19.6µg, lutein 19.6µg), vitamin D 10µg (400IU), vitamin E 13.4mg (20IU), vitamin C 150mg, thiamin (vitamin B1) 1.5mg, riboflavin (vitamin B2) 1.7mg, niacin (as niacinamide) 18mg, vitamin B6 50mg, folic acid 400µg, vitamin B12 4µg, biotin 35µg, pantothenic acid 7mg, calcium 500mg, iron 15mg, magnesium 200mg, zinc 15mg, iodine 150µg, boron 150µg, chromium 50µg, copper 2mg, manganese 2mg, selenium 70µg, choline 125µg, inositol 30µg.

🔳A nutritionally balanced composition to help ensure optimal nutrition before and during pregnancy and also during breastfeeding to benefit both mother and child.

🔳2 tablets per day with a meal.

Pharmacy only: Yes

PHARMATON CAPSULES
Boehringer Ingelheim Self Medication

PA No: 337/5/1

🔲Bottles of 30 or 100 capsules.

🔳Dimethylaminoethanol hydrogen tartrate (Pharmaton) 26mg, standardised ginseng extract G115 40mg, vitamin A 4,000IU, vitamin B1 2mg, vitamin B2 2mg, vitamin B6 1mg, vitamin B12 1µg, vitamin C 60mg, vitamin D 400IU, vitamin E 10mg, nicotinamide (PP) 15mg, calcium pantothenate 10mg, rutoside 20mg, iron 10mg, calcium 90.3mg, phosphorus 70mg, fluorine 0.2mg, copper 1mg, potassium 8mg, manganese 1mg, magnesium 10mg, zinc 1mg, choline, inositol and linolenic acid 66mg.

🔳As a supplement in the management of vitamin and mineral deficiencies due to the ageing process or to dietary restriction and, in cases of retarded convalescence, as a general tonic (e.g. during periods of mental and physical stress).

🔳Adults: 2 capsules for first 2-3 weeks; 1 at breakfast and 1 during lunch. Then 1 capsule daily at breakfast for a period of several months.

🔳Not recommended for children.

Not recommended for persons receiving other medication.

Pharmacy only: Yes

POKEMON MULTIVITAMIN
Nutricia Ireland Ltd

PA No: N/A

🔲Jars of 60 chewable flavoured tablets in a cardboard carton. Child resistant cap and tamper evident seal on lid.

🔳One tablet provides: Vitamin D 5µg, vitamin E 5mg, vitamin C 50mg, thiamin 0.7mg, riboflavin 0.9mg, niacin 11.5mg, vitamin B6 0.95mg, folic acid 125µg, vitamin B12 1µg, calcium 150mg, iron 5mg, magnesium 45mg, zinc 5mg, iodine 75µg, copper 0.4mg.

🔳Vitamin supplement.

🔳Adults and children: 1 tablet daily.

🔳This product contains food colourings that are unsuitable for children with a history of hyperactivity or allergy. This product contains iron, which, if taken in excess, may be harmful to young children.

Pharmacy only: No

Always Consult Your Pharmacist

POKEMON MULTIVITAMIN WITH EXTRA VITAMIN C
Nutricia Ireland Ltd

PA No: N/A

▣Jars of 60 chewable flavoured tablets in a cardboard carton. Child resistant cap and tamper evident seal on lid.

☑One tablet provides: Vitamin D 5µg, vitamin E 5mg, vitamin C 65mg, thiamin 0.7mg, riboflavin 0.9mg, niacin 11.5mg, vitamin B6 0.95mg, folic acid 125µg, vitamin B12 1µg, calcium 150mg.

▣Vitamin supplement.

☑Adults and children: 1 tablet daily.

❗This product contains colourings that are unsuitable for children with a history of hyperactivity or allergy.

Pharmacy only: No

POKEMON MULTIVITAMIN WITH IRON
Nutricia Ireland Ltd

PA No: N/A

▣Jars of 60 chewable flavoured tablets in a cardboard carton. Child resistant cap and tamper evident seal on lid.

☑One tablet provides: Vitamin D 5µg, vitamin E 5mg, vitamin C 50mg, thiamin 0.7mg, riboflavin 0.9mg, niacin 11.5mg, vitamin B6 0.95mg, folic acid 125µg, vitamin B12 1µg, calcium 150mg, iron 5mg.

▣Vitamin supplement.

☑Adults and children: 1 tablet daily.

❗This product contains colourings that are unsuitable for children with a history of hyperactivity or allergy. This product contains iron, which, if taken in excess, may be harmful to young children.

Pharmacy only: No

RUBEX MEGAVITES
Ricesteele Healthcare

PA No: N/A

▣Packs of 10, 30 or 100 capsules.

☑Vitamin A 2,500IU, thiamin 5mg, riboflavin 6mg, niacin 20mg, pantothenic acid as calcium salt 5mg, vitamin B6 8mg, vitamin B12 2µg, folic acid 5µg, biotin 2µg, choline 15mg, inositol 15mg, para-aminobenzoic acid 10mg, vitamin C 80mg, citrus bioflavonoid 10mg, vitamin D 250IU, vitamin E 10IU, calcium phosphate 50mg, iron 10mg, iodine 50µg, copper 200µg, potassium 5mg, magnesium 5mg, manganese 500µg, zinc 5mg, molybdenum 50µg, selenium 10µg, chromium 5µg, DL methionine 10mg, L-lysine 5mg, rutin 10mg, alfalfa extract 6.67mg, kelp powder 10mg, pollen powder 20mg, royal jelly 50mg, wheatgerm oil 50mg, siberian ginseng extract 50mg, oil of evening primrose 50mg, soya lecithin 50mg, garlic oil 200µg; carbohydrate 288.8mg, fat 425.5mg, protein 227.4mg, energy 25kj/6kcal.

▣Multivitamin and mineral supplement with evening primrose oil, ginseng and royal jelly to provide the essential micronutrients required by the body to maintain good physical and mental health. Can benefit those with irregular or poor eating habits.

☑Adults: 1 capsule daily with food or drink.

❗Not to be given to children under 14 yrs.

Do not exceed recommended dose.

Pharmacy only: Yes

If Symptoms Persist Consult Your Doctor

SANATOGEN GOLD
Roche Consumer Health

PA No: N/A

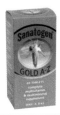

Packs of 30 or 60 tablets.

Beta carotene 400µg, biotin 0.15mg, boron 150µg, calcium 162mg, chloride 36.3mg, chromium chelated 25µg, copper 2mg, folic acid 400µg, iodine 150µg, iron 18mg, magnesium 100mg, manganese 2.5mg, molybdenum 25µg, niacin 20mg, nickel 5µg, pantothenic acid 10mg, phosphorus 109mg, potassium 40mg, selenium 25µg, silicon 2mg, tin 10µg, vanadium 10µg, vitamin A 800µg, vitamin B1 (thiamine hydrochloride) 1.5mg, vitamin B12 (cyanocobalamin) 6µg, vitamin B2 (riboflavin) 1.7mg, vitamin B6 (pyridoxine hydrochloride 2mg), vitamin C (ascorbic acid 60mg), vitamin D 10µg, vitamin E 20mg, vitamin K 25mg, zinc 15mg.

Complete multivitamin and multimineral supplement.

Adults: 1 daily.

Pharmacy only: Yes

SANATOGEN KIDS GOLD A-Z
Roche Consumer Health

PA No: N/A

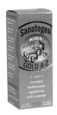

Packs of 30 or 90 strawberry flavoured chewable tablets. No artificial colours, flavours, preservatives, gluten, lactose, yeast or sugar.

Tricalcium phosphate, sorbitol, xylitol, mannitol, magnesium oxide, vitamin C, niacin compound, vitamin E compound, vitamin A compound, magnesium stearate, flavour enhancer (citric acid), vitamin B6 compound, riboflavin compound, beta carotene compound, flavouring, thiamin compound, zinc oxide compound, colour (iron oxide), sweetener (aspartame), biotin compound, folic acid compound, vitamin D compound, calcium pantothenate, vitamin B12 compound, potassium iodide.

Complete multivitamin and multimineral supplement. Helps maintain healthy bones, teeth and gums, eyes and skin and helps build a healthy immune system.

Children aged 3-12 yrs: Chew 1 tablet daily. For young persons over 12 yrs Sanatogen Gold for adults is recommended.

In case of excessive consumption, please consult your doctor.

Pharmacy only: Yes

SANATOGEN MULTIVITAMINS PLUS CALCIUM
Roche Consumer Health

PA No: N/A

Bottle of 30 white to off-white, biconvex, chewable tablets.

Vitamin A 750µg, vitamin B1 1.2mg, vitamin B2 1.6mg, niacin 18mg, folic acid 300µg, vitamin B6 2mg, vitamin B12 2µg, vitamin C 30mg, vitamin D2 2.5µg, vitamin E 5mg, calcium as tricalcium phosphate 92mg.

Multivitamin supplement providing vitamins and calcium which may be lost through missed meals, dieting, pregnancy, breastfeeding or as a result of medication; also strenghtens bones.

Adults: 1 tablet daily.

Children: Over 12 yrs: 1 tablet daily.

Pharmacy only: Yes

Always Read The Label

SANATOGEN MULTIVITAMINS PLUS IRON
Roche Consumer Health

PA No: N/A

Bottles of 30, 60 or 120 dark red, biconvex, chewable tablets.

Vitamin A 750µg, vitamin B1 1.2mg, vitamin B2 1.6mg, niacin 18mg, folic acid 300µg, vitamin B6 2mg, vitamin B12 2µg, vitamin C 30mg, vitamin D2 2.5µg, vitamin E 5mg, iron as ferrous fumarate 12mg.

Supplement supplying the full daily requirement of nutrients.

Adults: 1 tablet daily.

Children over 12 yrs: 1 tablet daily.

Pharmacy only: Yes

SEVEN SEAS ACTION PLAN 50+ ENERGY FORMULA
Seven Seas Ireland Ltd

PA No: N/A

Packs of 50 brown, oval capsules.

Vitamin C (ascorbic acid) 60mg, vitamin B1 (thiamine nitrate) 9mg, vitamin B2 (riboflavin) 2.5mg, niacin (nicotinamide) 30mg, vitamin B6 (pyridoxine HCl) 10mg, folic acid 300µg, vitamin B12 (prep) 10µg, pantothenic acid 10mg, iron 14mg, magnesium 100mg, zinc oxide 15mg, iodine 150µg, manganese sulphate 5mg, chromium amino acid chelate 200µg, Korean ginseng extract 100mg.

Multinutrient supplement for the maintenance of a healthy nervous system and muscle functions.

Adults: 1 capsule daily with liquid.

Pharmacy only: No

SEVEN SEAS ADVANCED FORMULA MULTIBIONTA COMPLETE MULTIVITAMIN WITH MINERALS & PROBIOTIC NUTRIENTS
Seven Seas Ireland Ltd

PA No: N/A

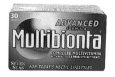

Packs of 30 or 60 enteric coated tablets.

Vitamin A (acetate preparation) 800µg, vitamin C (calcium ascorbate) 60mg, vitamin E (dl-alpha-tocopheryl acetate) 10mg, niacin (nicotinamide) 18mg, pantothenic acid 6mg, vitamin K1 (glucose trituration) 30µg, vitamin D3 5µg, vitamin B6 (pyridoxine HCl) 2mg, vitamin B1 (thiamine mononitrate) 1.4mg, vitamin B2 (riboflavin) 1.6mg, vitamin B12 (cyanocobalamine glucose trituration) 1µg, folic acid 200µg, iodine (potassium iodide) 150µg, biotin 0.15mg, molybdenum (sodium molybdate dihydrate) 25µg, calcium (tri calcium phosphate) 40mg, phosphorus 16mg, iron 14mg, magnesium 5mg, zinc oxide 15mg, copper (magnesium oxide) 2mg, manganese ((11) sulphate monohydrate) 2mg, silicon dioxide 2µg, chromium 25µg, selenium yeast 30µg, chloride 4.5mg, potassium 5mg, probiotic cultures 10 million, lactobacillus acidophilus PA 16/8, bifidobacterium bifidum MF 20/5, bifidobacterium longum SP 07/3.

Complete multivitamin and mineral supplement with probiotic nutrients to help maintain a healthy immune and digestive system.

Adults: 1 tablet daily with a cold drink.

Pharmacy only: No

SEVEN SEAS HALIBORANGE MULTIVITAMIN WITH CALCIUM
Seven Seas Ireland Ltd

PA No: N/A

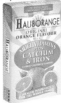

⬛Packs of 30 tablets.

☑Vitamin C 60mg, vitamin E 6mg, vitamin B12 2µg, vitamin B1 1.2mg, vitamin B2 1.5mg, vitamin B6 1mg, nicotinic acid 10mg, vitamin D 2.5µg, pantothenic acid 5mg, folic acid 300µg, calcium 135mg, iron 6mg, vitamin A 750µg.

❓Vitamin supplement.

☑Adults: 1 tablet daily.

Children: Over 3 yrs: 1 tablet daily.

Pharmacy only: No

SEVEN SEAS MULTIVITAMINS PLUS MINERALS FOR VEGETARIANS AND VEGANS
Seven Seas Ireland Ltd

PA No: N/A

⬛60 tablets in a plastic carton.

☑Calcium carbonate 200mg, vitamin C 90mg (ascorbic acid), maltodextrin, iron 14mg (ferrous fumarate), zinc sulphate 15mg, corn starch, vitamin E 20mg (dl-alpha-tocopheryl acid succinate), natural colouring (curcumin, titanium dioxide, copper chlorophyllin), cellulose, nicotinamide, hydroxypropylmethylcellulose, vitamin A acetate 800µg (prep.), silicon dioxide, vitamin B6 HCl 6mg, calcium pantothenate, thiamin mononitrate 2.45mg, vitamin B12 2.5µg (prep.), riboflavin 2.8mg, magnesium stearate, stearic acid (vegetarian), glycerin, folic acid 300µg, niacin 18mg, pantothenic acid 6mg.

❓Multivitamin and mineral supplement providing a comprehensive combination of 13 vitamins and minerals specially formulated so that people following a vegetarian or vegan diet can help maintain good health and vitality.

☑Adults: 1 tablet to be taken with liquid each day.

❗Do not exceed the stated dose.

Pharmacy only: No

SEVEN SEAS MULTI SPECTRUM MULTIVITAMINS & MINERALS
Seven Seas Ireland Ltd

PA No: N/A

⬛60 capsules.

☑Vitamin A (palmitate prep.) 800µg, vitamin C (ascorbic acid) 40mg, vitamin E (dl-alpha-tocopherol acetate) 20mg, vitamin D2 (prep.) 2.5µg, vitamin B12 (prep.) 2µg, vitamin B1 (thiamine HCl) 2.3mg, vitamin B2 (riboflavin) 2mg, vitamin B6 (pyridoxine HCl) 8mg, niacin (nicotinamide) 20mg, pantothenic acid 5mg, folic acid 300µg, biotin 0.0005mg, phosphorus 15mg, molybdenum 50µg, iodine 140µg, calcium 20mg, iron 12mg, inositol 1mg, copper 200µg, potassium 0.5mg, manganese 5µg, zinc 4mg, magnesium 0.5mg, choline (as bitartrate) 5mg.

❓Multivitamin and mineral supplement to help maintain general good health and well-being.

☑Adults: 1 capsule daily with liquid.

Pharmacy only: No

If Symptoms Persist Consult Your Doctor

SEVEN SEAS MULTI SPECTRUM MULTIVITAMINS & MINERALS WITH SIBERIAN GINSENG
Seven Seas Ireland Ltd

PA No: N/A

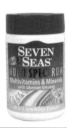

🔲60 capsules.

✔Vitamin A (palmitate prep.) 800µg, vitamin C (ascorbic acid) 40mg, vitamin E (dl-alpha-tocopheryl acetate) 20mg, vitamin D2 (prep.) 2.5µg, vitamin B12 (prep.) 2µg, vitamin B1 (thiamine HCl) 2.3mg, vitamin B2 (riboflavin) 2mg, vitamin B6 (pyridoxine HCl) 8mg, niacin (nicotinamide) 20mg, pantothenic acid 5mg, folic acid 12.5µg, biotin 0.0005mg, phosphorus 15mg, molybdenum 50µg, iodine 140µg, calcium 20mg, iron 12mg, inositol 1mg, copper 200ug, potassium 0.5mg, manganese 5µg, zinc 4mg, magnesium 0.5mg, choline (as bitartrate) 5mg, ginseng extract (from ginseng root 150mg) 30mg.

❓Multivitamin, mineral and ginseng supplement to help maintain general good health and vitality.

✏Adults: 1 capsule daily with liquid.

Pharmacy only: No

VIVIOPTAL
Pharma Global Ltd

PA No: 141/20/1

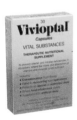

🔲Packs of 30 or 100 capsules.

✔Vitamins, lipotropic substances, mineral salts, trace elements and other bioactivators.

❓Vitamin and mineral supplement.

✏Adults and children over 14 yrs: Unless otherwise prescribed by physician, take 1 capsule during or after breakfast.

Pharmacy only: Yes

VIVIOPTAL JUNIOR
Pharma Global Ltd

PA No: 141/20/1

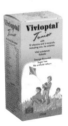

🔲250ml bottle of orange-flavoured, sugar-free liquid.

✔12 vitamins and 6 minerals including iron.

❓Nutritional supplement for children. Also suitable for adults with swallowing difficulties, if dose is doubled.

✏Children from 3 yrs: 5ml spoonful daily.

Older children (11 to 14 yrs): 10ml daily, or as advised by your doctor or pharmacist.

Pharmacy only: Yes

Always Read The Label

MULTIVITAMINS WITHOUT MINERALS

DECAVIT
Rowa Pharmaceuticals Ltd

PA No: 74/14/1

Packs of 30 and 60 orange-red, soft gelatin, oval capsules.

Vitamin A 1,455IU, vitamin D3 400IU, vitamin E 15mg, vitamin B1 2mg, vitamin B2 2mg, vitamin B6 2mg, vitamin B12 5µg, calcium pantothenate 10mg, folic acid 0.1mg, nicotinamide 20mg, ascorbic acid 70mg.

For the prevention of vitamin deficiency.

Adults: 1 daily or as directed.

Not recommended for children under 6 yrs.

Pharmacy only: Yes

OROVITE TABLETS
SSL Healthcare Ireland Ltd

PA No: 696/9/1

Packs of 25 or 100 tablets.

Thiamine hydrochloride 10mg, riboflavin 5mg, pyridoxine hydrochloride 5mg, nicotinamide 33.3mg, ascorbic acid 100mg.

For debility following febrile illness, infection or operation.

Adults: 1 tablet 3 times daily.

Not recommended for children under 12 yrs.

Pharmacy only: No

POWER HEALTH CHILDREN'S VITAMINS A, C AND D
Power Health Products Ltd

PA No: N/A

Cream-coloured, 13mm, round tablets.

Vitamin A 600µg, vitamin D 2.5µg and vitamin C 30mg.

Adults: 1 per day.

Children: 1 per day.

Pharmacy only: No

SANATOGEN KIDS A, C, D VITAMINS
Roche Consumer Health

PA No: N/A

Packs of 30 or 60 orange tasting chewable tablets. Available in 3 colours and flavours. Contains no artificial colours, flavours or preservatives. Gluten, yeast, lactose and sugar free.

400µg of vitamin A, 75mg vitamin C and 2.5µg vitamin D per tablet. Sorbitol, vitamin C, microcrystalline cellulose, magnesium stearate, natural flavourings, vitamin A compound, colour (riboflavin), colour (iron oxide), vitamin D compound, artificial sweetener (aspartame), acesulfame K.

Vitamin A, C and D supplement.

Children aged 3-12 yrs: Chew 1 tablet daily.

Whilst children are taking these tablets, no other vitamin supplement containing vitamins A and D should be taken except under medical supervision. Not suitable for a kosher diet.

Pharmacy only: Yes

Always Consult Your Pharmacist

SANATOGEN MULTIVITAMIN TABLETS
Roche Consumer Health

PA No: N/A

◻Packs of 30 or 60 orange-white speckled, biconvex,

chewable tablets.

◼Vitamin A 750µg, vitamin B1 1.2mg, vitamin B2 1.6mg, niacin 18mg, folic acid 300µg, vitamin B6 2mg, vitamin B12 2µg, vitamin C 30mg, vitamin D2 2.5µg, vitamin E 5mg.

❓Supplying multivitamins lost

when dieting, pregnant or breastfeeding or as a result of medication.

☑Adults: 1 tablet daily.

Children: Over 12 yrs: 1 tablet daily.

Pharmacy only: Yes

SEVEN SEAS HALIBORANGE A, C & D
Seven Seas Ireland Ltd

PA No: N/A

◻Packs of 60 or 120 orange-flavoured chewable tablets.

◼Vitamin C 30mg, vitamin D 2.5µg, vitamin A 750µg.

❓Vitamin supplement.

☑Adults: 1 tablet daily.

Children: Over 3 yrs: 1 tablet daily.

Pharmacy only: No

SEVEN SEAS HALIBORANGE MULTIVITAMIN ORANGE-FLAVOURED LIQUID
Seven Seas Ireland Ltd

PA No: N/A

◻250ml bottle of orange-

flavoured liquid.

◼Vitamin C (ascorbic acid) 15mg, vitamin E (dl-alpha-tocopherol acetate) 3mg, vitamin B1 (thiamin hydrochloride), vitamin B2 (riboflavin) 0.4mg, vitamin B6 (pyridoxine hydrochloride) 0.6mg, nicotinic acid (niacin) 5mg, vitamin D 5µg, pantothenic acid 3mg,

vitamin A 200µg.

❓Multivitamin supplement.

☑Adults: 10ml daily.

Children: Over 6 yrs: 10ml daily. 1 month-6 yrs: 5ml daily. Under 6 months: Mix dose into milk or diluted fruit juices.

Pharmacy only: No

SEVEN SEAS MINADEX CHILDREN'S VITAMINS A, C & D
Seven Seas Ireland Ltd

PA No: N/A

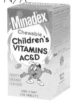

◻Packs of 100 orange, round, biconvex chewable tablets.

◼Vitamin C (ascorbic acid) 30mg, vitamin A acetate 500µg, vitamin D3 (cholecalciferol) 5µg.

❓Vitamin supplement.

☑Adults: 1 tablet daily.

Children: Over 3 yrs: 1 tablet daily.

Pharmacy only: No

If Symptoms Persist Consult Your Doctor

SEVEN SEAS MINADEX MULTIVITAMIN SYRUP
Seven Seas Ireland Ltd

PA No: 416/6/1

☐150ml bottle of orange-flavoured syrup.

☑Vitamin C (ascorbic acid) 35mg, vitamin E (dl-alpha-tocopherol acetate) 3mg, vitamin B1 (thiamin hydrochloride) 1.4mg, vitamin B2 (pyridoxine hydrochloride) 0.7mg, nicotinamide 18mg, vitamin A acetate 4,000IU, vitamin D3 (cholecalciferol) 400IU.

⚴For the prevention of vitamin A, B group, C, D and E deficiencies including use during convalescence from debilitating illness.

☑Children: From 6 months: 10ml daily mixed in feed or a drink.

Pharmacy only: No

SUPERTED VITAMINS A, C, D 50S
Perrans Distributors Ltd

PA No: N/A

☐Packs of 50 chewable, SuperTed-shaped tablets with a natural orange flavour.

☑Vitamin A 400µg (1,332IU),

vitamin D 5µg (200IU), vitamin C 30mg, sugar, sorbitol, maltodextrin, magnesium stearate, stearic acid, flavouring (natural orange), vitamin A (acetate prep. with antioxidant dl-alpha-tocopherol), vitamin D (as D3 prep.), colour (iron oxide).

⚴Children's vitamin supplement

providing vitamins A, C and D vital for sound growth, strong bones, healthy tissues and maintenance of the immune system.

☑Children: Over 3 yrs: Chew 1 tablet daily. Maximum 1 tablet in 24 hrs.

Pharmacy only: No

OTHER DIETARY SUPPLEMENTS

ABIDEC DROPS
Pfizer/Warner Lambert Consumer Healthcare

PA No: 823/30/1

☐25ml bottle and dropper graduated at 0.3ml and 0.6ml. Contains clear, yellow liquid

with a characteristic odour and taste.

☑Vitamin A 4,000IU, thiamine hydrochloride 1mg, riboflavin 0.4mg, pyridoxine hydrochloride 0.5mg, ascorbic acid 50mg, calciferol 400IU,

nicotinamide 5mg per 0.6ml.

⚴For the prevention of vitamin deficiencies.

☑Children: 1-12 yrs: 0.6ml daily. Under 1 yr: 0.3ml daily.

Pharmacy only: Yes

BUILD UP
Nestle Clinical Nutrition

PA No: N/A

☐Packs of 4 sachets containing a powdered supplement

available in vanilla, strawberry, natural, lemon and lime and chocolate flavours.

⚴Pre- and postsurgery, after trauma, fever, prolonged illness;

elderly patients.

☑Adults: 2-3 drinks daily.

Pharmacy only: Yes

Always Read The Label

CALOGEN
Scientific Hospital Supplies

PA No: N/A

◼250ml or 1L bottles available in neutral, strawberry and butterscotch flavours.

◪High fat energy supplement

providing 450kcals per 100mls.

❓For patients with high energy requirements. Specially indicated for patients with small appetites or on a low electrolyte diet.

☑Adults: 30mls x 3-4 times daily.

Children: 50mls daily (may need to dilute for children under 5 yrs).

Pharmacy only: Yes

CALSHAKE
Fresenius Kabi

PA No: N/A

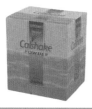

◼High energy, powdered, nutritional supplement. Vanilla, strawberry and banana flavours: 7 x 87g sachets; Chocolate flavour: 7 x 90g sachets.

☑When mixed with whole milk (240mls), Calshake provides 598kcal, 12g protein.

❓Developed to meet the requirements of patients with diseases characterised by

wasting, loss of appetite, taste fatigue and poor nutrition, e.g. cystic fibrosis, cancer and AIDS. Calshake is a suitable high energy food supplement for use in disease related malnutrition, malabsorption and other conditions requiring fortification with a fat/energy supplement.

☑Dosage to be advised by a clinician/dietitian.

Pharmacy only: Yes

CLINUTREN 1.5
Nestle Clinical Nutrition

PA No: N/A

◼Tetra brik containing a

1.5kcal supplement.

❓Pre- and postoperative and disease-related malnutrition, elderly patients, neurological

patients, undernourished patients.

☑Adults: 2-3 units daily.

Pharmacy only: Yes

CLINUTREN DESSERT
Nestle Clinical Nutrition

PA No: N/A

◼125g cup of high protein pudding available in vanilla, peach, caramel and chocolate

flavours.

☑Milk proteins, dried skimmed milk, gelatin (cocoa powder – chocolate).

❓Oral clinical nutrition of malnourished patients, patients at risk of malnutrition or patients lacking appetite.

☑Adults: 2-3/day (as snack or dessert).

❗Not to be prescribed to children under 1 yr.

No more than 80g protein intake per day (6 pots).

Pharmacy only: Yes

CUBITAN
Nutricia Ireland Limited

PA No: N/A

◼Nutritionally complete sip feed. Available in vanilla, strawberry and chocolate flavours.

☑Per 200ml: 250 kcal, 20g protein, 3.0g arginine. Contains higher levels of the vitamins, minerals and trace elements which have been shown to have a role in wound healing.

❓Cubitan is specially formulated to assist the healing of pressure sores in malnourished patients.

❗Not suitable for children under 3 yrs.

Pharmacy only: Yes

Always Consult Your Pharmacist

EFAMOL PURE EVENING PRIMROSE OIL
Nutricia Ireland Limited

PA No: N/A

🗌 Packs of 30 or 90 capsules.

☑ 2 capsules provide: Pure evening primrose oil 700mg, which provides 80mg GLA, vitamin E 10mg.

❓ Dietary supplement. Helps to maintain healthy looking skin.

☑ Adults: 2 capsules daily with liquid.

Children: As per adult dose.

Pharmacy only: No

EFAMOL PURE EVENING PRIMROSE OIL HIGH STRENGTH
Nutricia Ireland Limited

PA No: N/A

🗌 Packs of 30 capsules.

☑ 1 capsule provides: Pure evening primrose oil 700mg, which provides 80g GLA, vitamin E 10mg.

❓ Dietary supplement. Helps to maintain healthy looking skin.

☑ Adults: 1 capsule daily with liquid.

Children: As per adult dose.

Pharmacy only: No

EFAMOL PURE EVENING PRIMROSE OIL LEMON AND LIME LIQUID
Nutricia Ireland Limited

PA No: N/A

🗌 150ml amber glass bottle contained in a carton. Tamper evident lid.

☑ One of the richest sources of GLA. Pure EPO — 1,000mg (daily intake).

❓ For healthy looking skin.

☑ 1 tsp/day with food.

Pharmacy only: No

EFAMOL PURE EVENING PRIMROSE OIL (LIQUID)
Nutricia Ireland Limited

PA No: N/A

🗌 30ml amber glass bottle contained in a carton. Tamper evident lid.

☑ One of the most effective sources of gamma linolenic acid (GLA). Liquid EPO. $\frac{1}{4}$ tsp. (16 drops) provides: Pure evening primrose oil 1,000mg, which provides 80mg GLA.

❓ Dietary supplement for healthy looking skin.

☑ 16 drops per day with food ($\frac{1}{4}$ tsp approx.).

Pharmacy only: No

ENLIVE 240ML
Abbott Nutrition

PA No: N/A

🗌 240ml tetrapak with straw for sipping and pull tab for pouring. A refreshing, non-milk tasting nutritional supplement to sip. Available in orange, apple, lemon and lime and pineapple flavours.

☑ Per 240ml tetrapak: Energy: 300kcals, protein: 9.6g, fat: 0g, carbohydrate: 65.5g. Vitamins, minerals and trace elements. Gluten and lactose free.

❓ Enlive is a suitable supplement for patients who are malnourished or at risk of becoming undernourished. Preoperative and postoperative patients. Cancer cachexia, Crohn's disease, cystic fibrosis, inflammatory bowel disease, total gastrostomy and disease-related malnutrition.

❗ Not suitable for children under 1 yr.

Pharmacy only: Yes

If Symptoms Persist Consult Your Doctor

ENRICH PLUS
Abbott Nutrition

PA No: N/A

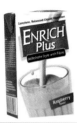

◻200ml tetrapak with straw for sipping and pull-tab for pouring. Enrich Plus is a nutritionally complete, high energy, milkshake-style sip supplement with a blend of fibre and FOS. Available in vanilla, chocolate, raspberry and banana flavours. Gluten and lactose free.

◼Per 200ml pack: 305kcal, 12.5g protein, a fibre blend selected to mimic the normal diet and containing FOS to help promote gut health. Fibre and FOS content: 5g (2.5g of each).

❓Enrich Plus is suitable for patients who are malnourished or at risk of becoming malnourished and need more fibre, e.g. constipated patients, such as the elderly, those with a physical disability and patients taking opioids (e.g. codeine, morphine). Also suitable for patients with diarrhoea.

◤Enrich Plus tetrapak 200mls twice or three times daily.

Pharmacy only: Yes

ENSURE PLUS 200ML
Abbott Nutrition

PA No: N/A

◻200ml tetrapak with straw for sipping and pull tab for pouring. A nutritionally complete high energy supplemental drink. Available in 12 flavours: fruits of the forest, raspberry, banana, coffee, orange, chocolate, blackcurrant, vanilla, strawberry, caramel, peach and neutral. Gluten and lactose free.

◼Per 200ml tetrapak: Energy: 300kcals, protein: 12.5g, fat: 10g, carbohydrate: 40g.

Vitamins, minerals, trace elements.

❓Ideal for patients who are malnourished or at risk of becoming malnourished. Preoperative and postoperative patients, poor wound healing, cancer cachexia, Crohn's disease, total gastrectomy and disease-related malnutrition.

❗Not suitable for children under 1 yr.

Pharmacy only: Yes

EPHYNAL
Roche Consumer Health

PA No: 50/57/4

◻Packs of 50 x 200mg or 100 x 50mg tablets.

◼Vitamin E (dl-alpha-tocopherol acetate) 50mg.

❓Vitamin E supplement.

◤Adults: Recommended daily intake 8-10mg. Increased dosage may be required in presence of large amounts of unsaturated fats in the diet. Intermittent claudication 400-600mg daily for 3 months or more.

Children and infants: 1-10mg/kg of bodyweight daily.

Pharmacy only: Yes

FLORESSE BODY BOOST STARFLOWER OIL
Roche Consumer Health

PA No: N/A

◻Pack of 30 capsules.

◼Vitamin C 10mg, thiamin 1.4mg, riboflavin 1.6mg, niacin 3mg, vitamin B6 2mg, folic acid 200µg, vitamin B12 1µg, pantothenic acid 6mg, starflower oil 500mg providing gamma-linolenic acid 115mg.

❓B complex vitamins help your body produce energy from food and keep your nervous system in good health. B vitamins cannot be stored in the body and a regular balanced intake is essential. Regular use will help maintain well-being.

◤Adults: 1 capsule daily. This may be increased to 2 capsules daily, especially prior to, or during, your monthly periods.

Pharmacy only: Yes

Always Read The Label

FLORESSE SKIN VITALITY STARFLOWER OIL WITH ANTI-OXIDANT VITAMINS
Roche Consumer Health

PA No: N/A

🖵Pack of 30 capsules.

🎽Vitamin E 2mg, vitamin C 10mg, starflower oil 500mg providing gamma-linolenic acid 115mg.

🛈Regular use helps keep your skin looking soft, smooth and supple. Rich in anti-oxidant vitamins, which help maintain healthy body cells and tissues and help revitalise, nourish and promote healthy skin. Starflower oil is a source of GLA which regulates cell growth and sustains healthy skin.

☑Adults: 1 capsule daily. This may be increased to 2 capsules daily, especially prior to, or during, your monthly periods.

Pharmacy only: Yes

FLORESSE STARFLOWER OIL 500MG
Roche Consumer Health

PA No: N/A

🖵Pack of 30 capsules.

🎽Vitamin E 2mg, starflower oil 500mg providing gamma-linolenic acid 115mg.

🛈Helps regulate the body's delicate chemistry and maintains healthy skin and joints. Vitamin E helps to maintain healthy skin, hair and nails.

☑Adults: If you are taking a GLA supplement for the first time, take 2-3 capsules daily for up to 12 weeks, after which daily intake may be reduced to 1-2 capsules to suit individual requirements.

Pharmacy only: Yes

FLORESSE STARFLOWER OIL 1,000MG ONE-A-DAY
Roche Consumer Health

PA No: N/A

🖵Packs of 30 capsules.

🎽Vitamin E 2mg, starflower oil 1,000mg providing gamma-linolenic acid (GLA) 230mg.

🛈Provides an extra boost of GLA throughout the month. Vitamin E helps maintain healthy skin, joints, hair and nails.

☑Adults: 1 capsule daily. If you are taking a GLA supplement for the first time, you may only require a lower dosage such as 500mg.

Pharmacy only: Yes

FORMANCE MOUSSE
Abbott Nutrition

PA No: N/A

🖵Ready to serve 113g pot. An energy-dense nutritional supplement, which has a semi-solid consistency. Available in vanilla, butterscotch and chocolate flavours.

🎽Per 113g pot: Energy 170kcals, protein 4g, fat 4.4g, carbohydrate 24.0g. FOS 1g. Vitamins and minerals.

🛈Formance Mousse is a nutritional supplement for patients who: require variety in their diet; have dysphagia; are malnourished or at risk of becoming malnourished; have fluid restrictions; are post CVA/stroke; are post-operative.

❗Not suitable for children under 1 yr.

Pharmacy only: Yes

Always Consult Your Pharmacist

FORTICREME
Nutricia Ireland Limited

PA No: N/A

◻A nutritionally balanced, high energy and protein dessert providing 201kcals per 125g.

Available in vanilla, forest fruit, coffee and chocolate flavours.

☑12.5g protein.

◻Creamy texture makes it ideal for patients with swallowing difficulties or for those patients

who are tired of liquid supplements.

❗Not suitable for infants under 1 yr.

Pharmacy only: Yes

FORTIFRESH
Nutricia Ireland Limited

PA No: N/A

◻200ml carton with straw. Nutritionally complete, high calorie, high protein, yoghurt-tasting sip feed. Gluten free. Available in blackcurrant,

peach, raspberry and orange flavours.

☑300kcals, 12g protein, 37.4g carbohydrate and 11.6g fat per pack. Complete in minerals, vitamins and trace elements.

◻For malnourished patients,

pre- and postoperative convalescence, cancer, dysphagia, disease-related malnutrition, elderly.

❗Not suitable for children under 3 yrs.

Pharmacy only: Yes

FORTIJUCE
Nutricia Ireland Limited

PA No: N/A

◻200ml carton with straw. A refreshing, juice-tasting, nutritionally complete, high energy sip feed. Gluten and lactose free. Available in blackcurrant, pineapple, peach and orange,

apple and pear, lemon and lime, apricot and forest fruits flavours.

☑300kcals, 8g protein, 67g carbohydrate per 200ml pack. Complete in minerals, vitamins and trace elements.

◻For malnourished patients, pre- and postoperative convalescence, cancer, dysphagia, disease-

related malnutrition, elderly. Particularly suitable for those tired of milk-tasting sip feeds.

❗Not suitable for children under 3 yrs. Use under medical/dietetic supervision for diabetic and renal patients.

Pharmacy only: Yes

FORTIMEL
Nutricia Ireland Limited

PA No: N/A

◻200ml carton with straw. Nutritionally balanced, high protein sip feed. Gluten free. Available in forest fruit, vanilla and strawberry flavours.

☑20g protein, 20.6g carbohydrate, 4.2g fat per carton.

◻Suitable for any condition where a high protein supplement is warranted: Wound healing, hypoproteinaemia, continuous

ambulatory peritoneal dialysis.

❗Not suitable for children under 3 yrs. Use under medical/dietetic supervision for renal and diabetic patients.

Pharmacy only: Yes

FORTISIP
Nutricia Ireland Limited

PA No: N/A

◻200ml carton with straw. Nutritionally complete high energy, high protein, milk-tasting sip feed. Gluten and lactose free. Available in chicken, mushroom, neutral, vanilla,

orange, strawberry, tropical fruit, toffee, chocolate and banana flavours.

☑300kcals, 12g protein, 36.8g carbohydrate, 11.6g fat per 200ml pack. Complete in vitamins, minerals and trace elements.

◻For malnourished patients,

pre- and postoperative convalescence, cancer, dysphagia, disease-related malnutrition, elderly. Suitable for diabetics once sipped slowly over 20 minutes.

❗Not suitable for children under 3 yrs.

Pharmacy only: Yes

If Symptoms Persist Consult Your Doctor

FORTISIP MULTI FIBRE
Nutricia Ireland Limited

PA No: N/A

■200ml carton with straw. Nutritionally complete, high calorie, high protein, fibre-enriched sip feed. Gluten and lactose free. Contains a unique blend of six different fibre sources. Available in orange, banana, chocolate, vanilla and strawberry flavours.

■300kcals, 4.5g fibre, 12g protein, 36.8g carbohydrate, 11.6g fat per 200ml pack. Complete in vitamins, minerals and trace elements.

■Suitable for all malnourished groups and especially suitable for patients with constipation or diarrhoea. Suitable for diabetics once sipped slowly over 20 minutes and monitor blood sugar levels.

■Not suitable for children under 3 yrs.

Pharmacy only: Yes

FRESUBIN ENERGY
Fresenius Kabi *(was Entera)*

PA No: N/A

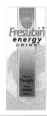

■200ml tetrabrik containing a 1.5kcal/ml, nutritionally complete and ready to use sip feed. Clinically free from lactose, cholesterol, purine and gluten. Available in vanilla, strawberry, vegetable soup, neutral, butterscotch, blackcurrant, chocolate-mint, banana, pineapple and orange flavours.

■Per 200ml carton: Protein 11.3g, carbohydrate 37.6g, fat 11.66g, vitamins, minerals, trace elements, flavouring, 300kcal.

■Fresubin Energy is suitable as a nutritional supplement or as a sole source of nutrition for patients who cannot or will not eat adequate quantities of foods and in particular patients who cannot tolerate large volumes.

■Not suitable for children under 1 yr.

Pharmacy only: Yes

FRESUBIN ENERGY FIBRE *(was Entera Fibre Plus)*
Fresenius Kabi

PA No: N/A

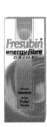

■200ml tetrapak containing a 1.5kcal/ml, high energy nutritionally complete and ready to use sip feed with fibre. Clinically free from lactose, cholesterol and purine. Gluten and carrageenan free. Available in vanilla, lemon, chocolate, strawberry, cappuccino and banana flavours.

■Per 200ml: 5g mixed source fibre (providing the benefits of both insoluble and soluble fibre), protein 11.3g, carbohydrate 37.6g, fat 11.6g, vitamins, minerals, trace elements, 300kcal.

■Fresubin Energy Fibre is suitable as a nutritional supplement or as a sole source of nutrition for patients who are unable or unwilling to eat adequate quantities of food to meet their nutritional requirements. As it is energy dense and enriched with dietary fibre it is particularly useful for patients who cannot tolerate a large volume and those who have, or who are at risk of, disturbances in bowel functions, e.g. diarrhoea or constipation.

■Not suitable for children under 1 yr. Use with care in children due to high fibre content. Use under medical supervision.

Pharmacy only: Yes

Always Read The Label

FRESUBIN ORIGINAL
Fresenius Kabi

PA No: N/A

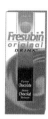

◼200ml Tetrapak of nutritionally complete sip feed available in 6 flavours: vanilla, chocolate, peach, mocha, nut and blackcurrant. Gluten and lactose free.

◼200kcal, 7.6g protein, 6.8g fat, vitamins, minerals and trace elements.

◼Suitable as a nutrition supplement or as a sole source of nutrition for patients who are unable or unwilling to eat adequate quantities of food to meet their nutritional requirements.

Pharmacy only: Yes

GEVRAL PROTEIN
Whitehall Laboratories Ltd

PA No: 37/22/2, 3, 4, 5

◼Box of 14 sachets containing fine, cream-coloured powder with orange, strawberry or custard flavour intended for dispersion in water or milk for oral administration to human beings.

◼Each sachet contains vitamin A palmitate 1,250IU, vitamin D 125IU, vitamin B1 1.25mg, vitamin B2 1.25mg, vitamin B6 0.125mg, vitamin B12 0.5µg, vitamin C 12.5mg, vitamin E 2.5IU, niacinamide 3.75mg, calcium pantothenate 1.25mg, calcium 160mg, phosphorus 170mg, elemental iron 2.5mg, lysine 0.5g, choline 10mg, inositol 12.5mg, copper 0.25mg, iodine 25µg, potassium 25mg, manganese 0.125mg, zinc 0.125mg, magnesium 0.25mg, soya protein isolate, carbohydrate, (from non-fat milk powder and sucrose) 6g, fat (not more than 2%), total protein 50%, sodium (not more than 1.2%), calories 57.

◼For the management of appropriate vitamin and mineral deficiencies.

◼Adults: 1 sachet daily.

◼Not recommended for patients with a known hypersensitivity to any of the constituents. The content of pyridoxine may interfere with the effects of concurrent levodopa therapy. Care should be taken in the concomitant use of this preparation with tetracyclines as iron salts diminish the absorption of tetracyclines. While children are taking this product, no other vitamin supplement containing vitamin A and D should be taken unless under medical supervision.

Pharmacy only: Yes

GLUCOSAMINE + CHONDROITIN
Intrapharma/Dugdale/Health Perception

PA No: N/A

◼Packs of 30 or 60 tablets.

◼Glucosamine sulphate 500mg, chondroitin sulphate 400mg, bioflavonoids 50mg and manganese 5mg.

◼To help maintain healthy joints.

Pharmacy only: Yes

G + C EFFERVESCENT 20S
Intrapharma/Dugdale/Health Perception

PA No: N/A

◼Tubes of 20 tablets.

◼Glucosamine sulphate KCl (salt free) 500mg, ester C 250mg.

◼An effervescent preparation to help maintain healthy joints.

Pharmacy only: Yes

Always Consult Your Pharmacist

HEALTHCRAFTS ACIDOPHILUS EXTRA 30S
Perrans Distributors Ltd

PA No: N/A

☐Pack of 30 capsules.

☑Dextrose, potato starch, capsule shell (gelatin, colour:

titanium dioxide), microcrystalline cellulose, bacterial culture (providing lactobacillus acidophilus and bifidobacterium bifidum), sucrose, magnesium stearate.

☑Take 1 capsule each day. Take with a glass of milk or water, or with a meal. Do not swallow capsules with hot

drinks, as heat kills bacteria.

❗Keep refrigerated.

Pharmacy only: No

HEALTHCRAFTS EVENING PRIMROSE OIL 500MG 2 X 30S
Perrans Distributors Ltd

PA No: N/A

☐Packs of 2 x 30 capsules.

☑Evening primrose oil 500mg, vitamin E 6mg, capsule shell (gelatin, glycerin).

❓Dietary supplement.

☑Adults: 1 capsule daily with food.

❗Consult doctor before use if

suffering from epilepsy.

Pharmacy only: No

HEALTHCRAFTS EVENING PRIMROSE OIL 1,000MG TWIN PACK 2 X 30S
Perrans Distributors Ltd

PA No: N/A

☐Packs of 2 x 30 capsules.

☑Evening primrose oil 1,000mg, vitamin E 6mg, capsule shell (gelatin, glycerin).

❓Dietary supplement.

☑Adults: 1 capsule daily with food.

❗Consult doctor before use if suffering from epilepsy.

Pharmacy only: No

HIGH STRENGTH GLUCOSAMINE 30S
Intrapharma/Dugdale/Health Perception

PA No: N/A

☐Jar of 30 tablets. Free from

preservatives, yeast, salt, starch, lactose and gluten.

☑Glucosamine sulphate KCl (salt free) 1,000mg, chondroitin sulphate (fish source) 800mg, bioflavanoids 100mg, manganese 10mg.

❓To help maintain healthy joints.

Pharmacy only: Yes

HIGH STRENGTH GLUCOSAMINE 60S
Intrapharma/Dugdale/Health Perception

PA No: N/A

☐30 blister packed tablets per box. Suitable for vegetarians and vegans.

☑Glucosamine sulphate KCl (salt free) 1,000mg, vitamin C 600mg, calcium carbonate 600mg, manganese 10mg

❓Could help maintain joint mobility.

Pharmacy only: Yes

If Symptoms Persist Consult Your Doctor

IDÉOS
Helsinn Birex Therapeutics Ltd
PA No: 737/1/1

Cartons of 4 tubes of 15 chewable tablets each. Calcium/vitamin D3 supplement.

Calcium carbonate 1,250mg, cholecalciferol 10mg, (corresponding to calcium 500mg and vitamin D3 400IU).

Vitamin D and calcium deficiency correction in the elderly. Also as an adjunct to specific therapy for osteoporosis.

Adults: 2 tablets to be chewed daily.

Not recommended for children.

Treatment with the digitalis glycosides or thiazide diuretics. Renal impairment/long-term use; check calcium excretion and plasma calcium.

Pharmacy only: Yes

MAXIJUL
Scientific Hospital Supplies
PA No: N/A

Maxijul Powder: 4 x 132g sachets, 200g tin or 2.5kg tub. Maxijul Liquid: 200ml tetrapak available in neutral, lemon and lime, blackcurrant and orange flavours.

Maxijul is a convenient, powder or liquid carbohydrate energy supplement. It can be easily added to sweet or savoury foods and drinks to enhance the energy content.

Maxijul Powder: 500kcals per 132g sachet. Maxijul Liquid: 400kcals per 200ml tetrapak.

For use in disease-related malnutrition or any condition requiring an additional energy source.

Use with caution in diabetes.

Pharmacy only: Yes

MAXISORB
Scientific Hospital Supplies
PA No: N/A

5 x 30g sachets. Versatile, high protein powder which can be made up into a milkshake or pudding. Available in strawberry, vanilla and chocolate flavours.

138kcals, 12g protein per 30g sachet.

Maxisorb is designed for those patients with high protein requirements, including disease-related malnutrition, dysphagia and renal disease.

Not suitable for infants under 1 yr.

Pharmacy only: Yes

NUTILIS
Nutricia Ireland Limited
PA No: N/A

225g tin of food and liquid thickener. Thickens food and drinks in 60 seconds and does not continue to thicken. 1 tablespoon = 8g Nutilis = 29kcals. Gluten and lactose free.

Modified maize starch.

For use in adults and children over 3 yrs who require thickened fluids and/or foods, e.g. those with dysphagia.

Add Nutilis to food or drink. Mix well with fork or whisk. Leave to stand for 60 seconds.

Pharmacy only: Yes

Always Read The Label

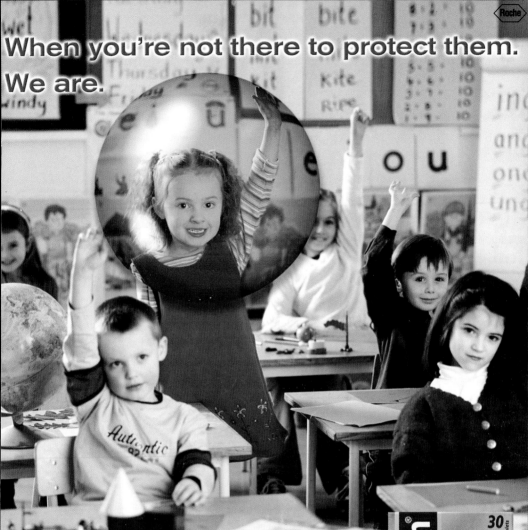

When you're not there to protect them. We are.

Taken first thing in the morning, sugar free Redoxon's high strength formula will help support your body's immune system. And a healthy immune system is what's needed to protect you and your family against infections such as colds and flu throughout the year.

Redoxon is packed with Vitamin C goodness and dissolves into a refreshing effervescent drink. Also suitable for children 6 years or older, Redoxon comes in three delicious flavours - orange, lemon and blackcurrant.

Added protection against infection.

REDOXON IS A ® REGISTERED TRADEMARK

ONLY AVAILABLE FROM YOUR PHARMACY. ALWAYS READ THE LABEL.

Roche

Redoxon 30 Tablets

EFFERVESCENT Tablets 1000mg

ORANGE FLAVOUR

Ascorbic Acid (Vitamin C) SUGAR FREE

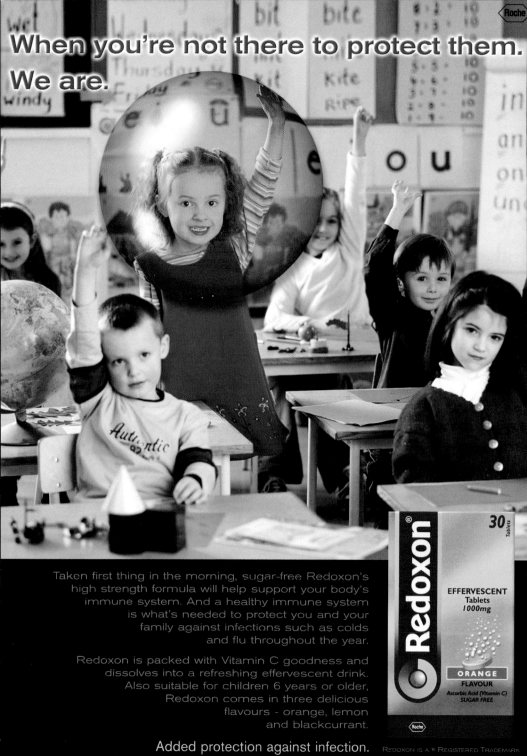

When you're not there to protect them. We are.

Taken first thing in the morning, sugar-free Redoxon's high strength formula will help support your body's immune system. And a healthy immune system is what's needed to protect you and your family against infections such as colds and flu throughout the year.

Redoxon is packed with Vitamin C goodness and dissolves into a refreshing effervescent drink. Also suitable for children 6 years or older, Redoxon comes in three delicious flavours - orange, lemon and blackcurrant.

Added protection against infection.

Redoxon

30 Tablets

EFFERVESCENT
Tablets
1000mg

ORANGE
FLAVOUR
Ascorbic Acid (Vitamin C)
SUGAR FREE

Roche

NUTRICIA EFALEX CAPSULES
Nutricia Ireland Limited

PA No: N/A

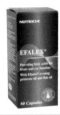

60 or 240 capsules in a jar in an outer cardboard carton. Tamper evident seal on jar.

2 capsules provide: Vitamin E 20mg, fish oil 588mg (providing docosahexaenoic acid (DHA) 120mg, arachidonic acid (AA) 10.5mg), evening primrose oil 280mg (providing gamma linolenic acid (GLA) 24mg), thyme oil 2mg.

Dietary supplement to safeguard the intake of fatty acids important for the brain and eye.

Adults and children aged 5 yrs and over: 4 capsules with food or drink.

Children aged 2-5 yrs: 2-4 capsules per day with food or drink. Capsules can be cut open and the contents mixed with food or drink.

Not suitable for children under 2 yrs.

If taking this product for the first time, then the above amounts should be doubled for the first 12 weeks with half the amounts being taken in the morning and half in the evening.

If using phenothiazine medication or with a history of epilepsy, consult doctor before using.

Pharmacy only: No

NUTRICIA EFALEX LIQUID
Nutricia Ireland Limited

PA No: N/A

150ml in a glass bottle in an outer cardboard carton. Tamper evident seal on bottle. Contains lemon and lime flavoured liquid.

1 tsp (5ml) provides: Vitamin E (natural source) 20mg, fatty acids (docosahexaenoic acid (DHA) 120mg, gamma linolenic acid (GLA) 24mg, arachidonic acid (AA) 10.5mg).

Dietary supplement to safeguard the intake of fatty acids important for the brain and eye.

Adults: 2 tsps (10ml) daily with food or drink.

Children: 2-5 yrs: 1 tsp (5ml) daily with food or drink.

5 yrs and over: 2 tsps (10ml) daily with food or drink.

Not suitable for children under 2 yrs.

If taking this product for the first time, then the above amounts should be doubled for the first 12 weeks with half the amounts being taken in the morning and half in the evening.

If using phenothiazine medication or with a history of epilepsy, consult doctor before using.

Pharmacy only: No

NUTRICIA EFAMOL® PMP™
Nutricia Ireland Limited

PA No: N/A

60 capsules in a jar in a cardboard carton. Tamper evident seal on jar. Evening primrose oil plus vitamins and minerals.

2 capsules provide: Vitamin E 20mg, vitamin C 60mg, niacin 12mg, vitamin B6 40mg, biotin 0.08mg, magnesium 40mg, zinc 4mg, Efamol Pure Evening Primrose Oil 1,000mg (providing GLA 80mg).

Dietary supplement to safeguard the intake of specific nutrients important for women during the female monthly cycle.

2 capsules daily with liquid.

If using phenothiazine medication or with a history of epilepsy, consult with doctor before using this product.

Pharmacy only: No

Always Consult Your Pharmacist

NUTRICIA EFANATAL®
Nutricia Ireland Limited

PA No: N/A

🔲60 capsules in a jar in a cardboard carton. Tamper evident seal on jar.

☑2 capsules provide: Natural source vitamin E 10mg, fish oil 500mg (providing docosahexaenoic acid (DHA) 125mg, arachidonic acid (AA) 9.4mg), Efamol Evening Primrose Oil 500mg (providing gamma linolenic acid (GLA) 60mg).

❓Dietary supplement to safeguard the intake of fatty acids required by mother and baby before, during and after pregnancy.

✅2 capsules daily with food or drink.

❗If using phenothiazine medication or with a history of epilepsy, consult doctor before using.

Pharmacy only: Yes

NUTRICIA MULTIFIBRE FORMULA
Nutricia Ireland Limited

PA No. N/A

🔲200g jar of powdered fibre in a cardboard carton. Tamper evident seal on jar.

☑Soy polysaccharide, alphacellulose, gum arabic, fructo-oligosaccharide, inulin, resistant starch.

❓Dietary supplement formulated to safeguard the intake of a variety of fibres for digestion and regularity.

✅Adults and children over 2 yrs: 1 scoop (9.5g) morning and evening. Mix 1 scoop with a glass of juice. Stir and drink immediately. Follow with a glass of juice or water.

❗Not suitable for children under 2 yrs.

Do not take in cases of intestinal obstruction.

Pharmacy only: Yes

PAEDIASURE TETRAPAK
Abbott Nutrition

PA No: N/A

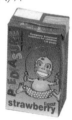

🔲200ml tetrapak with straw for sipping and pull-tab for pouring. Paediasure Tetrapak is a nutritionally complete, 1kcal/ml sip supplement. Available in strawberry, chocolate, banana and vanilla flavours. Gluten free.

☑5.6g protein, 10g fat, 22.4g carbohydrate, vitamins, minerals and trace elements.

❓Paediasure Tetrapak is nutritionally complete and specifically formulated for children aged 1-6 yrs who require a nutritional supplement, e.g. failure to thrive, short bowel syndrome, intractable malabsorption, bowel fistulae, pre-operative patients, dysphagia.

✅Paediasure Tetrapak 200ml twice daily.

❗Not suitable for children under 1 yr.

Pharmacy only: Yes

PEPTAMEN
Nestle Clinical Nutrition

PA No: N/A

🔲250ml recyclable steel can containing Peptide Bascel Isocaloric balanced complete liquid feed for enteral tube feeding and oral intake. Vanilla or unflavoured.

☑Water, maltodextrin, enzymatically hydrolysed whey protein, mct cornstarch, sunflower oil, vitamins, minerals and trace elements.

❓Used to give nutritional support in a readily absorbable form to patients with impaired digestion and/or absorption, i.e. in inflammatory disease, short bowel syndrome or pancreatic insufficiency.

✅Adults: 2,000ml/day.

❗Children: Not to be used for children under 1 yr.

Use under healthcare supervision.

Pharmacy only: Yes

If Symptoms Persist Consult Your Doctor

POLYCAL LIQUID
Nutricia Ireland Limited

PA No: N/A

▭200ml bottle of ready to use, high energy, carbohydrate-based drink. Available in neutral, orange, blackcurrant, lemon and apple flavours.

☑494kcals per 200mls.

❓Suitable for kidney failure, liver failure, fluid restricted diets, anyone unable to meet their energy requirements from normal food and drinks. Can be used for glucose tolerance tests.

Pharmacy only: Yes

POLYCAL POWDER
Nutricia Ireland Limited

PA No: N/A

▭400g tin of high energy, virtually tasteless powder. Can be added to sweet and savoury food and drink to enhance the energy content. Gluten and lactose free.

☑380kcals per 100g. 95g carbohydrate.

❓Any patients unable to meet their energy requirements from normal food; patients with kidney failure, liver failure and the following carbohydrate intolerances: lactose, galactose, fructose and sucrose, disorders of amino acid metabolism.

Pharmacy only: Yes

POWER HEALTH IRON AMINO ACID CHELATE 14MG
Power Health Products Ltd

PA No: N/A

▭Red/brown speckled, 8mm, round tablets.

☑70mg providing 14mg iron.

▨Adults: 1 per day.

Pharmacy only: No

PROTIFAR
Nutricia Ireland Limited

PA No: N/A

▭225g tin containing a concentrated protein powder. Gluten and lactose free. Virtually tasteless and can be added to sweet and savoury food or drinks.

☑370kcals, 88.5g protein per 100g.

❓Patients requiring high protein supplements, e.g. disease-related malnutrition, pre- and postoperatively, cancer cachexia and wound healing.

▨Mix with sufficient cold liquids to form a smooth paste then stir into food or drink.

Pharmacy only: Yes

PROVIDE XTRA
Fresenius Kabi

PA No: N/A

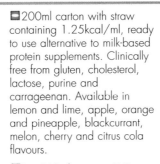

▭200ml carton with straw containing 1.25kcal/ml, ready to use alternative to milk-based protein supplements. Clinically free from gluten, cholesterol, lactose, purine and carrageenan. Available in lemon and lime, apple, orange and pineapple, blackcurrant, melon, cherry and citrus cola flavours.

☑Per 200ml: protein 7.5g, vitamins, minerals, trace elements, 250kcal.

❓Provide Xtra is a refreshing liquid, fruit-flavoured protein drink which can be used to supplement the diet of patients with increased protein requirements, malnutrition and milk protein intolerance. It is also a suitable alternative to the traditional, milk-based nutritional supplements for those patients who dislike/are tired of milk-based supplements.

❗Not suitable for children under 1 yr. To be used under medical supervision.

Pharmacy only: Yes

Always Read The Label

SCANDISHAKE MIX
Scientific Hospital Supplies

PA No: N/A

◻6 x 85g sachets.
Scandishake Mix is a high energy powdered supplement. Available in unflavoured, vanilla, strawberry and chocolate flavours.

☑Provides 600kcals, 12g protein when made up with 240ml whole milk.

❓It is a very useful supplement where there are increased energy requirements such as in cystic fibrosis, oncology and disease-related malnutrition.

☑Adults: 1-2 sachets/day.

Children: Under 5 yrs: ½ sachet and 240ml milk/day. 5+ yrs: 1 sachet and 240ml milk/day.

Pharmacy only: Yes

SEATONE 230MG 110S
Perrans Distributors Ltd

PA No: N/A

◻Packs of 110 capsules.

☑Stabilised, green-lipped mussel extract 230mg, gelatin.

❓Dietary supplement.

☑Adults: Up to 5 capsules daily with meals.

❗Not recommended for people with shellfish allergies.

Pharmacy only: No

SEATONE 350MG
Perrans Distributors Ltd

PA No: N/A

◻Packs of 30, 90 capsules.

☑Stabilised, green-lipped mussel extract 350mg, gelatin.

❓Dietary supplement

☑Adults: Up to 3 capsules daily with meals.

❗Not recommended for people with shellfish allergies.

Pharmacy only: No

SEATONE PLUS GLUCOSAMINE
Perrans Distributors Ltd

PA No: N/A

◻Packs of 90 capsules.

☑Stabilised, green-lipped muscle extract 200mg with glucosamine sulphate 150mg, gelatin.

❓Dietary supplement to help maintain the mobility of the joints. Glucosamine is an amino sugar that occurs naturally in the body and is involved in the rebuilding of healthy ligaments, tendons and cartilage.

☑Adults: Up to 3 capsules daily with meals.

❗Not recommended for people with shellfish allergies.

Pharmacy only: No

SELENIUM ACE
Intrapharma/Dugdale/Wassen International

PA No: N/A

◻Blister pack of 30 tablets (1 month's supply).

☑Each tablet contains: selenium 100µg, vitamin A 450µg, vitamin C 90mg, vitamin E 30mg.

❓Vitamin A is essential for growth, vision, and maintenance of mucous tissue. Vitamin C helps maintain healthy connective tissues and cell walls. Vitamin E stabilises cell membranes, protecting unsaturated fatty acids from oxidation.

☑1 tablet per day.

Pharmacy only: Yes

SELENIUM ACE EXTRA
Intrapharma/Dugdale/Wassen International

PA No: N/A

◻Blister pack of 30 tablets (1 month's supply).

☑Selenium 200mg, vitamin A 450mg, vitamin E 30mg, vitamin B6 2mg, vitamin C 90mg, manganese 3mg, alpha lipoic acid 15mg. Contains selenium in an organic form bound to yeast.

❓An antioxidant, vitamin and mineral supplement.

☑1 tablet per day.

Pharmacy only: Yes

Always Consult Your Pharmacist

SERENOA-C
Intrapharma/Dugdale/Wassen

PA No: N/A

Blister card of 30 tablets (1 month's supply).

Named after the herb *Serenoa repens* which is an extract of the Saw Palmetto palm berry. Vitamin D 2.5µg, vitamin B2 (riboflavin) 5mg, vitamin E 10mg, vitamin B6 5mg, manganese 2mg, vitamin C 30mg, magnesium 175mg, copper 0.5mg, vitamin B1 (thiamin) 5mg, zinc 5mg, selenium 25µg, chromium 25µg, *Serenoa repens* 160mg.

Vitamin and mineral supplement.

Adults: 1 tablet per day.

Pharmacy only: Yes

SEVEN SEAS 1,000MG EVENING PRIMROSE OIL PLUS STARFLOWER OIL
Seven Seas Ireland Ltd

PA No: N/A

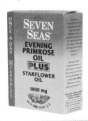

Packs of 30 clear, golden-yellow, oblong capsules.

Vitamin E 10mg, gamma-linolenic acid 130mg.

Helps to maintain a natural hormonal balance, healthy skin and supple joints.

Adults: 1-2 capsules once daily with liquid.

Pharmacy only: No

SEVEN SEAS HALIBORANGE VITAMIN C 1,000MG LEMON FLAVOUR
Seven Seas Ireland Ltd

PA No: 417/16/1

Tube of 20 effervescent tablets.

Vitamin C 1,000mg, sucrose, citric acid, sodium bicarbonate, flavours, maize starch, artificial sweeteners, glucose, syrup, colour.

Helps replace vitamin C lost through colds and flu and maintains good health.

Adults: 1 tablet dissolved in a glass of water to be taken up to twice daily.

Pharmacy only: No

If Symptoms Persist Consult Your Doctor

SEVEN SEAS HALIBORANGE VITAMIN C 1,000MG RUBY ORANGE FLAVOUR

Seven Seas Ireland Ltd

PA No: 417/16/1

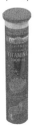

▣ Tube of 20 effervescent tablets.

▣ Vitamin C 1,000mg, sucrose, citric acid, sodium bicarbonate, flavours, maize starch, artificial sweeteners, glucose, syrup, colour.

▣ Helps replace vitamin C lost through colds and flu and maintains good health.

▣ Adults: 1 tablet dissolved in a glass of water to be taken up to twice daily.

Pharmacy only: No

SEVEN SEAS HÖFELS CARDIOMAX GARLIC TABLETS

Seven Seas Ireland Ltd

PA No: N/A

▣ Packs of 30 green, oval tablets.

▣ Garlic oil 4.5mg.

▣ Garlic oil supplement.

▣ Adults: 1 capsule daily with food or drink.

Pharmacy only: No

SEVEN SEAS HÖFELS ODOURLESS NEO GARLIC PEARLES

Seven Seas Ireland Ltd

PA No: N/A

▣ Packs of 30 odourless and tasteless capsules.

▣ Natural soya oil, gelatin, glycerine, silica, specially prepared garlic paste (0.4%, 2mg), natural colours (titanium dioxide, chlorophyll KK).

▣ Nutritional garlic supplement.

▣ Adults: 1 capsule daily.

Children: Over 3 yrs: As per adult dose.

Pharmacy only: No

SEVEN SEAS KOREAN GINSENG CAPSULES

Seven Seas Ireland Ltd

PA No: N/A

▣ 30 capsules in a plastic container.

▣ Korean ginseng root 600mg, soya bean oil, capsule shell (gelatin, glycerin), natural source colour (red iron oxide), Korean ginseng, hydrogenated vegetable fat, beeswax, emulsifier (lecithin).

▣ Korean ginseng supplement to help maintain natural energy, vitality and stamina.

▣ Adults: 1 capsule daily with liquid.

Pharmacy only: No

Always Read The Label

SEVEN SEAS ODOURLESS GARLIC PERLES
Seven Seas Ireland Ltd

PA No: N/A

⬜Packs of 60 clear oval capsules.

✅Garlic paste 2mg.

✅Adults: 1 capsule daily with liquid.

Pharmacy only: No

SEVEN SEAS PURE STARFLOWER OIL
Seven Seas Ireland Ltd

PA No: N/A

⬜Packs of 30 capsules.

✅Vitamin E (dl-alpha-tocopheryl acetate) 10mg, concentrated Starflower oil 500mg providing GLA 102mg.

❓Starflower oil and vitamin E supplement to help maintain healthy hair and skin and general good health.

✅Adults: 1-2 capsules daily with liquid.

Pharmacy only: No

THICK AND EASY
Fresenius Kabi

PA No: N/A

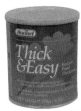

⬜8g sachet, 225g resealable tin and 10lb catering pack of instant food thickener, designed to thicken food and drinks. Stops thickening after 1 minute and retains consistency. Is fully digestible and releases 98% of available fluid after digestion. Gluten and lactose free. Suitable for diabetics.

✅18kcal/tbsp.

❓For patients with dysphagia. Can be added directly to hot and cold drinks to thicken consistency and prevent aspiration.

❗Not a nutritionally complete food. Not suitable for patients with maize starch intolerance.

Pharmacy only: Yes

THICK AND EASY THICKENED FRUIT JUICES
Fresenius Kabi

PA No: N/A

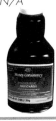

⬜Clear plastic 1.35L bottle with screw top containing a pre-thickened, ready to serve fruit juice mixed to the consistency of honey. Gluten and lactose free. Available in cranberry, orange and apple flavours.

✅Per 100ml: 58kcal, 14.5g carbohydrate, 64-78mg vitamin C.

❓Thick and Easy Thickened Fruit Juices are ready to serve fluids suitable for patients who have difficulty swallowing.

❗Not suitable for patients with maize starch intolerance.

Pharmacy only: Yes

WASSEN GLUCOSELENE
Intrapharma/Dugdale/Wassen

PA No: N/A

⬜Blister pack of 30 tablets.

✅Glucosamine sulphate 400mg, selenium 50µg, vitamin C, vitamin E, manganese, vitamin B6.

❓Joint action formula. Benefits active people and sports people who may be susceptible to joint injuries, older people whose glucosamine levels may have declined and people concerned about effects of wear and tear on their joints.

✅1 tablet per day.

Pharmacy only: Yes

VITAMIN C

HEALTHCRAFTS HI POTENCY VITAMIN C 1G
Perrans Distributors Ltd

PA No: N/A

▭Packs of 30 or 90 tablets.

☑Vitamin C 1,000mg, microcrystalline cellulose, rosehip powder 100mg, citrus bioflavonoids 50mg, hydrogenated vegetable oil, glazing agents (shellac, beeswax), magnesium stearate, silica.

⚅Vitamin C supplement to help maintain the health of tissues and organs. Ideal for those who lack fresh fruit and vegetables in their diets or are recovering from illness.

☑Adults: 1 tablet daily with food.

Children: As per adult dose.

Pharmacy only: No

HEALTHCRAFTS VITAMIN C 500MG TIME RELEASE 30S
Perrans Distributors Ltd

PA No: N/A

▭Packs of 30 tablets.

☑Vitamin C 500mg, dicalcium phosphate, hydroxypropylmethylcellulose, hydrogenated vegetable oil, tablet coating (hydroxypropylmethylcellulose, glycerin), colours (iron oxide, titanium dioxide), rosehip powder, magnesium stearate, methylcellulose.

⚅Vitamin C supplement to help maintain the health of tissue and organs. Ideal for those who lack fresh fruit and vegetables in their diets or are recovering from illness.

☑Adults: 1-2 tablets daily with food.

Pharmacy only: No

POWER HEALTH CHILDREN'S VITAMIN C
Power Health Products Ltd

PA No: N/A

▭Cream-coloured, speckled, 10mm, round tablets.

☑Vitamin C (as ascorbic acid) 60mg.

☑Children: 1 per day.

Pharmacy only: No

REDOXON EFFERVESCENT 1G
Roche Consumer Health

PA No: 50/7/3

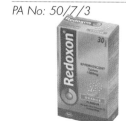

▭Cartons of 15 or 30 effervescent tablets in 3 flavours.

☑Vitamin C (ascorbic acid) 1,000mg.

⚅Redoxon provides added protection against infections like colds and flu. Maintenance of healthy bones, teeth, gums, skin and blood cells. Helps absorption of iron and functions as an antioxidant.

☑Adults: 1-3 tablets daily.

Children 4-12 yrs: ½ a tablet daily or as recommended by a physician.

Pharmacy only: Yes

If Symptoms Persist Consult Your Doctor

RUBEX CHEWABLE
Ricesteele Manufacturing

PA No: 95/8/3

Packs of 50 or 150 chewable, orange-flavoured tablets.

Ascorbic acid 250mg per tablet.

Prevention and treatment of ascorbic acid deficiency.

Adults: 2-4 tablets daily.

Children: 9-12 yrs: 1-2 tablets daily. 4-8 yrs: 1 tablet daily.

Ascorbic acid in doses greater than 1g daily should not be taken during pregnancy or by patients known to be at risk of hyperoxaluria.

Not suitable for diabetics.

Pharmacy only: Yes

RUBEX ORANGE, RUBEX LEMON
Ricesteele Manufacturing

PA No: Orange: 95/8/2; Lemon: 95/8/1

Rubex Orange packs of 10 or 24, and Rubex Lemon packs of 10 orange- or lemon-flavoured, effervescent tablets.

Ascorbic acid 1,000mg, 600mg glucose.

Prevention and treatment of ascorbic acid deficiency.

Adults: 1 tablet dissolved in water as required.

Ascorbic acid in doses greater than 1g daily should not be taken during pregnancy or by patients known to be at risk of hyperoxaluria.

Not suitable for diabetics.

Pharmacy only: Yes

RUBEX TABLETS
Ricesteele Manufacturing

PA No: 50mg: N/A; 100mg: 95/8/4; 200mg: 95/8/5; 500mg: 95/8/6

Packs of 100 x 50mg, 100mg, 200mg or 500mg white tablets.

Ascorbic acid 50mg, 100mg, 200mg or 500mg.

Prevention and treatment of ascorbic acid deficiency.

Adults: Up to 1,000mg daily or as directed by physician.

Ascorbic acid in doses greater than 1g daily should not be taken during pregnancy or by patients known to be at risk of hyperoxaluria.

Not suitable for diabetics.

Pharmacy only: Yes

SANATOGEN HIGH C 500MG
Roche Consumer Health

PA No: N/A

Bottles of 60 orange, flat, bevel-edged, chewable tablets embossed with the cross-section of a citrus fruit.

Vitamin C 500mg.

High dose vitamin C supplement used to replace vitamins used during colds and flu or when under stress. Helps maintain good health.

Adults: 1 tablet daily.

Pharmacy only: Yes

SEVEN SEAS CHEWABLE VITAMIN C
Seven Seas Ireland Ltd

PA No: 417/2/1

30 soft, cherry-coloured and flavoured gelatin capsules in a plastic container.

Vitamin C 250mg, fractionated coconut oil, xylitol, glycerin, gelatin, hard vegetable fat, modified starch, hydrogenated vegetable oil, flavouring (black cherry and cherry), emulsifier (lecithin), artificial sweeteners (aspartame and saccharine), natural source colours (red iron oxide and carmine red).

Vitamin C supplement to help maintain a healthy immune system and healthy teeth, gums, bones and blood vessels.

Adults: 1-2 capsules daily to be chewed or swallowed whole with a cold drink.

Pharmacy only: No

Always Read The Label

SEVEN SEAS HALIBORANGE HIGH STRENGTH VITAMIN C
Seven Seas Ireland Ltd

PA No: N/A

50 orange-flavoured, chewable tablets in a plastic container.

Vitamin E 10mg, vitamin C 500mg, natural bioflavonoids 20mg, sucrose, natural orange flavouring, vitamin E (dl-alpha-tocopherol acetate), magnesium stearate, artificial sweetener (aspartame).

Vitamin C supplement with natural bioflavonoids and vitamin E, to help maintain a healthy immune system.

Adults: 1-2 tablets, to be chewed daily.

Pharmacy only: No

SEVEN SEAS HALIBORANGE VITAMIN C 1,000MG LEMON FLAVOUR
Seven Seas Ireland Ltd

PA No: 417/16/2

Tube of 20 effervescent tablets.

Vitamin C 1,000mg, sucrose, citric acid, sodium bicarbonate, flavours, maize starch, artificial sweeteners, glucose, syrup, colour.

Helps replace vitamin C lost through colds and flu and maintains good health.

Adults: 1 tablet dissolved in a glass of water to be taken up to twice daily.

Pharmacy only: No

SEVEN SEAS HALIBORANGE VITAMIN C 1,000MG RUBY ORANGE FLAVOUR
Seven Seas Ireland Ltd

PA No: 417/16/1

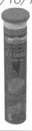

Tube of 20 effervescent tablets.

Vitamin C 1,000mg, sucrose, citric acid, sodium bicarbonate, flavours, maize starch, artificial sweeteners, glucose, syrup, colour.

Helps replace vitamin C lost through colds and flu and maintains good health.

Adults: 1 tablet dissolved in a glass of water to be taken up to twice daily.

Pharmacy only: No

SEVEN SEAS VITAMIN C PLUS CAPSULES
Seven Seas Ireland Ltd

PA No: 416/1/1

60 purple, oval capsules.

Vitamin C (ascorbic acid) 200mg, citrus bioflavonoids 10mg, blackcurrant concentrate 10mg.

Vitamin C supplement.

Adults: 1 capsule daily.

Pharmacy only: No

Always Consult Your Pharmacist

DRUGS PAYMENT SCHEME

Information

Under the Drugs Payment Scheme an individual or family pay a maximum of £42.00 (€53.33 euro) per month for all prescribed drugs, medicines or appliances used by that person or his or her family in that month.

Family expenditure covers the nominated adult, his or her spouse/partner and children under 18 years, or under 23 if in full-time education. A dependent with a physical or mental disability/illness living in the household, who does not have a medical card and who is unable to fully maintain himself/herself, may be included in the family expenditure regardless of age.

Medical card holders are entitled to prescribed drugs and medicines free of charge. Therefore, they are not eligible for this scheme.

You should register for this scheme by completing the registration form, which is available from pharmacies or from your health board, and returning it to your health board. The health board will then issue a plastic swipe card for each person named on the registration form. You should present this card whenever you have a prescription filled. It is intended that pharmacists will be able to access a central database to confirm if the £42.00 (€53.33) has been reached in any calendar month.

You can use the Drugs Payment Scheme along with a Long Term Illness Book.

Further information is available from your Health Board.

LONG TERM ILLNESS SCHEME

People who suffer from certain conditions, and who are not already medical card holders, may obtain the drugs, medicines and medical and surgical appliances for the treatment of that condition free of charge.

The conditions include:

- mental handicap
- mental illness (for people under 16 only)
- diabetes insipidus
- haemophilia
- cerebral palsy
- phenylketonuria
- epilepsy
- cystic fibrosis
- multiple sclerosis
- spina bifida
- muscular dystrophies
- hydrocephalus
- parkinsonism
- diabetes mellitus
- acute leukaemia

Once eligible, a person suffering from any of these conditions is issued with a Long Term Illness Book. This book lists the drugs and medicines for the treatment of their condition, which will be provided free of charge through their community pharmacist.

To apply for admission to the Long Term Illness Scheme, contact your local health board.

Important information about how to access your entitlements under current government schemes

MEDICAL CARD

A medical card issued by a local health board enables you to receive:

- free GP services
- prescribed drugs and medicines (with some exceptions)
- in-patient public hospital services
- out-patient services
- dental, optical and aural services
- medical appliances
- maternity and infant care services, and
- a maternity cash grant of £8 on the birth of each child.

When you qualify for a medical card, you will receive a plastic card (similar to a credit card). A medical card normally covers the applicant and his/her dependent spouse and children.

As of July 2001, all people over 70 are entitled to a medical card regardless of their means.

A full-time student aged 16-25, who is financially dependent on his/her parents, will only be entitled to a medical card if his/her parents hold a medical card. A student who is financially independent of his/her parents and who satisfies a means test in his/her own right may be entitled to a medical card. A student in receipt of Disability Allowance will generally be entitled to a medical card.

If you qualify for a medical card, you will be given a list of doctors and a Doctor's Acceptance Form. You pick a doctor from the list and ask the doctor to sign the Acceptance Form, which is then returned to the health board. Your medical card will show your doctor's name. The doctor you choose must generally have his/her practice within seven miles of where you live and must agree to accept you as a patient. It could happen that a doctor would be unwilling to take you on if, for example, he/she already has too many patients but this is not normally a problem.

Medical card holders are exempt from paying the Health Contribution. They may also be exempt from paying the school transport charges.

Rules

Persons with no income other than:

- Old Age Non-Contributory Pension (maximum)
- Deserted Wife's Allowance
- Infectious Diseases (Maintenance) Allowance
- Disability Allowance
- One-Parent Family Payment (max.)
- Widow's/Widower's (Non-Contributory) Pension (max.)
- Orphans (Non-Contributory) Pension (max.)
- Blind Person's Pension (max.)
- Supplementary Welfare Allowance

are eligible for a medical card. Hardship cases are dealt with individually on merit.

Important information about how to access your entitlements under current government schemes

---

252

In general, if you are getting the maximum rate of a means-tested payment, you will be granted a medical card without having to undergo a further means test. Medical cards are usually granted to children in foster care. Some people may be entitled to a medical card under EU regulations. Lone parents with dependants are assessed under the income limits for married people.

You can use your medical card for up to three months if you live temporarily in a different area. In this case, you can attend any GP in the area who is participating in the medical card scheme. If you are going to be away longer than three months, you should apply to the health board in that area for a medical card. If you move to a different part of your own health board area, you can apply to change your doctor.

Rates

Medical card income guidelines from 1 March 2001:

Weekly Income Limit (Gross less PRSI and Health Contribution)

Category	Aged under 66	Aged 66-69	Aged 70-79**	Aged 80+**
Single person living alone	£100.00 (€126.97)	£109.00 (€138.40)	£216.00 (€274.26)	£228.00 (€289.50)
Single person living with family	£89.00 (€113.01)	£94.00 (€119.36)	£187.00 (€237.44)	£195.50 (€248.23)
Married couple	£144.50 (€183.48)	£162.00 (€205.70)	£324.00 (€411.40)	£340.50 (€432.35)
Allowance for child aged under 16	£18.00 (€22.86)	£18.00 (€22.86)	£18.00 (€22.86)	£18.00 (€22.86)
Allowance for dependants aged over 16 (with no income)*	£19.00 (€24.13)	£19.00 (€24.13)	£19.00 (€24.13)	£19.00 (€24.13)

* This allowance is doubled where a child is in full-time education and is not grant-aided.

** The guidelines for people aged 70 and over were increased by one-third with effect from 1 March 2001. Patients who qualify for a medical card under the increased income limits for those aged 70 or over will be able to remain with their current GP only if that GP applies for a limited General Medical Services (GMS) contract.

How to apply for a medical card

- Get an application form and a list of participating doctors from the health centre or Community Care Office for your area.
- Complete the form and bring it to the doctor you have chosen from the list of participating doctors.
- If the GP accepts you as a patient, he/she signs the form.
- Your employer also has to sign the form and certify your earnings or, if you are claiming a social welfare payment, the form has to be stamped at the Social Welfare Local Office.
- Self-employed people have to submit their most recent Tax Assessment Form and audited accounts.

Important information about how to access your entitlements under current government schemes

BreastCheck – the National Breast Screening Programme

BreastCheck – The National Breast Screening Programme – is a major public health initiative that began in 1999. Funded by the Department of Health and Children, it aims to significantly reduce deaths from breast cancer in Ireland by detecting abnormalities early enough to improve prognosis and offer a wider choice of options for treatment.

Phase I of the National Breast Screening Programme began in February 2000 and offers screening to women in the Eastern, North Eastern and Midland Health Board regions through the following units:

- Eccles Unit, 36 Eccles St, Dublin 7 on the Mater Hospital campus
- Merrion Unit on the St Vincent's University Hospital campus
- Mobile mammography units.

Women aged between 50 and 64 years of age are invited for free mammography screening every two years. A register of women has been compiled in each health board area, but this is not complete, so women are invited to register themselves by contacting BreastCheck or picking up a registration form at their GP's surgery. Women on the register will receive an information leaflet and a letter asking for their consent. If the woman gives her consent, she will be sent an appointment to attend one of the units for a mammogram.

Phase II of the National Breast Screening Programme will extend mammography screening to the remaining health board regions.

For further information, or to register yourself for screening, contact BreastCheck, Corrigan House, Fenian Street, Dublin 2, Tel: (01) 676 2222, email: info@nbsp.ie, or register online on the website, www.breastcheck.ie.

Frequently Asked Questions

What is a mammogram?

A mammogram is a low dose X-ray of your breasts. It can pick up changes that are too small to be detected by touch alone. The smaller the lump the easier it is to treat.

What happens?

Your appointment takes about half an hour. All the staff are there to help you. You will be asked a few questions about your health and then asked to undress from the waist up (cubicles are provided for your privacy).

Each breast is placed between two special plates and pressure is applied to get the best possible X-ray. It may feel slightly uncomfortable – a bit like getting your blood pressure checked.

Helpful Hint: wear a top with a skirt or trousers – it makes it easier to undress.

How will I know my result?

The aim is to send the results to you by post within three weeks. Your GP will also receive a copy of the results. A very small percentage of women will be asked to come back.

What if I am asked to come back, is there something wrong?

Don't panic! The first X-ray may not have given a clear picture. Most queries raised by X-rays are not related to cancer.

> **Important information about how to access your entitlements under current government schemes**

How often should I be screened?

You will be invited to come back for screening every two years until you are 65. Even if your mammogram is normal, a very small number of breast cancers may not be seen on the mammogram. Therefore, even though you have been screened, be breast aware and look out for:

- Lumps or thickening in any part of the breast
- Puckering or dimpling of the skin
- A change in the shape or size of the breast
- Discharge from the nipple
- An inverted nipple (turned in on itself compared to how it used to be)
- A swelling in the armpit or above the breast.

NB If you have any worries go to your family doctor even if you have recently had a mammogram.

Important information about how to access your entitlements under current government schemes

CHILDHOOD VACCINATION FOR YOUR BABY

Information

A range of vaccinations against infectious diseases is available free of charge. These are widely publicised by the Health Promotion Unit of the Department of Health and if you have had a baby recently, you will find that you are sent information about the schedule automatically through the post. If you want further information, or have any concerns about vaccination, you can discuss these with your GP or public health nurse.

Vaccination is not mandatory, but it is strongly advised by the health authorities. The following are the vaccinations and tests that will be offered to you for your baby:

- The BCG provides protection against TB. It is administered in hospital if you have had your baby there, or in designated clinics by the Area Medical Officer, generally before your baby begins other vaccinations. Your public health nurse or the maternity hospital will be able to tell you the location of your nearest clinic.
- The Heel Prick Test. This test, done 3-5 days after birth, tests for metabolic disorders. It is administered by the midwife if you are still in hospital or by the public health nurse.
- The '5 in 1'. This vaccination provides protection against diphtheria, tetanus, whooping cough, polio and haemophilus influenza type B (Hib). You will need to take your baby to your GP at two months, at four months and again at six months for this vaccination. In July 2001, inactivated polio vaccine (IPV) replaced oral polio vaccination (OPV) and the five vaccines are now provided in combined form resulting in just one injection for your child.
- The 'MMR'. This vaccine provides protection against measles, mumps and rubella and is given by the GP when your child is 15 months old.
- The Meningitis 'C'. This provides protection against the 'C' strain of Meningitis and septicaemia (which causes about one-third of all meningitis/septicaemia illness in Ireland). The immunisation programme was introduced in Ireland in 2000 and a catch-up programme is currently being administered during 2001 to babies, young children, teenagers, students and young adults up to 22 years of age. It is available at the same time as the '5 in 1', if the child is under one year old, and in one single injection thereafter.

Booster injections of 4 in 1 and MMR are administered in primary school free of charge.

Contacts

Your Health Board will provide you with information on vaccination. The Health Promotion Unit has a range of leaflets on vaccination which are available in health centres, pharmacies, hospitals, GPs surgeries etc.

The Health Promotion Unit
Department of Health and Children
Hawkins House
Dublin 2
Tel: (01) 635 4000

Important information about how to access your entitlements under current government schemes

THE NATIONAL CERVICAL SCREENING PROGRAMME

Phase 1 of the Irish Cervical Screening Programme began in October 2000 in the Mid-Western Health Board region. Women aged 25-60 years in that region are invited to register with the Programme, which aims to ensure that women on the Register will automatically be invited by letter to attend for a free smear test at least every five years.

How will the register work?

- You will receive a letter from the Cervical Screening Register inviting you to a have your free smear test done
- You will visit your smeartaker, who gives you the information you need and performs a cervical smear test
- The cervical smears are sent to the cytology laboratory and are examined
- The result goes to your smeartaker and the Cervical Screening Register
- A letter will go to you from the Register with your results six weeks after your test
- Recall letters are sent out from the Register to you at the appropriate time.

There is very good evidence to suggest that a cervical screening programme leads to a reduction in cervical cancers.

How can I reduce my risk of getting cervical cancer?

Not everything is known yet about the cause of cervical cancer, but the following can reduce your risk:

- Have a regular smear test to pick up any early problems
- Stop smoking
- Visit your doctor if you have symptoms such as vaginal discharge, irregular vaginal bleeding, painful intercourse, bleeding after intercourse or bleeding following the menopause
- Practise safe sex using a condom or diaphragm.

What is the cervical smear test?

A cervical smear is a screening test done to look for early changes in the cells of the cervix – the neck of the womb – which, if not checked, could become cancer cells.

How common is cancer of the cervix?

Cancer of the cervix is the third most common female cancer. There is a lifetime risk that 1 in 25 Irish women will develop cancer of the cervix. It is not very common but it is very preventable.

Why should I be screened?

Screening could save your life, as it detects changes in cells that may become cancerous.

Who should have a cervical smear test?

All women between 25 to 60 years of age should have regular smear tests whether married, single, heterosexual or lesbian.

If you have had a total hysterectomy (womb removed) you do not usually need a cervical smear test but you should check with your doctor.

How is the cervical smear test done?

The smear test is a very simple procedure taking less than five minutes. It can be slightly uncomfortable. You will be asked to remove your clothes from the waist down and lie on the couch. The sample is taken by a doctor or nurse and then sent to be tested in the cytology laboratory.

Important information about how to access your entitlements under current government schemes

---

When is the best time to have your cervical smear test?

The best time to attend for your cervical smear test is mid-cycle or half way between periods.

If you have any unusual or abnormal bleeding, spotting or discharge do not wait for your smear test, contact your doctor.

Where can I have a cervical smear test?

You can have a cervical smear test from any of the following:
- Any GP
- Limerick Family Planning Clinic
- The Women's Health Clinic Newcastle West.
- Some Health Board Clinics.

It is especially important to have tests if you are over 35 and have never had a test.

How often will I be offered the test?

A minimum five yearly screening interval is advised with two smears to be taken within twelve months of entering the programme if you have never had a previous smear.

What happens when I've had my test?

You will receive a letter concerning your results within six weeks of your test.

There is a 1 in 10 chance that a smear result will mean going back to your doctor. Do not be alarmed if you are recalled.

What if my smear test is unsatisfactory?

If your smear is reported as being unsatisfactory it needs to be repeated within three months.

What if my smear test is not normal?

You may be required to have a repeat smear or more specialised tests. There are several treatments available and nearly all of them are done on an outpatient basis. It is very easy to treat the cells at this early stage before cancer develops.

The majority of smear tests are normal. Even a result that is not normal may not mean you have cancer. The earlier a change is found the easier it is to treat.

Are you on the register?

This is a FREE service to all women between the ages of 25 to 60 who are on the Register.

It is important to inform the cervical screening programme register of any change of name or address.

If you have any queries, contact the programme:
- Information Helpline: 1850 252 600 for the price of a local call.
- Email: icsp@mwhb.ie
- Post: Mid-Western Health Board, PO Box 161, Limerick.
- Website: www.icsp.ie

Important information about how to access your entitlements under current government schemes

PATIENT SUPPORT GROUPS

Age Action Ireland Ltd
30/31 Camden Street, Dublin 2
Tel: (01) 475 6989, Fax: (01) 475 6011, email: ageact@indigo.ie
A national non-governmental organisation that aims to improve the quality of life of the elderly by enabling them to live full, independent and satisfying lives.

Alcoholics Anonymous (AA)
109 South Circular Road, Leonard's Corner, Dublin 8
Tel: (01) 453 8998, Fax: (01) 453 7673, After Hours: (01) 679 5967, email: ala@indigo.ie
Alcoholics Anonymous is a fellowship of men and women who share their experience, strength and hope with each other that they may solve their common problem and help others to recover from alcoholism. The only requirement for membership is the desire to stop drinking. There are no dues or fees for AA membership.
Office hours: Mon-Fri 9.30am-5.00pm *After hours:* Mon-Fri 6.30pm-10.00pm
Sat-Sun 10.00am-10.00pm

Alzheimer Society of Ireland
Alzheimer House, 43 Northumberland Avenue, Dun Laoghaire, Co Dublin
Tel: (01) 284 6616, Fax: (01) 284 6030, email: alzheim@iol.ie
Support group for victims and families of those with Alzheimer's disease.

Arthritis Foundation of Ireland
1 Clanwilliam Square, Grand Canal Quay, Dublin 2
Tel: (01) 661 8188, Fax: (01) 661 8261, email: info@arthritis-foundation.com, website: www.arthritis-foundation.com
Furthers and funds research, education and arthritis care. Network of nation-wide branches.

Asthma Society of Ireland
Eden House, 15-17 Eden Quay, Dublin 1
Asthma Line: 1850 445464, Asthma Live Line: (01) 8788122, Tel: (01) 878 8511, Fax: (01) 878 8128, email: asthma@indigo.ie, website: www.asthmasociety.ie
A voluntary association of people with asthma and their families.
Asthma Live Line hours:
Monday & Friday 9.30am-1.00pm, Thursday 9.30am-5.30pm

Aware – Helping to Defeat Depression
72 Lower Leeson Street, Dublin 2
Tel: (01) 661 7208, Fax: (01) 661 7217, email: aware@webireland.ie, website: www.webireland.ie/aware, Depression Phone Line: (01) 6766166
Assists and supports those suffering from mood disorder and their families.

Brainwave – The Irish Epilepsy Association
249 Crumlin road, Dublin 12
Tel: (01) 455 7500, Fax: (01) 455 7013, email: brainwave@iol.ie
Information, education and counselling service.

Carers Association
St Mary's Community Centre, Richmond Hill, Rathmines, Dublin 6
Tel: (01) 497 4498, Fax: (01) 497 6108, Careline: 1800 240724
Founded in 1987. Information and advice service for carers.

Coeliac Society of Ireland
Carmichael House, North Brunswick Street, Dublin 7
Tel: (01) 872 1471, email: coeliac@iol.ie, website: www.iol/ie/~coeliac
Founded in 1970 to promote, safeguard and protect the interests of members in relation to coeliac disease.

Colostomy Care Group
Irish Cancer Society, 5 Northumberland Road, Dublin 4
Tel: (01) 668 1855, Fax: (01) 668 7599; email: admin@irishcancer.ie
Support for patients who have had or who are about to have surgery to treat cancer of the colon or rectum.

Cystic Fibrosis Association of Ireland
24 Lower Rathmines Road, Dublin 6
Tel: (01) 496 2433, Fax: (01) 496 2201, email: cfhouse@internet-ireland.ie, website: www.internet-ireland.ie/horizon/cf.html
Founded in 1963 to promote better treatment and further research into a cure for cystic fibrosis.

Diabetes Clinics
Beaumont Day Centre, Beaumont hospital, Beaumont, Dublin 9, Tel: (01) 809 2744
Eastern Regional Health Authority, Dr Steevens Hospital, Dublin 8, Tel: (01) 679 0700
Mater Day Centre, 30 Eccles St, Dublin 7, Tel: (01) 803 4620/803 4630
Our Lady's Hospital for Sick Children, Crumlin, Dublin 12, Tel: (01) 409 6121
Our Lady of Lourdes Hospital, Drogheda, Tel: (041) 983 7601
St James's Hospital, James's St, Dublin 8, Tel: (01) 453 7941
St Vincent's Diabetic Clinic, St Vincent's University Hospital, Elm Park, Dublin 4, Tel: (01) 269 4533, ext. 4527
Tallaght Hospital, Belgard Road, Tallaght, Dublin 24, Tel: (01) 414 2000/4143229

Diabetes Federation of Ireland
76 Lower Gardiner Street, Dublin 1
Tel: (01) 836 3022, Fax: (01) 836 5182
Represents the interests of people with diabetes.

Disability Federation of Ireland
2 Sandyford Office Park, Dublin 18
Tel: (01) 295 9344, Fax: (01) 295 9346, email: dfi@iol.ie, website: www.ireland.iol.ie/~dfi/
National umbrella body of organisations of and for people with disabilities.

Down Syndrome Ireland
1st Floor, 30 Mary Street, Dublin 1
Tel: (01) 873 0999, Fax: (01) 873 1064, email: dsi@eircom.net, website: www.downsyndrome.ie
National organisation of parents representing over 2,000 families.

Dyslexia Association of Ireland
1 Suffolk Street, Dublin 2
Tel: (01) 679 0276, Fax: (01) 679 0273, email: acld@iol.ie, website: www.acld-dyslexia.com
Promotes early and adequate diagnosis of dyslexia and appropriate tuition for both children and adults.

HADD Family Support Group
Carmichael Centre, North Brunswick Street, Dublin 7
Tel: (01) 874 8349
Help and support to children with attention deficit disorder and parents.

Headway Ireland - The National Head Injuries Association
101 Parnell Street, Dublin 1
Tel: (01) 872 9222, Fax: (01) 872 9590, email: services@headwayireland.ie
Promotes the development of services for people with brain injury, their families and carers.

Home Birth Association of Ireland
Triton Lodge, Nerano Road, Dalkey, Co Dublin
Tel: (01) 285 3264, email: hba@iol.ie, website: www.iol.ie/~hba
Voluntary organisation giving help and support to mothers considering home births.

Irish Association of Older People
Room B15, University College Dublin, Earlsfort Terrace, Dublin 2
Tel: (01) 475 0013, Fax: (01) 475 0010, email: iaop@oceanfree.net
Direct voice of older people, represents their interests and campaigns on their behalf.

Irish Cancer Society
5 Northumberland Road, Dublin 4
Tel: (01) 668 1855, Fax: (01) 668 7599, email: admin@irishcancer.ie
Founded in 1963. Funds research, welfare and information.

Irish Childbirth Trust – Cuidiú – Mother to Mother Support
Carmichael House, North Brunswick Street, Dublin 7
Tel: (01) 872 4501, Fax: (01) 295 4953
The ICT is a mother-to-mother, non-professional community-based group which aims to help women to have their babies happily and free from fear, and to prepare families for the experience of childbirth and parenthood.

Irish Haemophilia Society
Block C, Iceland House, Arran Court, Arran Quay, Dublin 7
Tel: (01) 872 4466, Fax: (01) 872 4494, email: haemophiliasociety@eircom.net, website: www.haemophilia-society.ie
Information and advice for those with haemophilia.

Irish Heart Foundation
4 Clyde Road, Ballsbridge, Dublin 4
Tel: (01) 668 5001, Fax: (01) 668 5896, email: info@irishheart.ie, website: www.irishheart.ie
Cork, Tel: (021) 450 5822, Fax: (021) 450 5374
Sligo, Tel: (071) 71002, Fax: (071) 71910
A voluntary organisation which aims to prevent heart and circulatory diseases.

Irish Hysterectomy Support Group
Margaret Hayes, 24 Tulip Court, Darndale, Dublin 17
Tel: (01) 847 3200
Established in 1984 by a group of women who had undergone hysterectomy ad saw the value of coming together to offer mutual support and share common problems.

Irish Kidney Association
Donor House, 156 Pembroke Road, Ballsbridge, Dublin 4
Tel: (01) 668 9788, Fax: (01) 668 3820, website: www.ika.ie
Support group for those with chronic renal failure.

Irish Osteoporosis Society
Emoclew, Batterstown, Co Meath
Tel/Fax: (01) 825 8159, email: crowleym@indigo.ie

Irish Society for Autism
Unity Buildings, 15-17 Lower O'Connell Street, Dublin 1
Tel: 874 4684, Fax: (01) 874 4224, email: autism@isa.iol.ie
Voluntary association of parents, friends and professionals providing support and services for autistic children and adults.

Irish Society for the Prevention of Cruelty to Children (ISPCC)
20 Molesworth Street, Dublin 2
Tel: (01) 679 4944, ChildLine: 1800 666666, Fax: (01) 679 1746, email: ispcc@ispcc.ie, website: www.ispcc.ie
Children's rights agency.

Irish Sudden Infant Death Association
Carmichael House, North Brunswick Street, Dublin 7
Tel: (01) 873 2711, Fax: (01) 872 6056, Free helpline: 1850 391391
Founded in 1976 to help and support bereaved parents after cot death.

ISANDS – Irish Stillbirth and Neonatal Death Society
Carmichael House, North Brunswick Street, Dublin 7
Tel: (01) 822 4688/872 6996
ISANDS is a support group for parents whose babies have died around the time of birth. They provide support and help to those who are recently bereaved and also to those who know their baby has died prior to delivery or is likely to live only a short time after birth.

La Leche League
30 Idrone Close, Knocklyon, Dublin 16
Tel/Fax: (01) 494 1279
International voluntary association. Promotes and assists breastfeeding mothers.

Meningitis Research Foundation
51 Cullenswood Road, The Triangle, Ranelagh, Dublin 6
Tel: (01) 496 9664, Fax: (01) 496 9656, email: meningitis@iol.ie, website: www.meningitis.org
Promotes awareness of meningitis and septicaemia in order to prevent death and disability.

Menopause Support Group
Tel: (01) 662 1497
Established in 1994 by the Dublin Well Woman Centre.

Migraine Association of Ireland
Coleraine House, Coleraine Street, Dublin 7
Tel: (01) 872 4137, Fax: (01) 872 4157, email: info@migraine.ie, website: www.migraine.ie

Miscarriage Association of Ireland
Carmichael House, North Brunswick Street, Dublin 7
Tel: (01) 873 5702, fax: (01) 873 5737
Support and information for those who have suffered loss through miscarriage.

Multiple Sclerosis Society of Ireland

The Royal Hospital, Donnybrook, Dublin 4
Tel: (01) 269 4599, Fax: (01) 269 3746, email: mssoi@iol.ie, website: www.ms-society.ie, Helpline: 1800 233233

Narcotics Anonymous

PO Box 1368, Cardiff lane, Dublin 2
Tel: (01) 830 0944 (24 hours)
Established in Ireland in 1983, helps addicts to any type of drug recover from addiction.

National Association for Deaf People

35 North Frederick Street, Dublin 1
Tel: (01) 872 3800, Fax: (01) 872 3816, email: nad@iol.ie
Voluntary, non-profit-making organisation that supports improved conditions and opportunities for deaf adults, children and their families.

National Association for the Mentally Handicapped of Ireland

5 Fitzwilliam Place, Dublin 2
Tel: (01) 676 6035, Fax: (01) 676 0517, email: info@namhi.ie, website: www.namhi.ie

National Association for Victims of Bullying

Frederick Street, Clara, Co Offaly
Tel: (0506) 31590
Supports and advises children, families and teachers. Counselling by phone or in private sessions.

National Council for the Blind of Ireland

PV Doyle House, 45 Whitworth Road, Drumcondra, Dublin 9
Tel: (01) 830 7033, SavePhone: 1850 334 3353, Fax: (01) 830 7787, email: ncbi@iol.ie, website: www.ncbi.ie
Founded in 1931. Aims to allow full independence and integration of people with visual impairment in Ireland.

Post Natal Distress Association of Ireland (PNDAI)

Carmichael House, North Brunswick Street, Dublin 7
Tel: (01) 872 7172, Fax: (01) 873 5735
Voluntary organisation providing information and support for those with postnatal depression.

Rape Crisis Centre

70 Lower Leeson Street, Dublin 2
Tel: (01) 661 4911, Fax: (01) 661 0873, Freephone 24 Hour counselling: 1800 778 888, email: rcc@indigo.ie, website: www.drcc.ie
Supports victims of rape and sexual assault.

Schizophrenia Ireland

38 Blessington Street, Dublin 7
Tel: (01) 860 1620, Fax: (01) 860 1602, Helpline: 1890 621631, email: schizi@iol.ie, website: www.iol.ie/lucia
Support, guidance and mutual help for sufferers and their families.

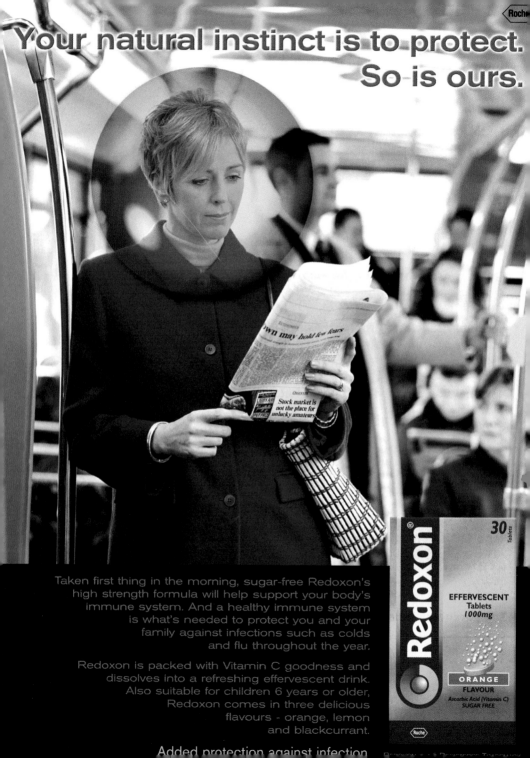

A

B

Sanatogen Multivitamins for Kids

Sanatogen Multivitamins for Kids

Sanatogen Multivitamins for Kids